ANGIOPLASTY, VARIOUS TECHNIQUES AND CHALLENGES IN TREATMENT OF CONGENITAL AND ACQUIRED VASCULAR STENOSES

Edited by **Thomas Forbes**

Angioplasty, Various Techniques and Challenges in Treatment of Congenital and Acquired Vascular Stenoses
Edited by Thomas Forbes

Published by InTech
Janeza Trdine 9, 51000 Rijeka, Croatia

Publishing Process Manager Adriana Pecar

Technical Editor Teodora Smiljanic

Cover Designer InTech Design Team

Additional hard copies can be obtained from orders@intechopen.com

Angioplasty, Various Techniques and Challenges in Treatment of Congenital and Acquired Vascular Stenoses, Edited by Thomas Forbes
p. cm.
ISBN 978-953-51-0084-3

For EU product safety concerns:
IN TECH d.o.o., Prolaz Marije Krucifikse Kozulić 3, 51000 Rijeka, Croatia,
info@intechopen.com or visit our website at intechopen.com.

Meet the editor

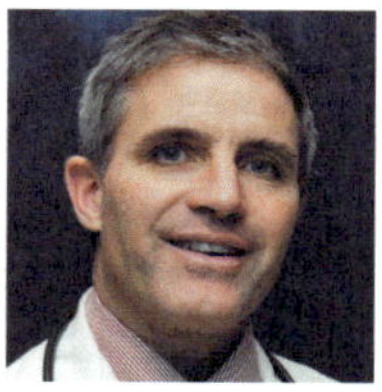

Dr Forbes' undergraduate, medical school, and residency training was completed at Creighton University/ University of Nebraska Medical Center in Omaha, Nebraska. He continued his Pediatric Cardiology training at Texas Children's Hospital/Baylor University Medical Center in Houston, Tx and completed a year in interventional cardiology training at Children's Memorial Hospital/Northwestern University in 1997. He joined Children's Hospital of Michigan/Wayne State University in the fall of 1997. His primary interest is in Congenital/Structural Interventional cardiology, authoring over 50 papers and 2 chapters in this area. He assisted in the development of the Genesis XD stent (Cordis, corp, Warren, NJ) and serves as the coordinating center for the Congenital Cardiovascular Interventional Study Consortium (CCISC), which is currently the largest Pediatric Interventional Consortium group in the world.

Contents

Preface

"To the patients whom we treat, allowing us to slowly convert the "art of medicine" into the "science of medicine".

Most interventional physicians believe that Andrea Gruentzig, who performed the first successful coronary angioplasty in 1977 in Zurich, Switzerland, began the era of less invasive intervention performed via the transcatheter route. At that time, in his first case, utilizing a *kitchen-built* catheter, he successfully performed dilation of an 80% lesion of a 3 mm section of the left anterior descending artery. He presented his first four coronary angioplasty cases at the "1977 American Heart Association" meeting and the rest, they say, was history. Fascinatingly, at the 10-year anniversary of the initial patient, the patient underwent elective repeat angiography which noted that the LAD narrowing remained almost perfectly expanded. Sadly, the German cardiologist, along with his wife, tragically died in a plane crash on October 27, 1985 at the young age of 46. If he was alive today, he would be amazed at the progress being made in the angioplasty arena for the treatment of congenital and acquired vessel stenosis. Dr. Gruentzig's initial foray into the coronary world served as the "launch pad" for the development of ideas and technology in the treatment of peripheral vascular lesions. For quite some time the treatment of coronary artery pathology has lead the way towards the development and treatment of other vascular lesions..

The past three decades has seen an explosion in interventional techniques to treat both congenital and acquired lesions in the vascular system. When I was first asked to edit this book on angioplasty, it came to my surprise that a similar book dealing with the techniques and issues of these congenital and acquired lesions had not been previously undertaken. Certainly individual chapters and reports have been written in these areas, though no formal book discussing the technical as well as current ongoing challenges in these areas have compiled in one setting.

In particular, the past decade has seen a significant advancement in balloon, wire, and catheter technology in the treatment of complicated congenital and acquired vascular lesions. This decade has born witness to the development of angioplasty procedures that many interventionalists had never imagined being able to treat via the transcatheter route, especially in the peripheral arena. The improvement of stent technology, especially regarding tracking capabilities of the newer generation stents, have played a significant role in the treatment of tortuous vascular lesions that otherwise were exclusively relegated to be treated in the surgical operating theater.

At first look, in reviewing the topics covered in this book, one's initial impression may be that this is a compilation of multiple different types of lesions and the treatment of these lesions. The common thread linking these procedures together relates to both the technology shared between disciplines, and the common techniques used to treat various lesions throughout the vascular system. A perfect example of this relates to chronic total obstructive lesions in the peripheral vascular system and the technique used to overcome technical challenges of a completely occluded coronary vessel.

One should not consider this textbook is a compendium of obscure interventional procedures. I believe that this textbook represents the greatest growth potential area in much of interventional cardiovascular medicine. For example, as techniques continue to improve regarding re-vascularization if distal extremities, especially in patients with peripheral vasculopathy secondary to diabetes, tens of thousands of patients will benefit from not having to undergo amputation procedures, or at least forestalling the amputation procedure until a much later time. The treatments, whether it be related to carotid stenosis, mesenteric ischemia, neural vascular spasm, or congenital vascular lesions, have the potential of reaching millions of patients every year.

This book also bridges issues related to complications or other challenges related to performing aggressive angioplasty procedures. Whether it be hyperperfusion syndrome following aggressive angioplasty or oxygen stress and altered function of platelets in patients with peripheral arterial vascular disease, not only do interventionalists need to be knowledgeable in the technique in performing an intervention, they also must have a strong understanding of what the potential ramifications are both on an anatomic and molecular level.

To end, this first edition on Angioplasty will hopefully inspire interventionalists to "cross-link" their experience with other interventionalists regarding the techniques used to treat complicated lesions. I personally feel that communication is the most important ally to overcoming challenges in both acquired and congenital vascular lesions. Hopefully this book will inspire this to occur between interventional radiologists, cardiologists, neurologists, and neurosurgeons. I would not be surprised, with the continued explosion of a technology in this area, that revision of this book will be required within the next 7-10 years. Finally, one would be remiss in not giving credit to Warner Forsmann for his insight in the catheterization procedure and, as previously mentioned, Andre Gruentzig in launching us into an interventional era for the treatment of vascular stenosis. On the shoulders of these two giants (and many others) we are able to proceed onto an exciting and changing world of interventional cardiology.

I would like to greatly acknowledge the authors of this book for their time in writing the chapters. Without their dedication to sharing their interventional expertise, this book would never come to fruition. I also would like to thank my lovely wife Marie who, without her dedication to raising nine children (myself included), I would never have had the remote possibility for being able to find the time to undertake this endeavor.

Dr. Thomas Forbes
Wayne State University / Children's Hospital of Michigan, Detroit
USA

1

Percutaneous Angioplasty and Stenting for Mesenteric Ischaemia

Emily He[1] and Stephen M. Riordan[2]
[1]*Gastroenterology Registrar, Gastrointestinal and Liver Unit Prince of Wales Hospital, Sydney*
[2]*Senior Staff Specialist, Gastrointestinal and Liver Unit, Prince of Wales Hospital Sydney, Australia and Professor of Medicine (Conjoint) University of New South Wales, Sydney Australia*

1. Introduction

Mesenteric ischaemia due to impaired arterial supply is an important cause of abdominal pain, especially in older patients with risk factors for vascular disease. Until recently, surgical revascularisation procedures such as endarterectomy and aorto-coeliac or aorto-mesenteric bypass grafting were the only available treatment options for patients with mesenteric ischaemia. However, reported rates of peri-operative major complications and mortality are high, influenced by a high prevalence of significant patient co-morbidities. Percutaneous angioplasty and stenting have been shown to be effective and safe alternatives to surgical revascularisation in high-risk patients with mesenteric ischaemia. Indeed, in high-surgical risk patients and in those with suitable lesions, such endovascular revascularisation has emerged as the primary treatment modality.

Here, we review current concepts in the diagnosis, treatment selection and outcomes for percutaneous angioplasty and stenting for patients with either chronic or acute mesenteric ischemia.

2. Chronic mesenteric ischaemia

Chronic mesenteric ischaemia (CMI) most commonly arises from atherosclerotic diseases of the mesenteric arteries. Other causes of CMI include aortic dissection, fibromuscular dysplasia, vasculitides and median arcuate ligament syndrome.

Atherosclerotic disease of the mesenteric arteries is estimated to occur in 17% of patients over the age 65 years (Hansen et al., 2004). Despite its prevalence, the majority of these patients are asymptomatic as a result of the extensive collateral circulation between the celiac trunk, superior mesenteric artery (SMA) and inferior mesenteric artery (IMA). Whether or not ischaemia ensues depends on the site of the stenosis or occlusion and the development or otherwise of collateral vessels (Loffroy et al., 2009). CMI typically occurs in patients who have SMA lesions in conjunction with lesions in either the celiac trunk or IMA. However, mesenteric ischaemia can also develop in patients with a single vessel lesion. Distal lesions are more likely to be symptomatic compared with more proximal arterial pathology due to the absence of an effective collateral circulation.

3. Clinical presentation

CMI commonly affects people over the age of 60 years, with women three times more likely to be affected than men (Hansen et al., 2004). Most patients have multiple cardiovascular risk factors and atherosclerotic complications in other vascular territories.
Classic symptoms of CMI include postprandial abdominal pain, fear of eating and significant weight loss. Patients may also present with persistent nausea and diarrhoea. These symptoms are non-specific and extensive investigations are generally undertaken to exclude other pathologies such as gastrointestinal or pancreatic malignancy.

4. Diagnosis

Duplex ultrasound is a useful, non-invasive screening test for mesenteric ischaemia (Moneta et al., 1993) (Table 1). Its accuracy is affected by operator experience and patient factors such as fasting status, body habitus and presence of bowel gas. CT-angiography and MR-angiography are of value in cases where duplex ultrasound is inconclusive (Cademartiri et al., 2008; Horton et al., 2007; Laissy et al., 2002). CT-angiography also provides excellent 3-D anatomical reconstruction to facilitate planning for endovascular revascularisation. Nevertheless, digital subtraction angiography remains the gold standard in evaluating the degree of stenosis in mesenteric vessels.

Vessel	Duplex criteria	Sensitivity	Specificity	Accuracy
SMA	PSV > 275cm/s	92%	96%	96%
Coeliac trunk	PSV > 200cm/s	87%	82%	82%

PSV: peak systolic velocity

Table 1. Duplex ultrasound criteria for detecting >70% stenosis in mesenteric vessels (from Moneta et al., 1993).

5. Treatment options

Treatment of symptomatic CMI is aimed at relieving symptoms and preventing progression to acute mesenteric ischaemia (AMI) and intestinal infarction. Prophylactic treatment of asymptomatic patients is controversial. The risk of progressing to AMI is greatest in patients with three-vessel disease with an estimated one third of these patients progressing to intestinal infarction if left untreated (Kolkman et al., 2004). The prognosis is relatively benign in those with single-vessel disease. In participants of the Cardiovascular Health Study who were found to have isolated coeliac trunk or mesenteric artery disease on duplex ultrasound, there was no increased risk of mortality, intestinal infarction or development of symptoms consistent with CMI over a median follow up period of 6.5years (Wilson et al., 2006).
The gold standard of treatment has traditionally been surgical revascularisation in the form of bypass, endarterectomy or embolectomy. Given that patients affected by CMI are generally malnourished, of advanced age and have multiple cardiovascular co-morbidities, there is considerable peri-operative mortality (0-17%) and morbidity (15-33%) associated with surgical revascularisation (Kougias et al., 2009).
Endovascular revascularisation is increasingly being offered to patients affected by CMI. In a large US registry study comprising of 5583 patients treated for CMI during the years 1988

to 2006 (Schermerhorn et al., 2009), the number of endovascular procedures steadily increased, surpassing all surgery for CMI in 2002. Endovascular revascularisation is associated with a lower in-hospital mortality and morbidity rate as well as shorter length of stay. Significantly lower rates of bowel resection, as well as fewer renal, cardiac and respiratory complications have been reported in patients who received endovascular revascularisation compared to surgically-treated counterparts (Table 2). A later analysis of published data concerning procedures performed between 2000 and 2009 similarly demonstrated a significantly reduced peri-operative complication rate in patients managed by endovascular therapy compared to surgery (Gupta et al., 2010).

	Endovascular revascularisation	**Surgical revascularisation**	**p-value**
Mortality	3.7%	15.4%	<0.001
Overall morbidity	20%	38%	<0.05
Bowel resection	3%	8%	<0.001
Cardiac events	0.7%	5.9%	<0.001
Respiratory events	0.3%	5.7%	<0.001
Acute renal failure	6.0%	10.5%	<0.05
LOS median (range), days	5 (0-94)	11 (1-135)	<0.001

Table 2. Mortality, morbidity, peri-operative complications and length of stay (LOS): endovascular revascularisation vs. surgical revascularisation. (adapted from Schermerhorn et al., 2009)

A serious potential complication of endovascular treatment is the precipitation of acute intestinal ischemia by plaque embolization or dissection of the artery. Standard catheter based salvage techniques such as stent deployment, embolectomy or thrombolysis are usually successful in treating these complications. Emergency laparotomy with mesenteric bypass and bowel resection is also used as salvage treatment. We recently reported the occurrence of splenic infarction complicating otherwise successful celiac artery stenting, presumably as a consequence of distal embolization of disrupted calcific plaque, with this complication representing a novel cause of abdominal pain post-procedure (Almeida & Riordan, 2008).

The most common procedural complication of endovascular therapy relates to the puncture site, manifesting as either haemorrhage or thrombosis. Haemorrhage is generally controlled with local pressure and/or injection of thrombin. Insertion of interventional sheaths in small arteries is associated with an increased risk of thrombosis. Rapid heparinization after sheath insertion is usually an adequate preventative measure.

Another important issue is the longer-term arterial patency rate in patients treated by endovascular means compared to those managed surgically. In a recent review of 328 patients undergoing endovascular treatment for chronic mesenteric ischaemia, the overall technical success rate was 91% and immediate symptomatic relief was achieved in 82% of patients (Kougias et al., 2007). Despite the initial success rate, approximately one third of patients (84/292) available for follow up developed restenosis over a mean follow up period of 26 months. The 30-day mortality rate was 3-5%. Clinical series comparing endovascular and surgical revascularisation have shown that long term patency rates and freedom from symptoms may be inferior in patients who have had endovascular revascularisation (Kougias et al., 2009; Atkins et al., 2007; Kasiragjan et al., 2001). Indeed, an analysis of all published literature comparing surgical and endovascular treatment options for CMI performed between 2000 and 2009 concluded that 5-year primary patency rates were 3.8 times greater in the surgical group (P<0.001), while freedom from symptoms at 5 years was 4.4 times greater in patients managed surgically compared to those treated with endovascular techniques (p<0.001) (Gupta et al., 2010).

6. Angioplasty vs stenting

There is general agreement that stenting is indicated for residual stenosis following primary angioplasty (defined as residual stenosis of 30% or more, or pressure gradient higher than 15mmHg), for ostial or eccentric lesions, or as a salvage procedure for acute dissection after angioplasty (Kougias et al., 2007). Balloon-expandable stents are preferred because of their accuracy and ability to generate considerable radial force. More distal or long lesions may be better suited to self-expandable stents given their flexibility (Loffroy et al., 2009).

Kougias et al (2007) reported that technical success was significantly higher with stenting compared with angioplasty alone (95% vs 83%, p=0.007), although the rate of restenosis was also higher in the stented subgroup, a finding that may have been biased by the inclusion of earlier studies where more primitive stents were used and peri-procedural anticoagulant and antiplatelet treatment regimens were not standardized. A recent case series demonstrated that long-term patency rate was higher in patients managed with primary stenting compared to angioplasty alone (Daliri et al., 2010).

7. Which vessel to treat

Literature from the surgical revascularisation setting has shown that complete revascularisation of the coeliac trunk and SMA is associated with improved long-term outcomes (Mateo et al., 1999; McAfee et al., 1992; Foley et al., 2000). The simultaneous treatment of two vessels prevents symptom recurrence in the event of restenosis in either artery. Improved graft patency and survival with complete reconstruction (McAfee et al., 1992), and a higher incidence of symptoms and graft failure with single vessel therapy (Foley et al., 2000) have each been demonstrated.

There is a tendency to treat fewer vessels when choosing endovascular revascularisation compared with surgical revascularisation (Kougias et al., 2009). The conventional approach to endovascular intervention is to treat SMA lesions in preference to celiac trunk or IMA lesions. There is conflicting evidence as to whether treatment of both SMA and celiac arteries will produce better long-term patency. A recent series by Peck et al indicated that two-vessel treatment resulted in lower symptomatic recurrences, improved patency and fewer re-interventions (Peck et al., 2010). On the other hand, Sarac et al. (2008) did not report any difference in 1 year patency between single-vessel and two-vessel treatment, while Malgor et al. (2010) similarly found in a study of longer follow-up of 3 years that two-vessel celiac artery and SMA stenting did not result in improved outcomes when compared with single-vessel SMA stent placement for CMI.

Traditionally, there has been a preference for treating stenotic rather than occlusive lesions by endovascular means. Although the presence of an occluded vessel is not an absolute contraindication to endovascular intervention, the practice in many centres is to convert from endovascular to open surgical revascularisation when an occlusion is found (Kasiragjan et al., 2001). Endovascular passage of guide wires and stents through totally occluded lesions is a technically challenging procedure and not without significant risks of vessel perforation or dissection. Although not statistically validated, the degree of difficulty is likely to increase with the length of occlusion. A theoretical concern also exists for plaque fragmentation and distal embolization, which also increases with the length of occlusion.

Although the efficacy of endovascular intervention in treating occluded mesenteric vessels is not well established, evolving endovascular technology with low-profile systems has now made recanalization of occluded vessels feasible. Landis et al. (2005) reported technical success and 1-year patency rates of 100% in 9 patients with mesenteric occlusion. A case series by Peck et al also indicated that patients with occluded SMA who underwent revascularisation had lower 3-year symptom recurrence rates, with three year patency rates of 90% for treated SMA occlusions versus 40% for untreated SMA occlusions (Peck et al., 2010). This difference however was not statistically significant, possibly due to the small numbers of patients studied.

8. Surveillance of vessel patency

There is a lack of uniformity in the follow up of patients who have received endovascular therapy for CMI. Although recurrence of symptoms is correlated with restenosis, this alone is not a reliable predictor of vessel patency, with sensitivity as low as 33% for detection of restenosis (McMillan et al., 1995). Failure to diagnose progressive disease in asymptomatic patients may result in the subsequent development of acute mesenteric thrombosis. This is a potentially fatal vascular emergency with overall mortality rate ranging from 32% to 65% (Park et al., 2002).

Abdominal duplex ultrasonography is the most commonly used method of surveillance due to its non-invasive nature. Although duplex ultrasonography has been validated in the diagnosis of mesenteric arterial stenosis (Zwolak et al., 1998), there is no current consensus on which velocity criteria should be used to define high-grade recurrent disease (Kasirajan et al., 2001; Armstrong et al., 2007; Fenwick et al., 2007). CT-angiography and MR-angiography are alternative modalities of imaging, although digital substraction angiography is generally considered the gold standard. There is a potential role for functional studies such as gastrointestinal tonometry to detect mesenteric ischemia and guide treatment (Otte et al., 2008).

9. Acute mesenteric ischemia

Acute mesenteric ischemia is associated with a daunting mortality rate of greater than 50% (Schermerhorn et al., 2009). Prompt diagnosis and institution of revascularisation therapy are crucial for a successful outcome.

Endovascular treatment for AMI was traditionally reserved for selected patients who have prohibitive operative risk, no clinical signs of peritoneal inflammation, or those with a contaminated peritoneal cavity and no autogenous vessel available for grafting (Loffroy et al., 2009). With evolving expertise and technological advancements in endovascular therapy, there has been an increase in the use of endovascular revascularisation for treatment of AMI. In the US registry study of 5237 patients treated for AMI, the outcomes of patients who were treated with endovascular intervention were compared to those who were treated with surgery (Schermerhorn et al., 2009). Patients who were treated with endovascular measures tended to have higher rates of cardiovascular comorbidities than those undergoing open surgical repair, including hypertension, peripheral vascular disease, coronary artery disease and chronic renal failure. Despite these unfavourable patient characteristics, mortality was significantly lower in the endovascular group compared with the surgical group (16% vs 39%, $p<0.001$).

In a recent retrospective, single centre case series of 70 patients with AMI, the largest such case series to date, Arthurs et al. (2011) demonstrated that the use of endovascular therapy as primary treatment for AMI produced lower complication rates and better outcomes (Arthurs et al., 2011). During a 9-year study period, endovascular therapy was initiated in 56 patients while surgical therapy was used in 24 patients. Overall, technical success for endovascular therapy was 87%. Failures in endovascular therapy were treated with embolectomy in 78% and revascularisation in 22%. Successful endovascular treatment resulted in a mortality rate of 36%, which was significantly lower compared with a rate of 50% in those treated surgically ($p<0.05$). Patients who failed endovascular treatment had a mortality rate of 50%, an outcome which was equivalent to that of traditional surgical therapy. Block et al. (2010) have also recently reported improved 30 day and long-term survival with endovascular revascularisation of the SMA compared to surgery in patients identified through the Swedish Vascular Registry from 1999 to 2006, although the need for prospective randomised data to confirm group differences was highlighted.

The general view that laparotomy is crucial for all patients with AMI to assess intestinal viability and perform resection as required has also recently been questioned. Arthurs et al. (2011) challenged this philosophy by performing laparotomy only on patients who had signs of peritoneal inflammation or deteriorated clinically following initial revascularisation. Over 30% of patients in the endovascular therapy group did not ultimately require laparotomy, thereby avoiding further physiologic insult to patients who are already critically ill.

Another important issue is to what extent ischaemia-reperfusion injury of the intestine, leading to microvascular injury and cellular necrosis and apoptosis, contributes to morbidity and mortality in patients in whom arterial revascularisation is attained and whether various recent advances in preventing or limiting this phenomenon described in the experimental situation can be translated clinically (Santora et al., 2011; Petrat & de Groot, 2011; Flessas et al., 2011).

10. Conclusions

There has been a recent paradigm shift in the treatment of mesenteric ischaemia. Whereas endovascular therapy was once reserved for the few patients who had prohibitive operative risks, it is now increasingly used for revascularisation of both chronic and acute mesenteric ischemia. Endovascular therapy is less invasive than open surgery, and is associated with lower peri-procedural morbidity and mortality. There is growing evidence that stenting may achieve better technical success and patency rates compared with angioplasty alone. The timing and choice of imaging modality for surveillance of vessel patency remains an important question for clinicians. Effective approaches to improving longer-term vessel patency rates following endovascular therapy are required, along with strategies to prevent ischaemia-reperfusion injury in those patients with acute mesenteric ischaemia in whom revascularisation is achieved.

11. References

Almeida JA, Riordan SM. Splenic infarction complicating percutaneous transluminal coeliac artery stenting for chronic mesenteric ischaemia. *Journal of Medical Case Reports* 2008; 2: 261.

Armstrong PA. Visceral duplex scanning: evaluation before and after artery intervention for chronic mesenteric ischemia. *Perspect Vasc Surg Endovasc Ther* 2007; 19: 386-92.

Arthurs ZM, Titus J, Bannazadeh M, et al. A comparison of endovascular revascularisation with traditional therapy for the treatment of acute mesenteric ischemia. *J Vasc Surg* 2011; 53:698-704.

Atkins MD, Kwolek CJ, LaMuraglia GM. Surgical revascularisation versus endovascular therapy for chronic mesenteric ischemia: a comparative experience. *J Vasc Surg* 2007; 45:1162-1171.

Block TA, Acosta S, Bjorck M. Endovascular and open surgery for acute occlusion of the superior mesenteric artery. Journal of Vascular Surgery 2010; 52 (4): 959-966.

Cademartiri F, Palumbo A, Maffei E, et al. Noninvasive evaluation of the celiac trunk and superior mesenteric artery with multislice CT in patients with chronic mesenteric ischemia. *Radiol Med* 2008; 113:1135-1142.

Daliri A. Grunwald C. Jobst B, et al. Endovascular treatment for chronic atherosclerotic occlusive mesenteric disease: is stenting superior to balloon angioplasty? *Vasa* 2010; 39: 319-24

Fenwick JL, Wright. Endovascular repair of chronic mesenteric occlusive disease: the role of duplex surveillance. *Aust N Z J Surg* 2007; 77:60-63

Flessas II, Papalois AE, Toutouzas K, Zagouri F, Zografos GC. Effects of lazaroids on intestinal ischemia and reperfusion injury in experimental models. Journal of Surgical Research 2011; 166: 265-274.

Foley MI, Moneta GL, Abou-Zamzam AM Jr, et al. Revascularisation of the superior mesenteric artery alone for treatment of intestinal ischemia. *J Vasc Surg* 2000;32:37-47

Gupta PK, Horan SM, Turaga KK, Miller WJ, Pipinos II. Chronic mesenteric ischemia: endovascular versus open revascularisation. Journal of Endovascular Therapy 2010; 17 (4): 540-549.

Hansen KJ, Wilson DB, Craven TE, et al. Mesenteric artery disease in the elderly. *J Vasc Surg* 2004;40:45-52

Horton KM, Fishman EK. Multidetector CT angiography in the diagnosis of mesenteric ischemia. *Radiol Clin North Am* 2007; 45:275-288

Kasirajan K, O'Hara PJ, Gray BH, et al. Chronic mesenteric ischemia: Open surgery versus percutaneous angioplasty and stenting. *J Vasc Surg* 2001;33:63–71

Kolkman JJ, Mensink PB, van Petersen AS, et al. Clinical approach to chronic gastrointestinal ischemia from "intestinal angina" to the spectrum of chronic splanchnic disease. *Scand J Gastroenterol Suppl* 2004; 241: 9-16.

Kougias P, El Sayed H, Zhou W, et al. Management of chronic mesenteric ischemia. The Role of Endovascular Therapy. *J Endovasc Ther* 2007; 14:395-405

Kougias P, Huyng TT, Lin PH. Clinical outcomes of mesenteric artery stenting versus surgical revascularisation in chronic mesenteric ischemia. *Int Angio.* 2009; 28(2):132-137.

Laissy JP, Trillaud H, Douek P. MR angiography: noninvasive vascular imaging of the abdomen. *Abdom Imaging* 2002; 27:488-506

Landis MS, Rajan DK, Simons ME, et al. Percutaneous management of chronic mesenteric ischemia: outcomes after intervention. *J Vasc Inter Radiol* 2005; 16:1319-1325

Loffroy R, Steinmetz E, Guiu B, et al. Role for endovascular therapy in chronic mesenteric ischemia. *Can J Gastroenterol* 2009; 23:365-373

Malgor RD, Oderich GS, McKusick MA, Misra S, Kalra M, Duncan AA, Bower TC, Glaviczki P. Results of single- and two-vessel mesenteric artery stents for chronic mesenteric ischemia. Annals of Vascular Surgery 2010; 24 (8): 1094-1101.

Mateo RB, O'Hara PJ, Hertzer NR, et al. Elective surgical treatment of symptomatic chronic mesenteric occlusive disease: early results and late outcomes. *J Vasc Surg* 1999; 29:821-31

McAfee MK, Cherry KJ Jr, Naessens JM, et al. Influence of complete revascularisation on chronic mesenteric ischemia. *Am J Surg* 1992; 164:220-4

McMillan WD, McCarthy WJ, Bresticker MR, et al. Mesenteric artery bypass: objective patency determination. *J Vasc Surg* 1995; 21: 729-740

Moneta GL, Lee RW, Yeager RA, et al. Mesenteric duplex scanning: a blinded prospective study. *J Vasc Surg* 1993; 17:79-84

Otte JA, Huisman AB, Geelkerken Rh, et al. Jejunal tonometry for the diagnosis of gastrointestinal ischemia. Feasibility, normal values and comparison of jejeunal with gastric tonometry exercise testing. *Eur J Gastroenterol Hepatol* 2008; 20:62-67

Peck MC, Conrad MF, Kwolek CJ, et al. Intermediate-term outcomes of endovascular treatment for symptomatic chronic mesenteric ischemia. *J Vasc Surg* 2010; 51:140-7

Petrat F, Ronn T, de Groot H.Protection by pyruvate infusion in a rat model of severe intestinal ischemia-reperfusion injury. Journal of Surgical Research 2011; 167 (2): e93-e101.

Santora RJ, Lie ML, Grigorev DN, Nasir O, Moore FA, Hassoun HT. Journal of Vascular Surgery 2010; 52 (4): 1003-1014.

Sarac TP, Altinel O, Kashyap V, et al. Endovascular treatment of steno tic and occluded visceral arteries for chronic mesenteric ischemia. *J Vasc Surg* 2008; 47:485-91

Schermerhorn ML, Giles KA, Hamdan AD, et al. Mesenteric revascularisation: management and outcomes in the United States, 1988-2006. *J Vasc Surg* 2009; 50:341-348

Wilson DB, Mostafavi K, Craven TE, et al. Clinical course of mesenteric artery stenosis in elderly Americans. *Arch Intern Med* 2006; 166:2095-100.

Zwolak RM, Fillinger MF, Walsh DB, et al. Mesenteric and celiac duplex scanning: a validation study. J Vasc Surg 1998; 27:1078-87.

2

Cerebral Hyperperfusion Syndrome After Angioplasty

D. Canovas[1], J. Estela[1], J. Perendreu[2], J. Branera[2], A. Rovira[3], M. Martinez[4] and A. Gimenez-Gaibar[5]

[1]*Department of Neurology*
[2]*Department of Interventional Radiologist*
[3]*Department of Neuroradiology*
[4]*Department of Intensive Care*
[5]*Department of Vascular Surgery*
Hospital de Sabadell, Barcelona
Spain

1. Introduction

Cerebral hyperperfusion syndrome (CHS) was first described by Sundt et al. (1981) as a clinical syndrome following carotid endarterectomy (CEA) characterized by headache, neurological deficit, and epileptic seizures that is not caused by cerebral ischemia.

This chapter deals with this uncommon but not exceptional complication of endovascular treatment of the arteries that supply the brain. We use the term carotid artery stenting (CAS) to refer to stenting of the internal carotid artery (ICA) because most publications are centered on this artery. Moreover, we include angioplasty without stent placement in the term CAS to facilitate reading comprehension because the relation between endovascular treatment and CHS is related to revascularization itself rather than to stent placement per se.

Given the high rate of ischemic brain disease in relation to carotid stenosis and the high prevalence of asymptomatic carotid stenosis, numerous publications discuss CHS in relation to CEA: the incidence in these series ranges from 0.3% to 2.2%. However, CAS has continually evolved in recent years to the point where, after more than 40 years' experience, it is considered an alternative to CEA. Furthermore, the development of new materials for stents, filters for distal protection, dual antiplatelet treatment, and the learning curve are minimizing the short- and long-term adverse effects of CAS.

Documented complications of CAS include cerebral embolism, hemodynamic compromise, vessel dissection, and early restenosis and occlusion, as well as the hyperperfusion syndrome we deal with in this chapter. Moreover, the spectacular increase in endovascular treatment has revealed that hyperperfusion syndrome can also occur after revascularization of other arteries, such as the vertebral arteries, the subclavian arteries, or even those located within the brain, mainly the middle cerebral artery (MCA).

In this chapter we will begin by discussing the pathophysiology, clinical presentation, and incidence of CHS in the different published series. We will then discuss the risk factors, diagnostic methods, and strategies for prevention and treatment. We will also discuss a condition that shares the same pathophysiology as CHS, contrast-induced encephalopathy, in which contrast agents crossing the blood-brain barrier have a toxic effect on the brain parenchyma, resulting in signs and symptoms similar to those of CHS. Given the larger number of publications about hyperperfusion after CEA and the obvious similarities in aspects like the pathophysiology and risk factors, we refer to CEA on numerous occasions in this chapter.

2. Pathophysiology

First, we must differentiate between the concept of hyperperfusion and CHS. In general, hyperperfusion is considered to occur when cerebral blood flow (CBF) in the revascularized territory increases by 100% or more with respect to the baseline values. In series by Ogasawara (2007) and Fukuda (2007), 16.7% to 28.6% of the patients with an increase in CBF 100% developed CHS. Moreover, a few cases of CHS in which CBF had increased less than 100% have been reported (Karapanayiotides et al, 2005; Henderson et al, 2001). Thus, other factors must be involved in CHS (Hosoda et al, 2003; Kaku et al, 2004; Ogasawara et al 2003; Suga et al, 2007; Yoshimoto et al, 1997).

All authors agree that it is very likely that there has to be damage to cerebral autoregulation, in other words, impaired cerebral vasoreactivity (CVR), for CHS to occur (Keunen et al, 2001).

Cerebral hemodynamics and CVR are individualized in each patient. This could be explained by the different extent of collateral circulation available and by the autoregulatory mechanisms of the cerebral circulation. The presence of sufficient collateral circulation has a key role in the preservation of CVR, and thus protects against CHS.

Similarly, other risk factors for CHS are low pulsatility index, severe ipsilateral and contralateral carotid disease, and an incomplete circle of Willis (Jansen et al, 1994; Reigel et al, 1987; Sbarigia et al 1993).

CVR makes it possible to keep blood pressure (BP) between acceptable limits (60 mmHg - 160 mmHg) through arteriolar vasodilatation or vasoconstriction in response to changes in carbon dioxide. This response is most pronounced in smaller arteries (diameter 0·5–1·0 mm), whereas arteries with a diameter of 2·5 mm or more like the ICA show no substantial change.

Regulation involves a myogenic and a neurogenic component. In myogenic autoregulation, increased intravascular pressure results in vasoconstriction of small arterioles at high systemic BP, but when BP exceeds the limit of myogenic autoregulation, the remaining autoregulation in small arteries is dependent on sympathetic autonomic innervation. As a result of sparse sympathetic innervation, the vertebrobasilar system is less protected than other regions of the brain, which explains why this system is more affected in entities like hypertensive encephalopathy. Impaired CVR results in failure of the arterial system to respond to a sudden increase in CBF and is usually due to severe vascular stenosis together with insufficient collateral blood flow. When these two factors coexist, cerebral perfusion is maintained by the maximum dilation of the arterioles. This prolonged vasodilation makes the vessels unable to respond with vasoconstriction when blood flow is increased, and especially when it is increased suddenly (Ascher et al, 2003; Jansen et al, 1994; Reigel et al, 1987; Tang et al, 2008 Sbarigia et al, 1993).

At the end of the 1990s, some surgical reports already suggested that patients with preoperative hemodynamic failure were at definite risk for CHS (Baker et al, 1998; Cikrit et al 1997; Yoshimoto et al, 1997) and that the presence of a critical stenosis in the ICA increased the risk of intracranial hemorrhage (ICH) (Jansen et al, 1994; Macfarlane et al, 1991; Ouriel et al, 1999; Sbarigia et al, 1993). Preoperative significant reduction in flow velocity compared with baseline values is indicative of hypoperfusion and is associated with postoperative hyperperfusion (Keunen et al, 2001).

Sudden revascularization brought about by angioplasty leads to dysfunction of the blood-brain barrier after the failure of arteriolar vasoconstriction. This results in transudation of fluid into the pericapillary astrocytes and interstitium, giving rise to vasogenic edema. This hydrostatic edema predominantly affects the vertebrobasilar circulation territory in both CHS and hypertensive encephalopathy, possibly as a result of regional variation in cerebral sympathetic innervation.

The most extreme form of this syndrome is bleeding, either ICH, which results in high morbidity and mortality, or subarachnoid hemorrhage (SAH), which has a better prognosis. The pathophysiology of the hemorrhage that results from revascularization might be different from that of CHS described by Sundt, et al (1981). Some authors (Karapanayiotides et al, 2005) prefer to call this entity "reperfusion syndrome" to emphasize the damage to tissues caused by simple reperfusion. Several investigators have analyzed the characteristics of this ICH when it appears in the first few hours and without prodromes, attributing it to the rupture of deep penetrating arteries as a result of the sudden normalization of the pressure of cerebral perfusion after angioplasty, similar to what occurs in hemorrhage due to hypertension (Buhk et al, 2006; Coutts et al, 2003).

Many cases of SAH after CAS have been reported (Abou-Chebl et al, 2004; Coutts et al, 2003; Hartmann et al, 2004; Ho et al, 2000; McCabe et al, 1999; Meyers et al, 2000; Morrish et al, 2000; Nikolsky et al, 2002; Pilz et al, 2006; Qureshi et al, 2002); these have a better prognosis than ICH.

It is logical to assume that CBF increases substantially after CAS in a severely stenosed carotid artery. However, studies show that the increase in CBF is actually related to impaired CVR. In a study by Hosoda et al (1998) CBF significantly increased on the first postoperative day in subjects with reduced preoperative CVR but not in those with normal preoperative CVR. Similarly, in a study of 23 patients, Ko et al (2005) were unable to demonstrate a relation between the degree of stenosis and the increase in CBF. In short, the degree of stenosis cannot be considered a key risk factor for CHS, although some series have taken it into account.

Ascher et al (2003) studied 455 patients undergoing CEA and found no relation between CHS and the severity of ipsilateral or contralateral carotid stenosis, arterial hypertension, or perioperative perfusion pressure. However, mean ICA volume flow and peak systolic velocity measured at the onset of symptoms in the 9 CHS cases were higher than in the remaining 446 cases.

In most cases of symptomatic carotid stenoses due to a hemodynamic mechanism CVR is also deficient, so it is logical to think that they will be more susceptible to developing CHS after revascularization (Brantley et al, 2009). However, in a study of 333 patients undergoing CAS, Karkos et al (2010) found no significant differences between symptomatic and asymptomatic patients.

Fukuda et al (2007) carried out an interesting study of CBF and cerebral blood volume (CBV) in 15 patients without contralateral carotid stenosis undergoing CEA. They observed a correlation between increased CBV and increased CBF after CEA on single-photon emission computed tomography (SPECT) and magnetic resonance imaging (MRI), with signs of hyperperfusion in seven patients (47%). Two of these seven patients developed

CHS, whereas none of the eight patients with normal CBV developed CHS. In this study, elevated preoperative CBV was the only significant independent predictor of post-CEA hyperperfusion.

The endothelial damage caused mainly by chronic hypertension in the small arteries may also be related to cerebral autoregulation (Skydell et al, 1987). In fact, some authors relate a history of stroke with a greater risk of CHS (Chamorro et al, 2000; McCabe et al, 1999).

Another important but not essential factor associated with CHS is high blood pressure. High blood pressure is the only factor we can treat, so it has become the principal target for prevention and treatment. Indeed, the pathophysiology of CHS is similar to that of hypertensive encephalopathy in which the blood-brain barrier ruptures as a consequence of severe hypertension. Furthermore, histologic changes like fibrinoid necrosis and petechial hemorrhage also occur in both hypertensive encephalopathy and CHS (Bernstein et al, 1984; Mansoor et al, 1996; Schwartz 2002; Vaughan & Delanty, 2000).

The mechanisms by which BP increases after carotid revascularization are poorly understood. The baroreceptor reflex might break down after receptor denervation after CEA or CAS, and hypertension accompanying this feature might increase cerebral perfusion which is more evident after bilateral carotid surgery (Ahn et al, 1989; Bove et al, 1979; Timmers et al, 2004) and is reported in 19% to 64% after CEA.

The stimulation of these baroreceptors in the carotid bifurcation during angioplasty can cause transient bradycardia and hypotension that can be followed by rebound hypertension. Other phenomena proposed to explain the high blood pressure include increased norepinephrine levels probably related to cerebral edema and increased intracranial pressure, the release of vasoactive neuropeptides, the use of anesthetic drugs, and perioperative stress (Bajardi et al, 1989; Benzel & Hoppens, 1991; Macfarlane et al, 1991; Towne JB & Bernhard, 1980; Skydell et al, 1987; Skudlarick & Mooring, 1982;).

Another possible mediator of impaired autoregulation in CHS is nitric oxide, which causes vasodilatation and can increase the permeability of cerebral vessels. Increased nitric oxide levels during clamping of the ICA and increased oxygen-derived free radicals produced during the restoration of cerebral perfusion are involved in endothelial dysfunction and deterioration of autoregulatory mechanisms after CEA (Suga et al, 2007). Several authors (Ogasawara et al, 2004; Saito et al, 2007) have reported that the degree of reactive oxygen species production after ischemia and reperfusion during CEA depends on the intensity of cerebral ischemia during ICA clamping.

Reactive oxygen species can play a role in the pathogenesis of post-CEA hyperperfusion, leading to widespread endothelial damage in the ipsilateral cerebral arteries and thereby increasing the risk of ICH in the early postoperative period. Furthermore, administering a free-radical scavenger can prevent CHS, providing additional support for this mechanism (Ogasawara et al, 2004).

Finally, an axon-like trigeminovascular reflex has been implicated in the pathophysiology of CHS (Macfarlane et al, 1991). The release of vasoactive neuropeptides from perivascular sensory nerves via axon reflex-like mechanisms has a significant bearing upon a number of hyperperfusion syndromes.

3. Clinical presentation

The typical clinical presentation of CHS combines symptoms due to ICH and those due to brain damage caused by vasogenic edema. The most common symptoms caused by ICH are headache, confusion, altered levels of consciousness, and sometimes vomiting. On the other hand, the edema usually manifests as a neurological deficit on the side of the untreated carotid artery, often associated with epileptic activity (seizures, usually starting as partial seizures). Arterial hypertension is the norm in patients that develop symptoms of CHS; however, it is important to remember that bradycardia and hypotension often occur initially after angioplasty due to stimulation of the baroreceptor reflex.

When a patient has symptoms of neurological deficit after angioplasty, the first diagnosis considered is embolic stroke from carotid plaque broken off during the procedure. Thus, CHS can mimic a stroke or transient ischemic attack (TIA), so it is important to take into account symptoms like headache, seizures, and altered mental status that can suggest CHS. Nevertheless, acute neurological deficit accompanied by headache or even seizures is obviously compatible with ICH, which can be ruled out only by neuroimaging.

Neurological deficit due to vasogenic edema is usually transitory, given the absence of ischemic infarction (Bernstein et al, 1984; Piepgras et al 1988; Reigel et al, 1987; Sundt et al, 1981; Solomon et al, 1986). Although the neurological symptoms can vary, the most common are visual or motor deficits and aphasia. Other, rarer, symptoms include psychotic alterations or mild cognitive deficit (Ogasawara et al, 2005).

Seizures are generally partial at first and sometimes become generalized later, although generalized seizures can also occur initially (Ho et al, 2000); in fact, even status epilepticus has been reported up to two weeks after the procedure (Kaku et al, 2004). One third of patients with CHS after CEA have seizures without hemiparesis, another third have hemiparesis without seizures, and another third have both (Bouri et al, 2011).

Curiously, the onset of symptoms after CEA and CAS differs. Symptoms usually do not appear until three to six days after CEA. In contrast, symptoms usually appear within a few hours of CAS. Ogasawara et al (2007) report that the incidence of CHS peaks six days after CEA and 12 hours after CAS. After reviewing 36 studies, Bouri et al (2011) concluded CHS peaks five days after CEA and the latest case occurred after 28 days.

The same is true of ICH, which appears 10.7 ± 9.9 days after CEA and 1.7 ± 2.1 days after CAS, peaking in the first 12 hours. Tan et al (2004) studied the appearance and onset of complications after CAS in 201 patients; they report 10 cases with TIA (4.9%), 5 of which occurred more than 48 hours after the procedure, and 8 strokes (3.9%), 5 of which occurred between 2 and 19 days after the procedure. Curiously, however, these authors found no cases of CHS.

The headache in CHS is usually moderate to severe and throbbing, similar to a migraine headache (Coutts et al, 2003), and it usually affects the same side as the artery treated.

Headache may be the only manifestation of CHS (Connolly 2000; Ouriel et al, 1999; Sbarigia et al, 1993), so occasionally it has been considered a diagnostic criterion. After CEA, headaches are reported in 20% of patients without CHS, in 59% of those with CHS, and in 84% of those with ICH (Bouri et al, 2011).

Postprocedural hypertension is a critical, though not essential, finding associated with CHS (Solomon et al, 1986; Schroeder et al, 1987; Ouriel et al 1999). Bouri et al review (2011) found that the mean systolic BP of CHS cases was 189 mmHg at presentation, and the proportion of patients with severe hypertension was significantly higher in patients who developed CHS after CEA than in those who did not.

Hypotension occurs immediately after CAS in 19% to 51% of patients. It is usually transient and rarely symptomatic, although it lasts longer than 24 hours in nearly 5% of patients. Bradycardia is also common, with an incidence of 3% to 37% in patients administered prophylactic atropine and of 20% to 60% in series with no use of prophylactic atropine. Increased age, symptomatic lesions, presence of ulceration and calcification, and carotid bulb lesions are significant predictors of bradycardia during CAS (Cayne et al, 2005; Lin et al, 2007; Pappada et al, 2006 & Taha et al, 2008).

Another complication with more dramatic consequences is ICH, which affects less than 1% of patients after CEA and between 0.36% and 4.5% after CAS. Generally, ICH has a poor prognosis, with a 37% to 80% mortality rate and a 20% to 30% risk of poor recovery in survivors after CEA (Piepgras et al,1988; Connolly 2000) and similar consequences after CAS.

4. Diagnosis

The diagnosis of CHS is based on the initial suspicion arising from the characteristic triad of headache, focal neurological deficit, and seizure after arterial revascularization. The differential diagnosis should include stroke and TIA. Seizures and altered consciousness favor the diagnosis of CHS. After the initial clinical suspicion, neuroimaging plays a crucial role because in addition to ruling out ischemic and hemorrhagic lesions it can reveal characteristic signs of hyperperfusion.

Given the widespread availability of CT, any acute neurological event after revascularization is usually studied with this technique. CT is most useful for ruling out hemorrhagic processes. Given that the initial symptoms of CHS can mimic stroke or TIA, CT can give us clues that argue against an ischemic stroke, because CT findings are usually normal after a TIA and are often normal within hours after a stroke. Diffusion MRI is the technique of choice to rule out acute ischemic stroke; MRI has shown that there are a greater number of embolic lesions up to 48 hours after CAS, although nearly all are asymptomatic (Rapp et al, 2007).

We will comment on two important aspects of neuroimaging studies. First, we will discuss their usefulness in the diagnosis of CHS, as apart from demonstrating typical findings like vasogenic edema (Case 1) they also enable CBF to be quantified (increases in CBF > 100% with respect to baseline values have been related to greater risk of developing CHS). Second, we will discuss the usefulness of these techniques in the evaluation of CVR, the key pathophysiological factor in CHS.

4.1 Diagnosing cerebral hyperperfusion

The imaging techniques that can demonstrate hyperperfusion are single-photon emission computed tomography (SPECT), positron emission tomography (PET), transcranial Doppler (TCD), CT and MRI. According to Penn et al (1995), xenon-enhanced CT is the best method for demonstrating hyperperfusion. Nevertheless, SPECT and TCD are the most common methods in the literature, followed by CT and MRI.

CT in CHS typically reveals ipsilateral sulcal effacement and cerebral edema immediately following the onset of symptoms; these findings are considered indirect signs of hyperperfusion. CT findings early after the onset of symptoms can be completely normal, even when SPECT shows hyperperfusion.

Without doubt, T2-weighted and FLAIR MRI sequences are more precise in demonstrating areas of cerebral edema, and diffusion-weighted MRI makes it possible to rule out hyperacute ischemic lesions.

However, normal findings on MRI do not exclude the presence of CHS. Both MRI and CT enable angiographic maps to be constructed to rule out arterial occlusions and perfusion maps can show local hyperemia. Karapanayiotides et al (2005) reported no abnormalities on diffusion-weighted MRI in patients with CHS after CEA, ruling out acute ischemia; however, perfusion sequences revealed differences in CBF between the hemispheres.

Hypoperfusion before revascularization and especially hyperperfusion (increase in CBF > 100% with respect to baseline values) after revascularization are conditions that are closely related with CHS. TCD is the method most often used to detect these conditions because it enables variations in CBF to be calculated in real time. TCD has many advantages and multiple indications in cerebral vascular disease (Alexandrov et al, 2010). TCD monitoring can provide direct and real-time information on MCA flow indicative of preoperative cerebral hypoperfusion, CVR, postoperative hyperperfusion, and emboli after CEA and CAS. Moreover, TCD is widely available, noninvasive, and reproducible. It is important to do a baseline study to enable flow velocities before and after revascularization to be compared (Dalman et al, 1999; Jansen et al, 1994).

Asher et al (2003) studied 455 patients undergoing CEA and reported a significant increase in mean ICA flow volume in all patients with CHS during the symptomatic period; moreover, after flow velocities return to normal, the symptoms of hyperperfusion disappear.

Diverse publications about patients undergoing CAS emphasize the role of TCD in detecting hemodynamic changes that make it possible to select patients with greater risk of developing CHS. For example, in one interesting study published recently, Kablak et al (2010) monitored both MCAs before and after CAS, finding a relation between ICH in 3 patients and an increase in peak systolic velocities in both MCAs after CAS. Fujimoto et al (2004) examined the changes in the MCA mean flow velocity measured by TCD before and 4 days after CEA. They reported a significant correlation between changes in mean flow velocity and changes in regional CBF; mean flow velocity increased more than 50% in all cases of CHS.

Some studies have used both TCD and SPECT to assess patients before and after revascularization. Recently, Iwata et al (2011) used these two techniques to study 64 patients and found 9 patients who fulfilled the clinical criteria for CHS. These authors relate CHS with decreased CVR and changes in MCA flow velocity after angioplasty.

Perfusion CT has also contributed to our understanding of CHS. Tseng at al (2009) used CT to study 55 patients with symptomatic stenoses >70% of the ICA, analyzing absolute values of CBV, mean transit time (MTT), and CBF. Three (5%) of 55 patients had CHS after CAS. The only significant factor related to the occurrence of CHS was MTT. An MTT cutoff of 3 seconds distinguished between the occurrence and absence of CHS. MTT prolongation is proportional to the degree of stenosis and decrease in blood flow (Maeda et al, 1999; Lythgoe et al, 2000; Soinne et al, 2003). Findings of decreased CBF together with MTT prolongation and a slight increase in CBV indicate that blood vessels are dilated, thus confirming that the autoregulation mechanism is impaired.

Several authors have examined the role of CT and MRI in demonstrating hyperperfusion (Adhiyaman & Alexander 2007; Imai et al 2005; Sundt et al, 1981). Multislice dynamic susceptibility contrast MRI or perfusion-weighted MRI can also be used in the preoperative assessment of CBF (Fukuda et al, 2007; Wiart et al 2000). Perfusion sequences, however, are not quantitative and can only help in the absence of contralateral ICA stenosis.

PET has also provided valuable information about CHS. Matsubara et al (2009) used PET to study patients before and after angioplasty. They found that the vascular reserve tended to improve gradually after CAS, while CBF, cerebral perfusion pressure, and cerebral metabolic rate of oxygen increased rapidly and peaked soon after CAS. These results suggest that a large discrepancy between rapidly increased CBF, perfusion pressure, and a small increase in vascular reserve in the acute stage after CAS could cause CHS.

Cerebral oxygen saturation can serve as an indirect measure of CBF. Clinically, regional cerebral oxygen saturation can be monitored using transcranial near-infrared spectroscopy, which enables noninvasive continuous real-time detection of changes in the ratio of oxyhemoglobin to deoxyhemoglobin in the frontal cortex, an indirect measure of cerebral oxygenation. Recently, a strong linear correlation was reported between increased transcranial regional cerebral oxygen saturation and increased CBF after CEA (Ogasawara et al, 2003). When compared with SPECT, the sensitivity and specificity of transcranial regional cerebral oxygen saturation for the detection of hyperperfusion were 100%. Transcranial near-infrared spectroscopy can demonstrate decreased cerebral oxygenation resulting from ICA clamping (Beese et al, 1998; Duncan et al, 1995; Kirkpatrick et al, 1995; Samra et al, 1996) and can predict post-CEA CHS. Matsumoto et al (2009) used transcranial near-infrared spectroscopy to study 64 patients undergoing CAS, two of whom developed CHS (diagnosed by increased CBF at SPECT the day after treatment). An increase in regional oxygen saturation > 24% three minutes after revascularization was associated with the development of CHS (with impaired CVR). In contrast, in patients without CHS, the normal upper limit of the change in regional oxygen saturation three minutes after revascularization was 10 %.

Oxygen saturation should be monitored for a prudential time because bradycardia and hypotension often occur with CAS and can occasionally lead to low initial values. As occurs in many studies, the small number of patients with CHS in this study does not allow clear conclusions to be drawn; nevertheless, given that transcranial near-infrared spectroscopy is noninvasive and easy to perform, it should be considered for monitoring patients at risk for CHS.

Alternative methods have been applied to identify risk factors for postoperative hyperperfusion, but their utility is not yet clearly established. Electroencephalography is used for neurological monitoring during CEA, but it is of low predictive value for CHS (Reigel et al, 1987). Nicholas et al (1993) reported that a postoperative increase in ocular blood flow greater than 204% measured by ocular pneumoplethysmography is associated with a high risk for CHS.

4.2 Diagnosing hemodynamic reserve

One strategy that is key to preventing CHS is the study of CVR, which is usually done by TCD and SPECT.

SPECT is sensitive for recognizing CHS, differentiating between ischemia and hyperperfusion, and identifying patients at risk for hyperperfusion after CEA (Hosoda et al, 2001; Naylor et al, 2003; Sfyroeras et al, 2006). Several studies using SPECT have demonstrated that decreased CVR using acetazolamide is a significant predictor of post-CEA hyperperfusion (Ogasawara et al, 2003; Yoshimoto et al, 1997).

Fewer studies have focused on patients undergoing CAS. Kaku et al (2004) published one of the first studies about predicting CHS with nuclear medicine techniques in patients undergoing CAS.

They measured resting CBF and CVR to acetazolamide to evaluate CVR, using split-dose [123I] iodoamphetamine SPECT before and 7 days after CAS in 30 patients with critical carotid stenosis. The 3 patients with hyperperfusion all had impaired CVR and asymmetrical carotid

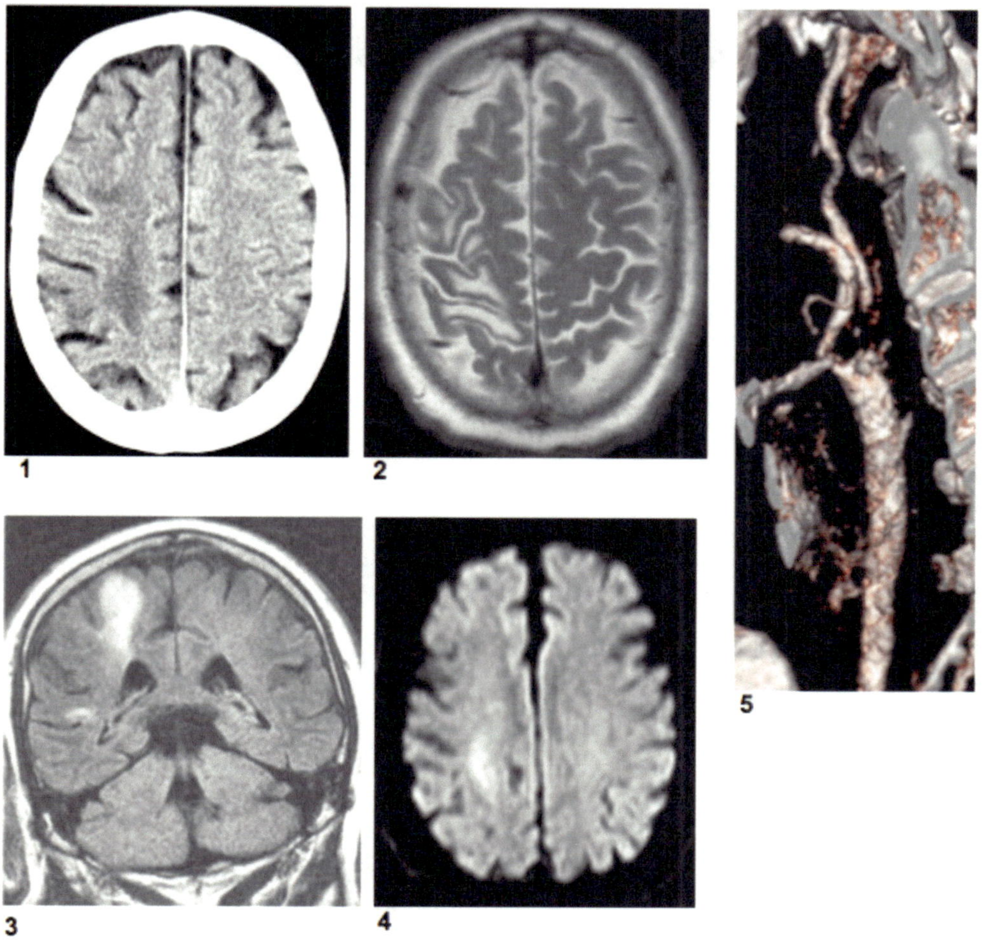

Case 1

A 71-year-old man with symptomatic pseudo-occlusion of the right ICA had a seizure with Todd´s paralysis six days after CEA. Neuroimaging showed vasogenic edema (1- CT, 2- Axial T2-weighted MRi, 3-Coronal FLAIR MRi, 4- Axial diffusion-weighted MRi, 5- CT angiography)

CBF. These authors determined that pretreatment resting CBF value, degree of carotid stenosis, and interval from the onset of ischemic symptoms were not significant risk factors. However, the high cost and limited availability of SPECT preclude its clinical use.

TCD has numerous advantages in diagnosing hemodynamic reserve: it is noninvasive, relatively simple, cheap, and reproducible, and it is risk free when the breath-hold and hyperventilation method is used. TCD enables CVR to be calculated using stimuli like hypocapnia (induced by breath holding or by inhalation of CO_2) or acetazolamide.

The response to these stimuli reflects the cerebral autoregulation capacity and thus makes it possible to determine which patients have a high risk of developing CHS (Sfyroeras 2006,

2009). However, TCD has some drawbacks. The absence of a cranial window makes TCD impossible in 15% of patients, mainly elderly women. Moreover, TCD is operator-dependent and the results also depend on anatomic variants, the degree of collateralization, and contralateral ICA occlusion or stenosis.
Table 1 shows the formulas to calculate the CVR using breath-holding and CO2 inhalation or acetazolamide. In the breath-hold method, patients are asked to hold their breath for at least 30 seconds during continuous MCA flow velocity monitoring; normal values are 1.2 +/- 0.6% / sec. In the hyperventilation/ breath-holding method, patients are asked to hyperventilate for 40 seconds followed by a breath-holding phase of at least 30 seconds. Flow velocity values under maximal hyperventilation and hypoventilation are compared; a relative difference greater than 15% argues against relevant impairment of CVR.

Breath-holding index (BHI)

$$BHI = \frac{V\ apnea - V\ baseline}{V\ baseline \times T\ apnea} \times 100$$

CO2 inhalation test/acetazolamide test

$$CVR = \frac{CO2/acetazolamide - V\ baseline}{Vbaseline} \times 100\%)$$

Table 1.

Chang et al (2009) used functional MRI to assess baseline CVR and changes in CBF after CAS. Although this small series of 14 patients had no cases of CHS, this study revealed that after CAS early CBF changes on the lesion side are more prominent in patients with impaired CVR. Therefore, baseline CVR might predict early CBF increase after CAS. New MRI techniques like dynamic susceptibility contrast MRI or perfusion-weighted MRI can determine CVR (Wiart et al, 2000).

5. Incidence and risk factors

This section reviews the incidence of CHS after CAS in the most relevant series included in PubMed from 2003 to April 2011. We focus on three aspects of CHS: extracranial CAS, angioplasty of intracranial arteries (including the ICA) with or without stenting, and cerebral hemorrhage, the most-feared complication of this treatment.

5.1 Extracranial carotid angioplasty

Most articles about CHS refer to CAS or CEA of the ICA because occlusive disease is more prevalent in these arteries than elsewhere. Bouri et al (2011) reviewed 36 studies of patients undergoing CEA and found 1% incidence of CHS and a 0.5% incidence of ICH.
In many CAS series, patients referred for endovascular treatment comprise a high-risk cohort of suboptimal candidates for conventional surgical management. This might partially

explain the greater number of complications, including CHS, in patients treated with CAS. Furthermore, the endovascular procedure is performed with stricter antithrombotic management, with anticoagulation and dual antiplatelet treatment that might lead to a higher rate of hemorrhagic events, although not all authors agree with this hypothesis (Abou-Chebl et al, 2004; Meyers et al, 2000). Table 2 lists risk factors for CHS, broken down into modifiable and non-modifiable factors.

Although procedural and midterm complication rates of CAS in elderly patients are acceptable, high age seems to be a possible risk factor for CHS (Kadkhodayan et al, 2007). Other risk factors often mentioned in the literature are severe (>90%) ipsilateral stenosis, impaired collateral flow secondary to advanced occlusive disease in other extracranial cerebral vessels or an incomplete circle of Willis, perioperative and postoperative hypertension, and the use of antiplatelet agents or other anticoagulants (Chamorro et al, 2000; Reigel et al, 1987; Sfyroeras et al 2008; Zahn et al, 2007).

Abou et al (2004) report a series of 450 patients undergoing CAS where 5 (1.1%) developed CHS, 3 of them developed ICH (0.67%), and 2 of them (0.44%) died. All the patients that developed CHS had stenoses >90%, contralateral stenoses >80%, and longstanding preprocedural hypertension. The authors calculate that in patients with these three conditions, the risk of developing CHS was 16%. Only 5.8% of the patients that did not develop CHS met these three criteria. The low incidence of CHS in this series might be due to the fact that CHS was not diagnosed in cases with headache and vomiting. Two of the cases of ICH appeared a few days after CAS and only one occurred immediately after the procedure.

Ogasawara et al (2007) published a series of 4494 patients revascularized with CEA or CAS. Of the 1596 patients treated with CEA, 30 (1.9%) developed CHS and 6 of these developed ICH (0.4% of the total). Of the 2898 patients treated with CAS, 31 (1.1%) developed CHS and 21 (0.7% of the total) of these developed ICH. In the group of patients treated with CEA but not in those treated with CAS, poor BP control after revascularization correlated with CHS. CHS and ICH ocurred significantly earlier after CAS than after CEA. The difference between the two procedures in terms of the timing of CHS onset may be explained as follows. First, the higher incidence of embolisms after CAS (Roh et al, 2005) might explain how a hemorrhagic transformation could occur after the resolution of the embolism in the tissue that was damaged; from a pathophysiological point of view, however, this would represent hemorrhagic infarction due to reperfusion rather than CHS. Second, the higher incidence of bradycardia and hypotension after the stimulation of the carotid baroreceptors during CAS (Mendelsohn et al, 1998; McKevitt et al, 2003; Qureshi et al, 1999) can favor cerebral ischemia and CHS after severe rebound hypertension (Abou-Chebl et al, 2007). In an earlier publication (Ogasawara et al, 2003), these authors suggested that SPECT findings of hyperperfusion continuing at least three days after revascularization predisposes to CHS.

In an excellent review of 9 studies of CAS comprising a total of 4446 patients, Moulakakis et al (2009) found the incidences of CHS and ICH were 1.16% (range, 0.44% - 11.7%) and 0.74% (range, 0.36% -4.5%), respectively. Table 3 shows the incidence of CHS and of ICH in the largest series published before 2010, including series of patients undergoing angioplasty of intracranial arteries.

In order to document the incidence of CHS after CAS and to determine possible predisposing factors, Sfyroeras et al (2009) studied 29 patients with CT, MRI, TCD including assessment of CVR, and SPECT before and after the procedure. A total of 5 patients developed adverse neurological events. Two of them developed CHS (6.9%); both had

exhausted CVR in the preoperative TCD examination. All studies that investigate CVR before treatment have found a relation between impaired CVR and the risk of CHS.
Brantley et al (2009) studied 482 patients, 7 (1.45%) of whom developed CHS after CAS. None had an ICH and all recovered within 6 to 24 hours. All had been classified as high risk for CEA, and CHS was more common in those with a previous TIA. The absence of ICH was probably related to the fact that 64% of the patients had asymptomatic stenoses. These authors found no significant relation between CHS and risk factors reported in other series like hypertension, high-grade ICA stenosis, and contralateral disease. The postprocedural BP in the CHS cohort tended to be higher than in the other patients, but this difference did not reach statistical significance.

Potential risk factors for CHS

Modifiable	Not modifiable
High blood pressure	Diminished CVR
Excessive administration of antithrombotic drugs	Hypertensive microangiopathy
Simultaneous revascularization of multiple vessels	Recent minor stroke
Use of high doses of volatile halogenated hydrocarbon anesthetics	Age >70 years
Recent (<3 months) contralateral CEA	High grade carotid artery stenosis
	Incomplete circle of Willis
	Contralateral carotid occlusion
	Poor collateral flow
	Increase in regional cerebral oxygen saturation >24%
	Diabetes mellitus, Hypertension
	Increase in perfusion >100%
	Preoperative hypoperfusion

Table 2.

Grunwald et al (2009) report a series of 417 patients treated with CAS in whom BP was meticulously controlled during the first 24 hours; furthermore, MRI was performed before and after the procedure in 269 cases. The mean degree of carotid stenosis was 87%, and 65% of the patients were symptomatic. Of the 10 (2.4%) patients who developed CHS, seven had excessive small vessel disease with old territorial infarcts or freshly demarked lesions. Small vessel disease is considered a risk factor for CHS because it impairs the capacity of these arteries to contract. Curiously, none of these patients had severe hypertension. In three cases, ICH occurred within a few hours of CAS, and all of these had extensive microvascular changes and impaired collateral blood flow due to high-grade stenosis (>80%) of the contralateral ICA. However, 23% of the patients that did not develop CHS also had high-grade stenosis of the contralateral ICA. On MRI, all had increased signal intensity in the subarachnoid space on the same side as the stented ICA, which resolved within 3–5 days.
Curiously, this study was unable to demonstrate a relation between CHS and factors like postprocedural hypertension, advanced age, degree of ipsilateral stenosis, or contralateral disease.
Regarding prior stroke as a risk factor for CHS, many authors have found that diseases like diabetes mellitus or longstanding pre-existing hypertension in which microangiopathy affects the endothelium of small vessels predispose to hyperperfusion and CHS (Chamorro et al, 2000; McCabe et al, 1999; Naylor et al, 2003; van Mook et al, 2005).

Tietke et al (2010) analyzed the outcomes of 358 patients treated with CAS using small closed-cell stents without distal protection. The peri-interventional and 30-day mortality/stroke rate was 4.19% (15/358). These events included 3 deaths, 5 CHS (comprising one death by a secondary fatal ICH), one SAH and 7 ischaemic strokes. All but one of the patients with CHS had an initial stenosis of >90%; the remaining patient had an initial stenosis of 50% to 70% and was the only one with CHS without ICH. The patient who died was the only woman with CHS and she also had an occluded contralateral ICA. Most complications occurred in initial symptomatic patients (5.36%).

The risk of CHS related to the type of protection (proximal or distal) has not been thoroughly studied. Pieniazek et al. (2004) compared the complications in 135 patients undergoing CAS, 42 with proximal protection and 93 with distal protection, but only one case of CHS developed.

Bilateral carotid stenoses are generally treated in two separate stenting procedures to minimize hemodynamic impairment from stimulation of the carotid sinus baroreceptor reflex (severe bradycardia, hypotension) and the risk of CHS. As we explained in section 2 (pathophysiology), the baroreceptor reflex might break down after receptor denervation after CEA or CAS; this is more common after bilateral carotid surgery, and accompanying hypertension might increase the risk of CHS.

Author / Year	**Patients**	**CHS (%)**	**ICH (%)**
Meyers / 2000	140	7 (5%)	1 (0.7%)
Coutts / 2003	44	3 (6.8%)	2 (4.5%)
Abou / 2004	450	2 (0.44%)	3 (0.67%)
Kaku / 2004	30	1 (3.33%)	0%
Imai / 2005	17	2 (11.7%)	2 (11.7%)
du Mesnil de Rochemontn / 2006	50	1 (2%)	0%
Kablak-Ziembicka / 2006	92	2 (2.2%)	2 (2.2%)
Abou / 2007	836	8 (0.96%)	3 (0.36%)
Ogasawara / 2007	2989	31 (1.1%)	21 (0.7%)
Sfyroeras / 2008	29	2 (7%)	0%
Brantley / 2009	482	7 (1.5%)	0%
Grunwald / 2009	417	7 (1.7%)	3 (0.7%)
Tietke et al (2010)	358	4 (1.1%)	1 (0.27%)
Karkos et al (2010).	316	10 (3%)	0%

Table 3. Incidence of hyperperfusion syndrome, and intracranial hemorrhage after CAS in the reviewed series from 2003 to 2010

Few studies have addressed the subject of simultaneous bilateral CAS. Henry et al. (2005) reported a series of 17 patients who underwent simultaneous bilateral CAS and 40 patients who underwent bilateral CAS in a staged manner (among these 40 patients 10 underwent the second procedure 24 hours after the first, while the other 30 underwent the second procedure from 2 days to 2 months after the first). Two cases of CHS occurred, one each group, although the patient in the simultaneous treatment group who developed CHS died. Lee et al. (2006) found no CHS in a series of 27 patients who underwent bilateral CAS. Diehm et al. (2008) studied patients treated with bilateral CAS with at least one month between procedures and reported no significant differences in complications compared to patients treated with unilateral CAS.

An interesting study that deals with pseudo-occlusive carotids was published by Choi et al (2010). These authors analyze the outcome after CAS in 48 patients with nearly occlusive stenosis of the ICA. The procedural success rate was 98% and a good outcome at six months (modified Rankin scale ≤2) was achieved in 44 patients (92%). Four (8%) patients developed CHS.

Another interesting article was published by Karkos et al (2010). They studied the complications in the first 30 days in 333 angioplasties in 316 patients, 35% of whom had symptomatic carotid disease. Perioperative neurological events included stroke in 6 patients (1.8%), TIA in 15 (4.5%), and CHS in 10 (3.0%). The incidence of CHS did not differ between the group of patients with symptoms and those without. Bradycardia was noted in 48 patients (14%) and hypotension in 45 (13%), and two of these patients (0.6%) required admission to the intensive care unit for hemodynamic instability. Curiously, the only factors related to increased morbimortality were hyperlipidemia and current or previous smoking.

5.2 Angioplasty in intracranial arteries

As is to be expected, fewer studies have addressed CHS in relation to intracranial angioplasty because this procedure is newer than angioplasty in extracranial arteries. In this section, we will discuss the most interesting series and cases of patients treated with this technique. In 2000, Meyers et al reported the first SAH due to stenosis of the intracranial vertebral artery. In their series of 140 patients treated with CAS (including 10 intracranial carotids, 14 intracranial vertebral arteries, 4 basilar arteries, and 1 MCA), the incidence of CHS was 5% (7 of 140 patients, 5 carotids and 2 vertebral arteries), one with ICH and another with SAH. Importantly, six patients (85%) were symptomatic with crescendo TIAs before treatment, and these symptoms were probably related to impaired CVR. The first case of CHS with ICH after intracranial MCA angioplasty was reported by Liu et al in 2001.

One of the first series of patients undergoing intracranial CAS was published by Terada et al (2006). These authors reported 106 procedures in 99 patients (57 patients had intracranial ICA stenosis, 23 had MCA stenosis, and 19 had vertebrobasilar stenosis). The ICA stenosis involved the petrous or cavernous in 47 cases (24 patients were treated with angioplasty and 23 with stenting). Four hemorrhagic complications occurred in 106 procedures. One patient had SAH and the other 3 cases had the following characteristics: severe stenosis with poor collateral flow, low perfusion with CVR damage on SPECT, appearance of ICH between 30 minutes and 16 hours after the procedure, and patient age greater than 70 years. The rate of ICH directly related to CAS was 3%. In two of three cases, CHS was strongly suspected from the SPECT findings. In the nonhemorrhagic group, hemodynamic compromise was found in 27 of 47 (57%) patients.

It is important to remember that hemorrhage caused by vessel injury is also a possible mechanism of hemorrhagic complications. For instance, in the patient with SAH in Terada et al (2006) studies, wall dissection, perforation of the vessel wall by the guidewire, or rupture of a tiny aneurysm located at the distal part of ICA were not completely ruled out.
Rezende et al (2006) reported a case of CHS after stenting for intracranial vertebral stenosis. They point out the significant hemodynamic component due to the absence of the contralateral vertebral artery and collateral supply from the carotid territory.
More recent articles about intracranial angioplasty show more promising results. Guo et al (2010) implanted 53 self-expanding stents with a technical success rate of 98%. Complications included SAH (1.9%) and occlusion (3.8%), but there were no cases of CHS.
Zhang et al (2008) reported the first case of ICH after CAS in both vertebral arteries with stenosis >90%. The flow velocity of both vertebral arteries measured by TCD increased more than 100% and high BP coincided with the abrupt onset of ICH three hours after the procedure.
In conclusion, the factors involved in the development of CHS after intracranial procedures seem similar to those involved in extracranial procedures, and the results of intracranial angioplasty are very promising.

5.3 Intracranial hemorrhage after angioplasty

ICH is the severest form of CHS and it has the worst prognosis (Case 2). The low incidence of ICH and the small number of patients in the various series reported precludes clear conclusions about the risk factors involved, although presumably they are the same as those involved in CHS. The first question is whether ICH is an extreme consequence of CHS or whether it has a distinct pathophysiology. Numerous mechanisms are possible: CHS, hemorrhagic diathesis caused by antiplatelet and anticoagulation therapy after stenting, hemorrhage around or in a recent infarction or other associated lesion (including hypertensive ICH), or rupture of an intracranial aneurysm.
In an interesting article published in 2003, Coutts et al try to narrow the definition of CHS. After studying 129 patients treated with CEA and 44 treated by CAS, these authors postulate that three different syndromes can occur in relation to hyperperfusion: acute focal edema, acute hemorrhage, and delayed classic presentation described for Sundt et al (1981). One of their patients had ICH three hours after CAS in the absence of high BP or symptoms suggestive of hyperperfusion. Other authors like Buhk et al (2006) argue for the existence of two distinct syndromes: first, classic CHS, in which symptoms of ipsilateral, frontotemporal, or retro-orbital headache, neurological deficit, and sometimes seizures typically begin between the fifth and seventh days after revascularization, and second, a more dramatic clinical presentation with ICH considered as damage due to reperfusion (Imparato et al, 1984; Takolander & Bergqvist 1983). In many of the cases published, ICH occurred within a few hours of the procedure and predominantly affected the basal ganglia; furthermore, all the patients in these cases presented with a high-grade stenosis. Therefore, the pathophysiology of this type of ICH might differ from that of CHS, being closer to that of hypertensive ICH, in this case due to rupture of small perforating arteries in the basal ganglia after acute exposure to suddenly normalized perfusion pressure after angioplasty of a high grade stenosis.
Brantley et al (2009) reported a patient with a nearly occlusive ICA stenosis who developed a fatal ipsilateral ICH immediately after the intervention; ICH was due to hemorrhagic conversion of a prior stroke.

The incidence of ICH after CEA in the series published ranges between 0.2% and 0.7% (Piepgras et al, 1988; Pomposelli et al, 1988; Solomon et al, 1986; Wilson & Ammar, 2005), whereas the incidence of ICH after CAS is higher (Timaran et al, 2009), reaching 5% in some series.
Schoser et al (1997) reported the first case of ICH after CAS, a 59-year-old woman with severe stenosis of the left ICA who developed putaminal hemorrhage on the third day after the procedure. CT showed an ipsilateral border zone infartion.
McCabe et al (1999) reported the first fatal case of ICH after CAS, a man with severe stenosis who developed ICH within hours of CAS without any prodromes. Mori et al (1999) reported a similar case in which ICH affected the basal zones with ventricular and subarachnoid extension. Both cases had signs of microangiopathy, which is associated with increased risk of ICH (Chamorro et al, 2000; McCabe et al, 1999).

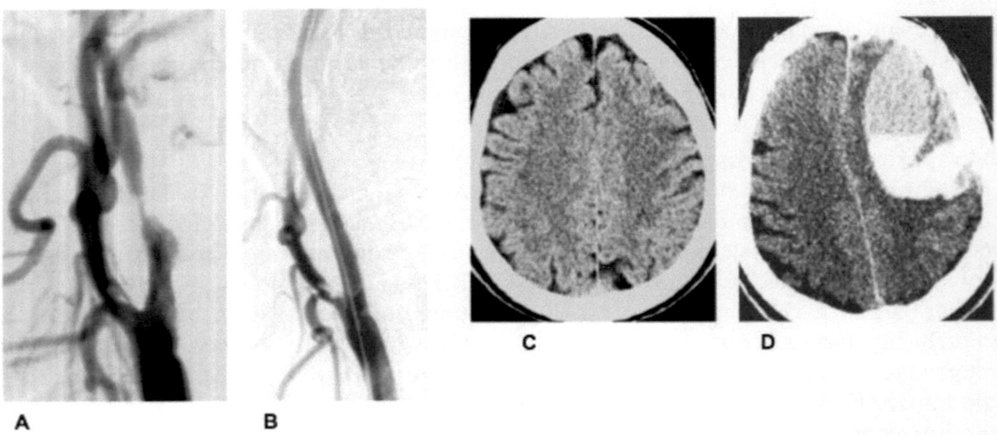

Case 2

1- Angiogram showing 95% stenosis of the left ICA in a patient with occlusion of the right ICA.
2- Angiogram after left CAS.
3- No lesions were discernible on the pre-treatment CT .
4- CT 24 hours later shows extensive hematoma in the left frontal lobe
(Courtesy of Dr. Carlos Castaño).

Tan and Phatouros (2009) reviewed 170 patients treated with CAS, 4 (2.3%) of whom developed CHS, one of these with cerebral edema, one with petechial hemorrhage, and two with ICH, which was fatal in one case. All developed CHS within six hours of the procedure and all had stenoses of the internal carotid >95%. Both patients who developed ICH had been treated within three weeks after an ischemic event.
Morrish et al (2000) observed a 4.4% incidence of ICH after 104 CAS in 90 patients; the mean ICA stenosis was 95% in those who developed ICH. In two of the patients, who died, ICH involved the basal ganglia. In this series, the incidence of ICH may have been increased due to a high dose of heparin and the absence of distal protection, given that recent ischemia is a risk factor for ICH.

Matsuo et al (2000) reported two cases of ICH, one of which affected the basal ganglia the day after CAS. The fatal ICH reported by Abou et al (2004) appeared at the level of the basal ganglia one hour after CAS. Finally, the series of 161 patients reported by Koch et al (2002) included a single case of fatal ICH after CAS in a severely stenosed ICA. Kablak et al (2010) reported 3 (1.4%) cases ICH among 210 patients, one of whom had SAH. In their study, increased systolic velocity in both MCAs was a clear risk factor, and one of the three patients had occlusion or severe stenosis of the contralateral carotid.
In addition to impaired CVR, the most widely accepted risk factors are insufficient intracranial collateralization and signs of cerebral microangiopathy. We know that hypertensive encephalopathy does not consist only of periventricular demyelination but possibly also includes small areas of perivascular hemorrhage that can be associated with higher risk of developing ICH. It also seems that the severity of the stenosis plays an important role, as most patients in the literature have severe stenosis.

6. Contrast-induced encephalopathy

Neurotoxicity from contrast agents is a rare but well-known complication of diagnostic and therapeutic procedures that employ these agents.
Leptomeningeal enhancement is often reported after CAS due to the abrupt increase in blood flow even when this does not cause symptoms (Wilkinson et al, 2000). Nevertheless, some authors purport that this phenomenon represents the extravasation of contrast material toward the subarachnoid space; Bretschneider and Strotzer (2000) reported 11 cases, some of which were related to hypoxic brain damage. Ekel et al (1998) reported a case of contrast enhancement mimicking SAH, and Mamourian et al (2000) used an animal model to demonstrate that contrast material can cross into the cerebrospinal spinal fluid in sufficient concentration to alter the appearance of the subarachnoid space on MRI. Dangas et al (2001) reported a case of contrast-induced encephalopathy after CAS in an 82-year-old man with a TIA and 90% stenosis in the right carotid. Immediately after CAS, this patient presented confusion and left hemiparesis in the territory of the right carotid. CT showed marked cortical enhancement and edema of the right cerebral hemisphere. The patient improved rapidly and by day 2 was completely recovered; MRI found no cortical edema and normal sulci.
Canovas et al (2007) published a case of extravasation of contrast material immediately after the rupture of the balloon in a woman with a very calcified plaque (Case 3) in whom the pressure of the balloon reached 8 atmospheres. The pressure of the balloon probably magnified the hemodynamic effect, making the extravasation of the contrast material very aggressive and giving rise to a clinical picture identical to an embolic stroke of the MCA. As in other cases reported in the literature, this patient's condition improved and the imaging findings were normal after 48 h.
Contrast-induced encephalopathy should be differentiated from the classical CHS described Sundt et al (1981), although it probably has a similar pathophysiology. A high dose of contrast agent may result in acute breakdown of the blood-brain barrier, allowing the contrast material to enter the brain and resulting in the acute development of a dramatic clinical presentation. The higher osmolality of ioxaglate compared with blood may in turn produce fluid extravasation and cerebral edema. The prognosis is usually excellent, as is evidenced by other recently published cases occurring after endovascular procedures (Guimaraens et al, 2010, Fang et al, 2009; Paúl et al, 2009).

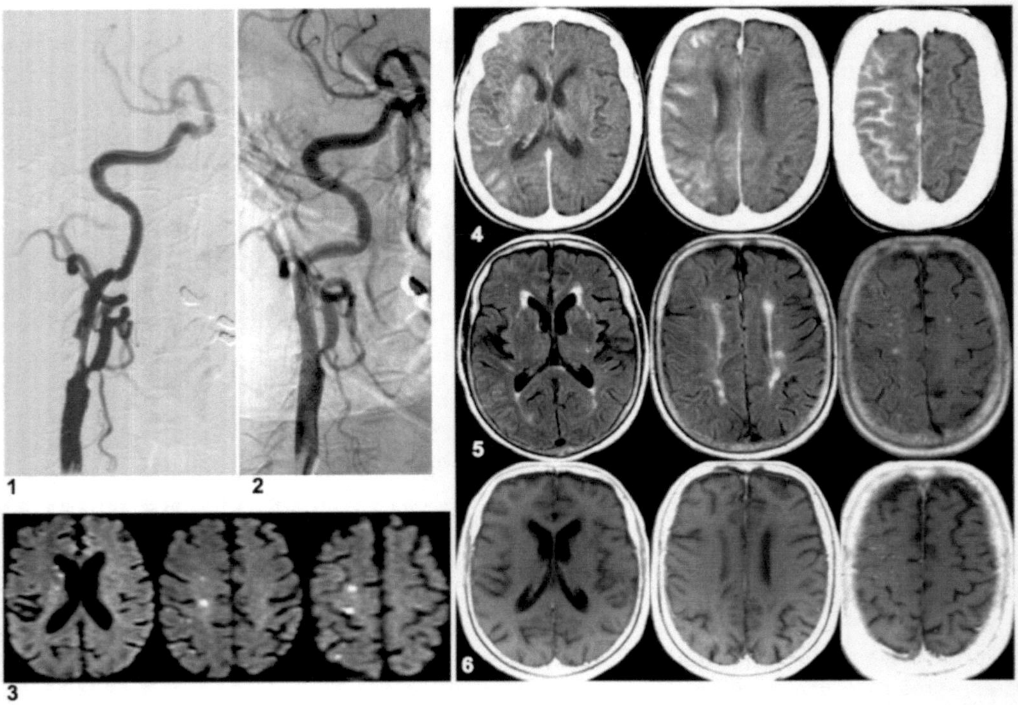

Case 3

1- Angiogram before left CAS showing 70% stenosis of the left ICA
2- Angiogram after left CAS
3- Axial diffusion-weighted MRi showing ipsilateral silent ischemic lesions
4- CT with extravasation of the contrast
5- Axial FLAIR MRi
6- Axial T1-weighted MRi

7. Prevention and treatment

It is crucial to identify patients with risk factors for developing hyperperfusion so that preventive measure can be taken during and after revascularization. In the previous section, we discussed the factors most commonly considered to increase this risk, and in this section we discuss the most interesting preventive strategies.

There is a consensus that the most important risk factors are severely impaired CVR and deficient collaterality (severe ipsilateral stenosis, impaired collateral flow, occlusive disease in other extracranial cerebral vessels, and incomplete circle of Willis). Other proposed factors include advanced age, perioperative and postoperative hypertension, and the use of antiplatelet agents or other anticoagulants. Thus, we should concentrate our efforts on the factors in which we can intervene. Regarding preventive measures before the procedure, we will discuss the assessment of CVR as the primary measure and we will also examine the usefulness of assessing the supra-aortic trunks and the circle of Willis. Regarding preventive measures during and after the procedure, we will focus on detecting cerebral hyperperfusion and thus on the importance of strict, prolonged BP control and appropriate antithrombotic management.

As we discussed in the Diagnosis section, various options are available for assessing CVR. Probably the most widely available option is TCD, which has many advantages and enables us to measure cerebral flow at rest and under certain stimuli (breath-holding, inhalation of CO2, intravenous acetazolamide administration). The simplest and most noninvasive TCD test is breath-holding with or without hyperventilation (see the Diagnosis section). Therefore, the first preventive measure that is recommended before revascularization is CVR assessment using TCD (Sfyroeras 2006, 2009).

It would also be advisable to do a thorough MRI study of the supra-aortic trunks and of the circle of Willis as well as a study of the cerebral parenchyma using FLAIR, T2-weighted, and diffusion sequences to detect hyperacute lesions and small-vessel disease, which are also related to increased risk of CHS. As mentioned in the Diagnosis section, CVR can also be assessed by SPECT, CT, and MRI, although these approaches are more expensive and less widely available.

Again, TCD is very useful for monitoring cerebral flow during revascularization procedures. In patients undergoing CEA, TCD can detect increases in MCA flow velocity greater than 100% during the intervention, thus alerting to a situation of risk. Likewise, TCD monitoring during CAS and probably in the hours after the procedure can help select high risk patients (Dalman et al, 1999; Fujimoto et al, 2004; Kablak et al, 2010; Jansen et al, 1994; Iwata et al, 2011; Sfyroeras et al, 2009).

Strict control of hypertension is one of the preventive measures that has received the most attention. Most Investigators recommend strict control of BP in the postoperative period to prevent ICH after CEA (Ahn et al, 1989; Bernstein et al, 1984; Bove et al, 1979; Buhk et al, 2006; Hosoda et al, 2001; Ko et al, 2005; Roh et al, 2005; Safian et al, 2006; Tang et al, 2008) and after CAS, as we will see below.

It has been suggested that even BP in the normal range may be deleterious in patients at high risk for CHS (Piepgras et al, 1988; Ouriel et al, 1999; Jorgensen & Schroeder, 1993).

Regarding strict control of BP, Abou-Chebl et al (2007) published an interesting study that analyzed the presence of CHS and ICH in 836 patients treated with CAS. These authors maintained BP $< 140/90$ mmHg in patients with lower risk and BP $< 120/80$ mm Hg in patients with a treated stenosis $\geq 90\%$, contralateral stenosis $\geq 80\%$, and hypertension (i.e., risk factors for CHS). They conclude that comprehensive management of arterial hypertension can lower the incidence of ICH and CHS in high-risk patients following CAS, without additional complications or prolonged hospitalization. The strict control of BP must be maintained until CVR is restored, and this interval varies among patients. Thus, the use of TCD to assess the recovery of CVR can probably help guide antihypertensive therapy (Buhk 2006).

Bando et al (2001) reported a stroke patient with a 90% stenosis of the intracranial left vertebral artery treated with CAS. Immediately after the procedure, hyperperfusion was detected by SPECT and TCD. The patient recovered from CHS quickly after a week's antihypertensive therapy.

Brus-Ramer et al (2010) published an interesting case of a patient treated with CAS who developed signs of hyperperfusion detected by TCD and depicted on angiography as hyperintense punctate foci potentially representing small dilations in the vascular territory of stented arteries. Lowering BP by 40% probably prevented CHS; thus, in high risk patients, aggressive BP management during and after CAS can prevent potentially serious sequelae.

Another aspect that remains to be determined is the most appropriate type of drugs for these patients. In this context, it seems logical that drugs that have no direct effects on CBF and those that give some degree of cerebral vasoconstriction could be beneficial. Drugs like nitroprusside and calcium antagonists that increase CBF should be avoided. The ß 1-adrenergic antagonists (beta-blockers) reduce BP with little effect on intracranial pressure within the autoregulatory range, although they can exacerbate the bradycardia that can occur after CAS.

The mixed alpha-adrenergic antagonist and ß -adrenergic antagonist labetalol, which has no direct effects on CBF and decreases the cerebral perfusion pressure and mean arterial pressure by about 30% compared with baseline, has successfully been used in CHS after CEA (Halliday et al, 2004). The alpha 2-adrenergic agonist clonidine, which is commonly used after CEA (associated with raised cranial and plasma catecholamine concentrations), has the advantage of decreasing CBF.

General anesthesia is often unnecessary for CAS. However, when general anesthesia is required, it is important to use anesthetics that do not increase CBF. Studies of CBF during surgery have shown that high doses of volatile halogenated hydrocarbon anesthetics may lead to the development of CHS (Skydell et al, 1987). Isoflurane is the volatile anesthetic of choice in neurosurgery because it results in less pronounced vasodilation than other halogenated anesthetics at equipotent doses. The effects of isoflurane on cerebral metabolic rate and autoregulation are dose dependent, with impairment of CVR at high doses. Propofol has been used in patients with CHS, it normalizes CBF, probably because of its effects on cerebral metabolism (Kaisti et al, 2003).

Safety concerns have been raised about the effects of anticoagulants and antiplatelet agents and the risk of ICH following CEA, but no causal link has been found (Ouriel et al, 1999; Penn et al, 1995). Likewise, no association between these drugs and ICH has been found in patients undergoing CAS (Abou et al, 2003), although some studies have reported higher incidences of ICH, probably related to higher than usual doses of anticoagulants (Meyers et al, 2000 ; Morrish et al, 2000).

Levy et al (2002) propose an interesting preventive strategy consisting of performing angioplasty in two phases, with posterior stent collocation. These authors published a series of 8 cases of intracranial vertebral stenosis with good outcomes despite one case of arterial dissection that required stenting. Yoshimura et al (2009) also used two-step endovascular treatment in high risk patients with impaired CVR. These authors first performed angioplasty with a small balloon (3 mm), and once hyperperfusion improved on SPECT about one month later they performed a second, definitive angioplasty with stent placement. None of the 9 patients treated with the two-step approach had problems related with hyperperfusion (one required stenting for a dissected artery), whereas 5 of the 9 patients in the control group had hyperperfusion and one had status epilepticus related to CHS.

Additional efforts to reduce the risk of ICH may include limiting the duration of balloon inflation and employing emboli-prevention devices, as these practices have been related to ischemia with posterior development of ICH (Jansen et al, 1994; Sakaki et al, 1992; Sundt et al 1981).

An important, somewhat controversial factor is the optimal interval between stroke and revascularization. We know that an extensive ischemic lesion represents a greater risk of damage due to reperfusion. Furthermore, classically a six-week interval was recommended to avoid treatment complications. However, studies like the NASCET show that the benefits of carotid revascularization are greatest in the first two weeks after the event, and the subgroup of patients with less risk for early revascularization are those with small ischemic lesions and mild neurologic impairment (Keldahl et al, 2010). A recent (<3 months) contralateral CEA is an additional potential risk factor for CHS and should also be considered in the timing of surgery (Ascher et al, 2003). Very few studies have addressed the use of CAS in hyperacute strokes, but those that have report good safety outcome (Miyamoto et al, 2008; Setacci et al 2010).

Some authors (Henry et al, 2005; Lee et al, 2006) claim that treatment of both carotid arteries is feasible in carefully selected patients, either in the same procedure or in two procedures separated by an interval of one day; these authors report safety and complication rates comparable to those of large published series in high-risk patients. Nevertheless, careful monitoring of the patient, blood pressure, and heart rate is mandatory to avoid complications related to CHS.

Owing to the presence of free radicals during reperfusion and their relation to post-ischemic hyperperfusion, substances like edaravone have been investigated. Edaravone inhibits lipid peroxidation and vascular endothelial cell injury, improving edema cerebral and tissue injury. Pretreatment with edaravone decreased the incidence of hyperperfusion after CEA as measured by SPECT (Ogasawara et al, 2004).

Once CHS occurs, aggressive measures to lower BP are imperative. As there are no data from randomized trials comparing the optimal perioperative management protocol for patients with CHS due to the rarity of this complication, we must focus on controlling BP, reducing cerebral edema, and, according to some authors, temporarily withdraw antithrombotic therapy. Treatments for cerebral edema include adequate sedation, hyperventilation, and administration of mannitol or hypertonic saline. Evidently, there are no data to support these treatments in CHS. Corticosteroids and barbiturates have also been used in CHS.

There are no available data recommending prophylactic use of anticonvulsant therapy in patients undergoing carotid revascularization; however, in the presence of seizures, treatment with anticonvulsants is indicated.

In conclusion, assessing CVR before treatment and monitoring CBF velocities during and after the procedure can help select the patients who need strict control of BP to prevent CHS. The optimal BP remains to be determined, but BP should be lowered to below the baseline after luminal gain with stenting to prevent secondary injury. Despite the lack of a precise BP target, lowering systolic BP to at least 20% to 30% below baseline values seems critical, particularly in patients with critical stenosis and above all in patients with impaired CVR. Labetalol and clonidine seem to be the most appropriate drugs for BP control in this context.

To determine when discharge is safe after CAS, patients should be divided into two groups. One group includes asymptomatic, hemodynamically stable patients with low comorbidity who could be discharged after 6 h of observation, according to some authors. These patients should be treated using a hemostatic closure device for the arterial puncture. The other group includes older patients with associated comorbidity, mainly those with altered renal function, those that require anticoagulation, and those with altered BP or bradycardia. Finally, it is recommendable to warn the family about symptoms that call for re-evaluation, especially seizures, neurological deficit, and headaches associated with hypertension.

8. Abbreviations

CHS: Cerebral Hyperperfusion Syndrome
CBF: Cerebral Blood Flow
CBV: Cerebral blood volume
CT: Cranial tomography
CVR: Cerebral Vasoreactivity
HTA: hypertension
ICA: Internal Carotid Artery
ICH: Intracranial Hemorrhage
MMT: mean transit time
MCA: Middle Cerebral Artery
MRi: magnetic resonance imaging,
PET: Positron Emission Tomography
TCD: transcranial doppler
TIA: Transient Ischemic Attack
SAH: Subarachnoid hemorrhage
SPECT: Single-photon emission computed tomography

9. References

Abou-Chebl, A.; Yadav, JS.; Reginelli, JP.; Bajzer, C.; Bhatt D & Krieger DW: Intracranial hemorrhage and hyperperfusion syndrome following carotid artery stenting: risk factors, prevention, and treatment. J Am Coll Cardiol 43:1596–1601, 2004

Abou-Chebl, A.; Reginelli, J.; Bajzer, CT & Yadav JS. Intensive treatment of hypertension decreases the risk of hyperperfusion and intracerebral hemorrhage following carotid artery stenting. Catheter Cardiovasc Interv 2007 69:690–696

Adhiyaman, V & Alexander, S. Cerebral hyperperfusion syndrome following carotid endarterectomy. QJM 2007; 100: 239-44.

Ahn, SS.; Marcus, DR & Moore, WS. Post-carotid endarterectomy hypertension: association with elevated cranial norepinephrine. J Vasc Surg 1989; 9: 351-60.

Alexandrov, AV.; Sloan, MA.; Tegeler, CH.; Newell, DN.; Lumsden, A.; Garami, Z.; Levy, CR.; Wong, LK.; Douville, C.; Kaps, M & Tsivgoulis G; for the American Society of Neuroimaging Practice Guidelines Committee. Practice Standards for Transcranial Doppler (TCD) Ultrasound. Part II. Clinical Indications and Expected Outcomes. J Neuroimaging. 2010 Oct 26.

Al-Mubarak, N.; Roubin, GS.; Vitek, JJ.; Iyer, SS.; New, G & Leon MB: Subarachnoidal hemorrhage following carotid stenting with the distal-balloon protection. Catheter Cardiovasc Interv 54: 521–523, 2001 Ascher, E.; Markevich, N.; Schutzer, RW.; Kallakuri, S.; Jacob, T & Hingorani, AP. Cerebral hyperperfusion syndrome after carotid endarterectomy: predictive factors and hemodynamic changes. J Vasc Surg 2003; 37: 769–77.

Bajardi, G.; Ricevuto, G.; Grassi, N & Latteri, M. Arterial hypertension alter carotid endarterectomy. Minerva Chir 1989; 15; 44: 1115-7.

Baker, CJ.; Mayer, SA.; Prestigiacomo, CJ.; Heertum, RLV & Solomon, RA. Diagnosis and monitoring of cerebral hyperperfusion after carotid endarterectomy with single photon emission computed tomography: case report. Neurosurgery 1998; 43: 157–161

Bando, K.; Satoh, K.; Matsubara, S.; Nakatani, M & Nagahiro, S. Hyperperfusion phenomenon after percutaneous translumi nal angioplasty for atherosclerotic stenosis of the intracranial vertebral artery. Case report. J Neurosurg 2001; 94: 826 830.078. 49:933–938

Beese, U.; Langer H.; Lang, W & Dinkel, M. Comparison of near-infrared spectroscopy and somatosensory evoked potentials for the detection of cerebral ischemia during carotid endarterectomy. Stroke 1998; 29: 2032–2037. Benzel, EC & Hoppens, KD. Factors associated with postoperative hypertension complicating carotid endarterectomy. Acta Neurochir (Wien) 1991; 112: 8-12.

Bernstein, M.; Ross Fleming, JF & Deck, JH. Cerebral hyperperfusion after carotid endarterectomy: a cause of cerebral hemorrhage. Neurosurgery 1984; 15: 50-6.

S. Bouri, A.; Thapar, J.; Shalhoub, G.; Jayasooriya, A.; Fernando, I.J.; Franklin & Davies,AH. Hypertension and the Post-carotid Endarterectomy Cerebral Hyperperfusion Syndrome. Eur J Vasc Endovasc Surg (2011) 41, 229-237

Bove, EL.; Fry, WJ.; Gross, WS & Stanley, JC. Hypotension and hypertension as consequences of baroreceptor dysfunction following carotid endarterectomy. Surgery 1979; 85: 633-7.

Brantley, HP.; Kiessling, JL.; Milteer, HB Jr & Mendelsohn, FO. Hyperperfusion syndrome following carotid artery stenting: thelargest single-operator series to date. J Invasive Cardiol 2009 21(1):27–31

Bretschneider, T & Strotzer, M. Leptomeningeal Enhancement and Extravasation of Contrast Medium into de CSF Space? Stroke 2000, 31 (9) 2275-76.

Brus-Ramer, M; Starke, RM, Komotar, RJ & Meyers, PM. Radiographic evidence of cerebral hyperperfusion and reversal following angioplasty and stenting of intracranial carotid and middle cerebral artery stenosis: case report and review of the literature. J Neuroimaging 2010 Jul; 20(3): 280-3. Epub 2009 Feb 13.

Buhk, JH.; Cepek, L & Knauth, M. Hyperacute intracerebral hemorrhage complicating carotid stenting should be distinguished from hyperperfusion syndrome. AJNR Am J Neuroradiol 2006; 27: 1508-13.

Cánovas, D, Perendreu, J; Rovira, A & Estela J. Extravasation of contrast medium after carotid stent with brain infarction symptoms. Neurologia 2007 Apr; 22(3): 187-90.

Cayne, NS.; Faries, PL & Trocciola, SM et al. Carotid angioplasty and stent-induced bradycardia and hypotension: Impact of prophylactic atropine administration prior carotid endarterectomy. J Vasc Surg 2005 41:956–961

Chamorro, A.; Vila, N.; Obac, V.; Macho, J & Blasco, J. A case of cerebral hemorrhage early after carotid stenting. Stroke 2000. 31: 792–793.

Chang, TY; Liu, HL; Lee, TH; Kuan, WC, Chang, CH; Wu, HC, Wu, TC & Chang YJ. Change in cerebral perfusion after carotid angioplasty with stenting is related to cerebral vasoreactivity: a study using dynamic susceptibility-weighted contrast-enhanced MR imaging and functional MR imaging with a breath-holding paradigm. AJNR Am J Neuroradiol 2009 Aug;30(7):1330-6. Epub 2009 May 27.

Christos D, Karkos.; Dimitrios G, Karamanos.; Konstantinos, O.; Papazoglou Filippos, P.; Demiropoulos Dimitrios, N.; Papadimitriou Thomas, S & Gerassimidis. Thirty-

Day Outcome Following Carotid Artery Stenting: A 10- Year Experience from a Single Center. Cardiovasc Intervent Radiol (2010) 33:34–40

Choi, BS.; Park, JW.; Shin, JE.; Lü, PH.; Kim, JK.; Kim, SJ.; Lee, DH.; Kim, JS.; Kim, HJ & Suh, DC. Outcome evaluation of carotid stenting in high-risk patients with symptomatic carotid near occlusion. Interv Neuroradiol. 2010 Sep; 16(3):309-16. Epub 2010 Oct 25.

Cikrit, DF.; Dalsing, MC & Harting, PS, et al. Cerebral vascular reactivity assessed with acetazolamide single photon emission CT scans before and after carotid endarterectomy. Am J Surg 1997; 174: 193–197

Coutts, SB.; Hill, MD & Hu, WY. Hyperperfusion syndrome: toward a stricter definition. Neurosurgery 2003;53:1053-60.

Dalman, JE.; Beenakkers, IC & Moll, FL, et al. Transcranial Doppler monitoring during carotid endarterectomy helps to identify patients at risk of postoperative hyperperfusion. Eur J Vasc Endovasc Surg. 1999; 18: 222-227.

Dangas G, Monsein LH, Laureno R, Peterson MA & Laird JR. Transient contrast encephalopathy after carotid artery stenting. J Endovasc Ther. 2001 Apr; 8 (2): 111-3

Diehm N, Katzen BT, Iyer SS, White CJ, Hopkins LN & Kelley L; BEACH investigators. Staged bilateral carotid stenting, an effective strategy in high-risk patients - insights from a prospective multicenter trial. J Vasc Surg. 2008 Jun;47(6):1227-34. Epub 2008 Apr 28.

Duncan, LA.; Ruckley, CV & Wildsmith, JA. Cerebral oxime- try: a useful monitor during carotid artery surgery. Anaesthesia 1995;50: 1041–1045.

Eckel, TS.; Breiter, SN & Monsein, LH. Subarachnoid contrast enhancement after spinal angiography mimicking diffuse subarachnoid hemorrhage. AJR Am J Roentgenol. 1998; 170: 503-5

Fang, HY; Kuo, YL & Wu CJ. Transient contrast encephalopathy after carotid artery stenting mimicking diffuse subarachnoid hemorrhage: a case report. Catheter Cardiovasc Interv 2009 Jan 1; 73(1):123-6.

Fujimoto, S.; Toyoda, K.; Inoue, T.; Hirai, Y.; Uwatoko, T & Kishikawa K, et al. Diagnostic impact of transcranial color-coded real-time sonogra- phy with echo contrast agents for hyperperfusion syndrome after carotid endarterectomy. Stroke 2004; 35: 1852-6.

Fukuda, T.; Ogasawara, K.; Kobayashi, M.; Komoribayashi, N.; Endo, H & Inoue T, et al. Prediction of cerebral hyperperfusion after carotid endarterectomy using cerebral blood volume measured by perfusion- weighted MR imaging compared with single-photon emission CT. AJNR Am J Neuroradiol 2007; 28: 737-42.

Guimaraens, L; Vivas, E; Fonnegrea, A; Sola, T; Soler, L; Balaguer, E; Medrano, J; Gandolfo C & Casasco A.. Transient encephalopathy from angiographic contrast: a rare complication in neurointerventional procedures. Cardiovasc Intervent Radiol 2010 Apr;33 (2):383-8. Epub 2009 Jun 6.

Halliday, A.; Mansfield, A & Marro, J. et al. Prevention of disabling and fatal strokes by successful carotid endarterectomy in patients without recent neurological symptoms: randomised controlled trial. Lancet 2004; 363: 1491–502.

Hartmann, M.; Weber, R.; Zoubaa, S.; Schranz, C & Knauth M: Fatal subarachnoid hemorrhage after carotid stenting. J Neuroradiol 31:63–66, 2004

Henderson, R.; Phan, T.; Piepgras, D & Wijdicks, E. Mechanisms of intracerebral hemorrhage after carotid endarterectomy. J Neurosurg 2001;95: 964 -9.

Henry M, Gopalakrishnan L, Rajagopal S, Rath PC, Henry I & Hugel M. Bilateral carotid angioplasty and stenting. Catheter Cardiovasc Interv. 2005 Mar;64(3):275-82.

Ho, DS.; Wang, Y.; Chui, M.; Ho, SL & Cheung, RT. Epileptic seizures attributed to cerebral hyperperfusion after percutaneous transluminal angioplasty and stenting of the internal carotid artery. Cerebrovasc Dis. 2000 Sep-Oct; 10 (5): 374-9.

Hosoda, K.; Fujita, S.; Kawaguchi, T.; Shose, Y.; Shibata, Y & Tamaki, N. Influence of degree of carotid artery stenosis and collateral pathways and effect of carotid endarterectomy on cerebral vasoreactivity. Neurosurgery 1998; 42: 988–995

Hosoda, K.; Kawaguchi, T.; Shibata, Y.; Kamei, M.; Kidoguchi, K & Koyama, J, et al. Cerebral vasoreactivity and internal carotid artery flow help to identify patients at risk for hyperperfusion after carotid endarterectomy. Stroke 2001; 32: 1567-73

Hosoda, K.; Kawaguchi, T & Ishii, K, et al. Prediction of hyperperfusion after carotid endarterectomy by brain SPECT analysis with semiquantitative statistical mapping method. Stroke 2003; 34: 1187–1193.

Imai, K.; Mori, T.; Izumoto, H.; Watanabe, M & Majima K. Emergency carotid artery stent placement in patients with acute ischemic stroke. AJNR Am J Neuroradiol 2005;26:1249-58.

Imparato, AM.; Riles, TS & Ramirez, AA. Early complications of carotid surgery. Int Surg 1984; 69; 223-29

Iwata T, Mori T, Tajiri H, Nakazaki M. Predictors of hyperperfusion syndrome before and immediately after carotid artery stenting in single-photon emission computed tomography and transcranial color-coded real-time sonography studies. Neurosurgery. 2011 Mar; 68 (3): 649-55; discussion 655-6.

Jansen, C.; Sprengers, AM & Moll, FL et al. Prediction of intracerebral haemorrhage after carotid endarterectomy by clinical criteria and intraoperative transcranial Doppler monitoring. Eur J Vasc Surg. 1994; 8: 303-308.

Jansen, C.; Sprengers, AM.; Moll, FL.; Vermeulen, FE.; Hamerlijnck, RP.; van Gijn, J & Ackerstaff RG. Prediction of intracerebral haemorrhage after carotid endarterectomy by clinical criteria and intraoperative transcranial Doppler monitoring: results of 233 operations. Eur J Vasc Surg 1994; 8: 220-5.

Jorgensen, LG & Schroeder TV. Defective cerebrovascular autorregulation alter endarterectomy. Eur J Vasc Surg 1993; 7: 370-9

Karapanayiotides, T.; Meuli, R.; Devuyst, G.; Piechowski-Jozwiak, B.; Dewarrat, A & Ruchat, P, et al. Postcarotid endarterectomy hyperperfusion or reperfusion syndrome. Stroke 2005;36: 21-6.

Kaisti, KK.; Langsjo, JW & Aalto S, et al. Effects of sevoflurane, propofol, and adjunct nitrous oxide on regional cerebral blood flow, oxygen consumption, and blood volume in humans. Anesthesiology 2003; 99: 603–13.

Kadkhodayan, Y.; Cross, DT.; Derdeyn, CP & Moran, CJ. Carotid angioplasty and stenting in the elderly. Neuroradiology. 2007 Nov; 49 (11): 933-8. Epub 2007 Jul 27.

Kablak-Ziembicka, A.; Przewlocki, T.; Pieniazek, P.; Musialek, P.; Tekieli, L.; Rosławiecka, A.; Motyl, R.; Zmudka, K.; Tracz, W & Podolec, P. Predictors of cerebral reperfusion injury after carotid stenting: the role of transcranial color-coded Doppler ultrasonography. J Endovasc Ther. 2010 Aug; 17(4): 556-63.

Kaku, Y.; Yoshimura, S & Kokuzawa J. Factors predictive of cerebral hyperperfusion after carotid angioplasty and stent placement. AJNR Am J Neuroradiol 2004; 25: 1403–1408.

Keldahl, M & Eskandari, M. Timing of carotid surgery after acute stroke. Expert Rev Cardiovasc Ther 2010 vol. 8 (10) pp. 1399-403

Keunen, R.; Nijmeijer, HW.; Tavy, D.; Stam, K.; Edelenbosch, R & Muskens, E et al. An observational study of preoperative transcranial Doppler examinations to predict cerebral hyperperfusion following carotid endarterectomies. Neurol Res 2001; 23: 593-8.

Kirkpatrick, PJ.; Smielewski, P.; Czosnyka, M.; Menon, DK & Pickard, JD. Near-infrared spectroscopy use in patients with head injury. J Neurosurg 1995; 83: 963–970.

Ko, NU.; Achrol, AS.; Chopra, M.; Saha, M.; Gupta, D & Smith, WS, et al. Cerebral blood flow changes after endovascular treatment of cerebro- vascular stenoses. AJNR Am J Neuroradiol 2005; 26: 538-42.

Ko, NU,; Achrol, AS.; Martin, AJ.; Chopra, M.; Saloner, DA.; Higashida, RT & Young WL. Magnetic resonance perfusion tracks 133Xe cerebral blood flow changes after carotid stenting. Stroke 2005; 36: 676-8.

Lee YH, Kim TK, Suh SI, Kwon BJ, Lee TH, Kwon OK, Han MH, Lee NJ, Kim JH & Seol HY. Simultaneous Bilateral

Carotid Stenting under the Circumstance of Neuroprotection Device. A Retrospective Analysis. Interv Neuroradiol. 2006 Jun 15;12(2):141-8. Epub 2006 Jul 31.

Levy, EI.; Hanel, RA.; Bendok, BR.; Boulos, AS.; Hartney, ML.; Guterman, LR.; Qureshi, AI & Hopkins LN. Staged stent-assisted angioplasty for symptomatic intracranial vertebrobasilar artery stenosis. J Neurosurg. 2002 Dec; 97 (6): 1294-301.

Lin, PH.; Zhou, W.; Kougias, P.; El Sayed, HF.; Barshes, NR & Huynh TT . Factors associated with hypotension and bradycardia after carotid angioplasty and stenting. J Vasc Surg 2007. 46:846–854

Liu, AY.; Do, HM.; Albers, GW.; Lopez, JR.; Steinberg, GK & Marks, MP: Hyperperfusion syndrome with hemorrhage after angioplasty for middle cerebral artery stenoses. AJNR Am J Neuroradiol 22:1597–1561, 2001.

Lythgoe, DJ. Ostergaard, L & William, SC et al. Quantitativeperfusion imaging in carotid artery stenosis using dynamic susceptibility contrast-enhanced magnetic resonance imaging. Magn Reson Imaging. 2000;18:1Y11.

Macfarlane, R.; Moskowitz, MA.; Sakas, DE.; Tasdemiroglu, E.; Wei, EP & Kontos, HA. The role of neuroeffector mechanisms in cerebral hyperperfusion syndromes. J Neurosurg 1991;75:845-55.

Maeda, M.; Yuh, WT & Ueda T, et al. Severe occlusive carotid artery disease: hemodynamic assessment by MR perfusion imaging in symptomatic patients. AJNR Am J Neuroradiol. 1999; 20:43Y51.

Mamourian, AC.; Hoopes, PJ & Lewis LD. Visualization of intravenously administered contrast material in the CSF on fluid-attenuated inversion- recovery MR images: an in vitro and animal-model investigation. AJNR Am J Neuroradiol. 2000; 21: 105-111.

Mansoor, GA.; White, WB.; Grunnet, M & Ruby, ST. Intracerebral hemorrhage after carotid endarterectomy associated with ipsilateral fibrinoid necrosis:a consequence of the hyperperfusion syndrome? J Vasc Surg 1996;23:147- 51.

McKevitt, FM.; Sivaguru, A.; Venables, GS.; Cleveland, TJ.; Gaines, PA & Beard JD, et al: Effect of treatment of carotid artery stenosis on blood pressure: a comparison of hemodynamic disturbances after carotid endarterectomy and endovascular treatment. Stroke 34: 2576–2581, 2003

Matsubara, S.; Moroi, J.; Suzuki, A.; Sasaki, M.; Nagata, K.; Kanno, I & Miura, S. Analysis of cerebral perfusion and metabolism assessed with positron emission tomography before and after carotid artery stenting. Clinical article. J Neurosurg. 2009 Jul; 111 (1):28-36.

Masuo, O.; Terada, T & Matsumoto, H, et al. Haemorrhagic complication following percutaneous transluminal angioplasty for carotid stenosis. Acta Neurochir (Wien) 2000; 142: 1365-68

Matsumoto, S.; Nakahara, I.; Higashi, T.; Iwamuro, Y.; Watanabe, Y.; Takahashi, K.; Takezawa, AM & Kira, JI. Near-infrared spectroscopy in carotid artery stenting predicts cerebral hyperperfusion syndrome. Neurology 2009; 72: 1512–1518

McCabe, DJ.; Brown, MM & Clifton, A. Fatal cerebral reperfusion hemorrhage after carotid stenting. Stroke 1999; 30: 2483-86

Mendelsohn, FO.; Weissman, NJ.; Lederman, RJ.; Crowley, JJ.; Gray, JL & Phillips, HR, et al: Acute hemodynamic changes during carotid artery stenting. Am J Cardiol 82: 1077–1081, 1998

du Mesnil de Rochemont, R.; Schneider, S.; Yan, B.; Lehr, A.; Sitzer, M & Berkefeld, J. Diffusion-weighted MR imaging lesions after filter- protected stenting of high-grade symptomatic carotid artery stenoses. AJNR Am J Neuroradiol 2006; 27: 1321-5.

Meyers, PM.; Phatouros, CC & Higashida, RT. Hyperperfusion syndrome after intracranial angioplasty and stent placement. Stroke 2006; 37: 2210–2211

Meyers, PM.; Higashida, RT.; Phatouros, CC.; Malek, AM.; Lempert, TE.; Dowd, CF & Halbach, VV: Cerebral hyperperfusion syndrome after percutaneous transluminal stenting of the craniocervical arteries. Neurosurgery 47: 335– 343, 2000.

Meyer, SA.; Gandhi, CD.; Johnson, DM.; Winn, HR & Patel, AB. Outcomes of carotid artery stenting in high-risk patients with carotid artery stenosis: a single neurovascular center retrospective review of 101 consecutive patients. Neurosurgery. 2010 Mar; 66 (3): 448-53; discussion 453-4.

Miyamoto, N.; Naito, I.; Takatama, S.; Shimizu, T.; Iwai, T & Shimaguchi H. Urgent stenting for patients with acute stroke due to atherosclerotic occlusive lesions of the cervical internal carotid artery. Neurol Med Chir (Tokyo) 2008 Feb; 48(2): 49-55; discussion 55-6.

van Mook, WN.; Rennenberg, RJ.; Schurink, GW.; van Oostenbrugge, RJ.; Mess, WH.; Hofman, PA & de Leeuw, PW. Cerebral hyperperfusion syndrome. Lancet Neurol 2005; 4: 877-88.

Mori, T.; Fukuoka, M & Kazita K. Intraventricular hemorrhage after carotid stenting. J Endovasc Surg 1999; 6: 337- 41

Morrish, W.; Grahovac, S.; Douen, A.; Cheung, G.; Hu, W & Farb, R, et al: Intracranial hemorrhage after stenting and angioplasty of extracranial carotid stenosis. AJNR Am J Neuroradiol 21: 1911- 1916, 2000

Moulakakis, KG.; Mylonas, SN.; Sfyroeras, GS & Andrikopoulos, V. Hyperperfusion syndrome after carotid revascularization J Vasc Surg 2009; 49: 1060-8

Naylor, AR.; Evans, J.; Thompson, MM.; London, NJ.; Abbott, RJ.; Cherryman, G & Bell PR. Seizures after carotid endarterectomy: hyperperfusion, dysautoregulation or hypertensive encephalopathy? Eur J Vasc Endovasc Surg. 2003 Jul; 26 (1): 39-44.

Nicholas, GG.; Hashemi, H.; Gee, W & Reed JF. The cerebral hyperperfusion syndrome: diagnostic value of ocular pneumoplethysmography. J Vasc Surg 1993; 17: 690-95.

Nikolsky, E.; Patil, CV & Beyar, R. Ipsilateral intracerebral hemorrhage following carotid stent-assisted angioplasty: a manifestation of hyperperfusion syndrome, a case report. Angiology 53: 217–223, 2002

Ogasawara, K.; Konno, H.; Yukawa, H.; Endo, H.; Inoue, T & Ogawa, A. Transcranial regional cerebral oxygen saturation monitoring during carotid endarterectomy as a predictor of postoperative hyperperfusion. Neurosurgery 2003; 53: 309- 314.

Ogasawara, K.; Yukawa, H & Kobayashi, M et al. Prediction and monitoring of cerebral hyperperfusion after carotid endarterectomy by using single-photon emission computerized tomography scanning. J Neurosurg 2003; 99: 504 -10

Ogasawara, K.; Inoue, T.; Kobayashi, M.; Endo, H.; Fukuda, T & Ogawa, A. Pretreatment with the free radical scavenger edaravone prevents cerebral hyperperfusion after carotid endarterectomy. Neurosurgery. 2004 Nov; 55(5): 1060-7.

Ogasawara, K.; Yamadate, K.; Kobayashi, M.; Endo, H.; Fukuda, T.; Yoshida, K et al: Postoperative cerebral hyperperfusion associated with impaired cognitive function in patients undergoing carotid endarterectomy. J Neurosurg 102:38–44, 2005

Ogasawara, K.; Sakai, N.; Kuroiwa, T.; Hosoda, K.; Iihara, K & Toyoda, K et al. Japanese Society for Treatment at Neck in Cerebrovascular Disease Study Group. Intracranial hemorrhage associated with cerebral hyperperfusion syndrome following carotid endarterectomy and carotid artery stenting: retrospective review of 4494 patients. J Neurosurg 2007; 107:1130-6.

Ouriel, K.; Shortell, CK.; Illig, KA.; Greenberg, RK & Green, RM. Intracerebral hemorrhage after carotid endarterectomy: incidence, contribution to neurologic morbidity, and predictive factors. J Vasc Surg 1999; 29: 82-7.

Pappada, G.; Beghi, E.; Marina, R.; Agostoni, E.; Cesana, C.; Legnani, F.; Parolin, M.; Petri, D & Sganzerla, EP hemodynamic instability after extracranial carotid stenting. Acta Neurochir (Wien) 2006. 148:639–645

Paul, L; Vicente, JM; Pastorín, & Casasco, A.. A case of temporary nonthrombotic hemiplegia and aphasia due to neurotoxicity from angiographic contrast material? Radiol 2009 Nov-Dec; 51(6):614-7. Epub 2009 Oct 22.

Penn, AA.; Schomer, DF.; Steinberg, GK.; Imaging studies of cerebral hyperperfusion after carotid endarterectomy. Case report. J Neurosurg. 1995 Jul; 83(1): 133-7.

Pieniazek P, Kabłak-Ziembicka A, Przewłocki T, Musiałek P, Moczulski Z, Motyl R, Frasik W, Leśniak-Sobelga A,

Zmudka K & Tracz W. Carotid artery stenting with proximal or distal brain protection: early outcome. Kardiol Pol. 2004 Sep;61 Suppl 2: II48-56.

Piepgras, DG.; Morgan, MK.; Sundt, TM Jr.; Yanagihara, T & Mussman, LM. Intracerebral hemorrhage after carotid endarterectomy. J Neurosurg 1988;68:532-6.

Pilz, G.; Klos, M.; Bernhardt, P.; Schöne, A.; Scheck, R & Höfling, B: Reversible cerebral hyperperfusion syndrome after stenting of the carotid artery, two case reports. Clin Res Cardiol 95:186–191, 2006

Pomposelli, FB.; Lamparello, PJ & Riles, TS, et al. Intracranial hemorrhage alter carotid endarterectomy. J Vasc Surg 1988; 7: 248-55

Qureshi, AI.; Luft, AR.; Sharma, M.; Janardhan, V.; Lopes, DK & Khan, J et al: Frequency and determinants of postprocedural hemodynamic instability after carotid angioplasty and stenting. Stroke 30:2086–2093, 1999

Qureshi, AI.; Saad, M.; Zaidat, OO.; Suarez, JI.; Alexander, MJ & Fareed, M et al: Intracerebral hemorrhages associated with neurointerventional procedures using a combination of antithrombotic agents including abciximab. Stroke 33:1916–1919, 2002

Rapp, JH.; Laura Wakil, BA.; Rajiv Sawhney.; Xian Mang Pan.; Midori, A.; Christine Glastonbury, Y.;, Sheila Coogan & Max Wintermark. Subclinical embolization after carotid artery stenting: New lesions on diffusion-weighted magnetic resonance imaging occur postprocedure. J Vasc Surg 2007; 45: 867-74.

Renliang Zhang, Guangyi Zhou, Gelin Xu & Xinfeng Liu. Posterior Circulation Hyperperfusion Syndrome after Bilateral Vertebral Artery Intracranial Stenting. Ann Vasc Surg 2009; 23: 686.e1 686.e5

Reigel, MM.; Hollier, LH.; Sundt, TM Jr.; Piepgras, DG.; Sharbrough, FW & Cherry, KJ. Cerebral hyperperfusion syndrome: a cause of neurologic dysfunction after carotid endarterectomy. J Vasc Surg 1987; 5: 628-34.

Reigel, MM.; Hollier, LH.; Sundt, TM Jr.; Piepgras, DG.; Sharbrough, FW & Cherry KJ. Cerebral hyperperfusion syndrome: a cause of neurologic dysfunction after carotid endarterectomy. J Vasc Surg 1987;5:628-34.

Roh, HG.; Byun, HS.; Ryoo, JW.; Na, DG.; Moon, WJ.; Lee, BB & Kim DI. Prospective analysis of cerebral infarction after carotid endarterectomy and carotid artery stent placement by using diffusion-weighted imaging. AJNR Am J Neuroradiol 2005;26:376-84.

Safian, RD.; Bresnahan ,JF.; Jaff, MR.; Foster, M.; Bacharach, JM & Maini B et al; CREATE Pivotal Trial Investigators. Protected carotid stenting in high-risk patients with severe carotid artery stenosis. J Am Coll Cardiol 2006; 47:2384-9.

Samra, SK.; Dorje, P.; Zelenock, GB & Stanley, JC. Cerebral oximetry in patients undergoing carotid endarterectomy under regional anesthesia. Stroke 1996; 27: 49–55.

Saito,H.; Ogasawara, K.; Komoribayashi, N.; Kobayashi, M.; Inoue, T & Otawara, Y, et al: Concentration of malondialdehyde modified low-density lipoprotein in the jugular bulb during carotid endarterectomy correlates with development of postoperative cognitive impairment. Neurosurgery 60:1067–1073, 2007

Sbarigia, E.; Speziale, F.; Giannoni, MF.; Colonna, M.; Panico, MA & Fiorani P. Post-carotid endarterectomy hyperperfusion syndrome: preliminary observations for identifying at-risk patients by transcranial Doppler sonography and the acetazolamide test. Eur J Vasc Surg 1993; 7: 252-6.

Schoser, BG.; Heesen, C & Eckert, B et al. Cerebral hyperperfusion injury after percutaneous transluminal angioplasty of extracranial arteries. J Neurol 1997; 244: 101-04

Schwartz RB. Hyperperfusion encephalopathies: hypertensive encephalopathy and related conditions. Neurolog 2002; 8: 22-34.

Setacci, C.; de Donato, G.; Chisci, E & Setacci, F. Carotid artery stenting in recently symptomatic patients: a single center experience. Ann Vasc Surg. 2010 May; 24 (4): 474-9. Epub 2009 Nov 4.

Sfyroeras,GS; Karkos, CD; Arsos, G; Liasidis, C; Dimitriadis, AS; Papazoglou, KO & Gerassimidis, TS. Cerebral hyperperfusion after carotid stenting: a transcranial doppler and SPECT study. Vasc Endovascular Surg 2009 Apr-May; 43(2): 150-6. Epub 2008 Sep 30.

Sfyroeras, GS.; Karkos, CD & Gerassimidis, TS. Cerebral perfusion patterns in patients with extracranial carotid atherosclerosis and the impact of carotid stenting. A review. J Cardiovasc Surg (Torino) 2008. 49:497–502

Sfyroeras, G.; Karkos, CD.; Liasidis, C.; Spyridis, C.; Dimitriadis, AS.; Kouskouras, K & Gerassimidis, TS. The impact of carotid stenting on the hemodynamic parameters and cerebrovascular reactivity of the ipsilateral middle cerebral artery. J Vasc Surg. 2006 Nov; 44(5):1016-22; discussion 1022.

Sfyroeras, GS.; Karkos, CD & Gerassimidis, TS. Cerebral perfusion patterns in patients with extracranial carotid atherosclerosis and the impact of carotid stenting. A review. J Cardiovasc Surg (Torino) 2008. 49:497–502

Sharp, S.; Stone, J & Beach, R. Contrast agent neurotoxicity presenting as subarachnoid hemorrhage. Neurology. 1999; 52: 1503–1505.

Skudlarick, JL & Mooring, SL. Systolic hypertension and complications of carotid endarterectomy. South Med J 1982; 75: 1563-5,1567.

Skydell, JL.; Machleder, HI.; Baker, JD.; Busuttil, RW & Moore WS. Incidence and mechanism of post-carotid endarterectomy hypertension. Arch Surg 1987; 122: 1153–55.

Solomon, RA.; Loftus, CM.; Quest, DO & Correll, JW. Incidence and etiology of intracerebral hemorrhage following carotid endarterectomy. J Neurosurg 1986;64:29-34.

Sticherling, C.; Berkefeld, J & Auch-Schwelk, W et al. Transient bilateral cortical blindness after coronary angiography. Lancet. 1998; 351: 570.

Soinne, L.; Helenius, J & Tatlisumak, T et al. Cerebralhemodynamicsin asymptomatic and symptomatic patients with high-grade carotid stenosis undergoing carotid endarterectomy. Stroke. 2003;34: 1655Y1661.

Solomon, RA.; Loftus, CM.; Quest, DO & Correll, JW. Incidence and etiology of intracerebral hemorrhage following carotid endarterectomy. J Neurosurg 1986;64:29-34.

Suga, Y.; Ogasawara, K & Saito, H et al. Preoperative cerebral hemodynamic impairment and reactive oxygen species produced during carotid endarterectomy correlate with de- velopment of postoperative cerebral hyperperfusion. Stroke 2007; 38: 2712–2717.

Sundt, TM Jr.; Sharbrough, FW.; Piepgras, DG.; Kearns, TP.; Messick, JM Jr & O'Fallon, WM. Correlation of cerebral blood flow and electroencephalographic changes during carotid endarterectomy: with results of surgery and hemodynamics of cerebral ischemia.

Tang, SC.; Huang, YW.; Shieh, JS.; Huang, SJ.; Yip, PK & Jeng, JS. Dynamic cerebral autoregulation in carotid stenosis before and after carotid stenting. J Vasc Surg 2008; 48: 88-92.

Tan GS & Phatouros CC. Cerebral hyperperfusion syndrome post-carotid artery stenting. J Med Imaging Radiat Oncol. 2009 Feb;53(1):81-6.

Taha, MM.; Toma, N.; Sakaida, H.; Hori, K.; Maeda, M.; Asakura, F.; Fujimoto, M.; Matsushima, S & Taki, W. Periprocedural hemodynamic instability with carotid angioplasty and stenting. Surg Neurol. 2008 70:279–286

Tietke, MWK.; Kerby, T.; Alfke, H.; Riedel, C.; Rohr, A.; Jensen, U.; Zimmermann, P.; Stingele, R & Jansen, O. Complication rate in unprotected carotid artery stenting with closed-cell stents. Neuroradiology (2010) 52:611–618

Timaran, CH.; Veith, FJ.; Rosero, EB.; Modrall, JG.; Valentine, RJ & Clagett, GP. Intracranial hemorrhage after carotid endarterectomy and carotid stenting in the United States in 2005. J Vasc Surg. 2009 Mar;49 (3): 623-8.

Takolander RJ, Bergqvist D. Intracerebral hemorrhage after internal carotid endarterectomy. Acta Chir Scand 1983; 149: 215-20

Timmers, HJ.; Wieling, W.; Karemaker, JM & Lenders, JW. Baroreflex failure: a neglected type of secondary hypertension. Neth J Med 2004; 62:151-5.

Towne, JB & Bernhard, VM. The relationship of postoperative hypertension to complications following carotid endarterectomy. Surgery 1980; 88:575-80.

Vaughan CJ & Delanty N. Hypertensive emergencies. Lancet 2000;356: 411-17.

Wiart, M.; Berthezène, Y.; Adeleine, P.; Feugier, P.; Trouillas, P.; Froment, JC & Nighoghossian, N. Vasodilatory response of border zones to acetazolamide before and after endarterectomy: an echo planar imaging dynamic susceptibility contrast-enhanced MRI study in patients with high-grade unilateral internal carotid artery stenosis. Stroke 2000; 31: 1561-5.

Wilkinson, I.;. Griffiths, P.; Hoggard, N.; Cleveland & Trevor. Unilateral Leptomeningeal Enhancement After Carotid Stent Insertion Detected by Magnetic Resonance Imaging. Stroke 2000 31 (4) 848-51

Wilson, PV & Ammar, AD. The incidente of ischemic stroke versus intracerebral hemorrhage alter carotid endarterectomy: a review of 2452 cases. Ann Vasc Surg 2005; 19; 1-4

Yasuhiko Kaku.; Shin-ichi Yoshimura & and Jouji Kokuzawa. Factors Predictive of Cerebral Hyperperfusion after Carotid Angioplasty and Stent Placement. AJNR Am J Neuroradiol 25:1403–1408, September 2004

Ying-Chi Tseng.; Hui-Ling Hsu.; Tsong-Hai Lee.; I-Chang Hsieh & Chi-Jen Chen, Prediction of Cerebral Hyperperfusion Syndrome After Carotid Stenting: A Cerebral Perfusion Computed Tomography Study. J Comput Assist Tomogr & Volume 33, Number 4, July/August 2009

Yoshimoto, T.; Houkin, K.; Kuroda, S.; Abe, H & Kashiwaba, T. Low cerebral blood flow and perfusion reserve induce hyperperfusion after surgical revascularization: case reports and analysis of cerebral hemodynamics. Surg Neurol 1997; 48:132–138.

Yoshimura, S.; Kitajima, H.; Enomoto, Y.; Yamada, K.; Iwama, T. Staged angioplasty for carotid artery stenosis to prevent postoperative hyperperfusion. Neurosurgery. 2009 Mar;64(3 Suppl):122-8; discussion 128-9.

Zahn, R.; Ischinger, T & Hochadel, M et al. Carotid artery stenting in octogenarians: results from the ALKK Carotid Artery Stent (CAS) Registry. Eur Heart J 2007. 28:370–375

3

Below the Knee Techniques: Now and Then

Daniel Brandão[1,2], Joana Ferreira[1,2],
Armando Mansilha[3,4] and António Guedes Vaz[1]
[1]*Angiology and Vascular Surgery Department*
Vila Nova de Gaia / Espinho Hospital Center
[2]*Department of Biochemistry, Faculty of Medicine of the University of Porto*
[3]*Angiology and Vascular Surgery Department; São João University Hospital, Porto*
[4]*Faculty of Medicine of the University of Porto*
Portugal

1. Introduction

Critical Limb Ischemia (CLI) is defined as the presence of ischemic rest pain for more than two weeks or ischemic tissue loss associated with an absolute ankle pressure less than 50 mmHg or great toe pressure less than 30 mmHg (Norgren et al., 2007). Patients with CLI experience high amputation rates, significant morbidity and cardiovascular events exceeding those in patients with symptomatic coronary heart disease (Varu et al., 2010). In spite of recent developments in revascularization techniques and wound care centers, amputations continue to be performed, partly because patients with CLI are referred late to vascular surgeons (Varu et al., 2010). However, revascularization when compared with amputation have an overall lower perioperative mortality and enhanced long-term survival (Brosi et al., 2007; Varu et al., 2010). However, CLI is associated with multisegmental complex arterial lesions and consequently with high rates of revascularization failure (Allie et al., 2009). Specific features of the tibial vessels, such as the small caliber, the remote location, the slow flow of the distal bed, and the need of preserving runoff capacity, make this vascular territory particularly challenging for endovascular treatment (Blevins and Schneider, 2010). Meanwhile, continued technical improvements and very encouraging results have changed the paradigm of CLI therapy, until recently based on vein graft bypass. As so, the endovascular approach is, nowadays, the first-line modality for limb-threatening ischemia for a majority of authors (Allie et al., 2009; DeRubertis et al., 2007).

2. Epidemiology

CLI is a global epidemic, with high clinical, social and economic costs (Adam et al., 2005; Allie et al., 2009; Brosi et al., 2007). Its incidence in the United States (US) is estimated to be 50-100 per 10 000 every year (Adam et al., 2005). It affects 1% of the population aged 50 and older and the incidence roughly doubles in the over 70 age group (Allie et al., 2009). The prevalence of CLI is also higher in diabetic patients and its prognosis is even worst in this population: one of every four diabetics will face CLI within his/her lifetime, and a diabetic is at 7 to 40 times greater risk of an amputation than a non-diabetic (Allie et al., 2009). As so, it is expected that the incidence of CLI would rise significantly with the current aging population and the expected increase in inactivity, obesity and consequently in diabetes (Allie et al., 2009; van Dieren et al., 2010). As a result and despite advances in medical therapies, the number of patients needing lower limb revascularization for severe limb ischemia will probably increase in the near future (Adam et al., 2005). Moreover, the diagnosis of CLI remains a predictor of poor survival and outcomes (Varu et al., 2010): the overall mortality in these patients approaches 50% at 5 years and 70% at 10 years (Varu et al., 2010). Within one year of being diagnosed with CLI, 20% to 25% will die and 40% to 50% of the diabetics will experience an amputation (Allie et al., 2009; Kroger et al., 2006). The economic impact of CLI is considerable. It has been assessed that the total cost of treating CLI in the US is $10 to $20 billion per year (Allie et al., 2009). The cost of follow-up, long-term care, and treatment for an amputee who remains at home has been estimated at $49,000 per year compared to only $600 to $800 per year after limb salvage (Allie et al., 2009). It is estimated that just a 25% reduction in amputations could save $2.9 to $3.0 billion yearly in US healthcare costs (Allie et al., 2009). Despite the facts noted above, CLI is still poorly understood, infrequently reported and inconsistently treated (Allie et al., 2009).

3. The arterial lesions in patients with critical limb ischemia

CLI is highly predictive for failure of both primary and secondary patency, as a result of the increased prevalence of advanced lesion severity and treatment complexity (DeRubertis et al., 2007). There is several indicators of lesion severity in these patients: (1) increasing TASC grade (mostly C and D lesions); (2) multilevel intervention; (3) general involvement of tibial arteries in diabetic patients; (4) diffusely diseased tibial arteries (combination of long stenoses and occlusions; (5) reduced outflow bed (DeRubertis et al., 2007; Graziani et al., 2007; Ihnat and Mills, 2010).

4. Revascularization in CLI patients

4.1 Bypass surgery approach

Historically, infrainguinal autogenous saphenous vein bypass surgery has been considered the gold-standard therapy for CLI, with long-term anatomical patency, clinical durability and high limb salvage rates (Adam et al., 2005; Allie et al., 2009; Varu et al., 2010). The Pomposelli's classic report of more than 1000 pedal bypasses over a decade documented a 10-year primary patency rate of 37.7% and limb salvage rates of 57.8% (Pomposelli et al., 2003). Regrettably, most of these single center series were reported in optimal surgical candidates with favorable anatomy and adequate autogenous vein conduits (Allie et al., 2009). Furthermore, the durability of the vein graft may rely on routine ultrasonography surveillance, frequently leading to repeated prophylactic re-interventions and relevant resource utilization (Adam et al., 2005; Varu et al., 2010). Unfortunately an adequate vein is often unavailable and the long-term results of bypasses constructed with prosthetic graft are clearly much less satisfactory (Adam et al., 2005). The good results of infrainguinal surgery are not applicable to contemporary CLI patients who seldom have favorable anatomy and recurrently have poor autogenous conduits (Allie et al., 2009). Additionally, the *real world* CLI patients are frequently very elderly and have numerous medical issues, significantly increasing the mortality and morbidity associated with infrainguinal bypass (Allie et al., 2009; Brosi et al., 2007). Consequently the open surgery option could come at the cost of high morbidity and mortality, as well as substantial resource use (Adam et al., 2005).

Abou-Zamzam et al. analyzed the functional outcomes after surgery in CLI patients (Abou-Zamzam et al., 1997). This report aimed at identifying the *ideal* post-infrainguinal bypass results from CLI patient's functional perspective (Abou-Zamzam et al., 1997). The patient who survived the intervention, had his wounds healed at 6 months, was living independently and completely mobile, was defined as the *ideal functioning* patient (Abou-Zamzam et al., 1997). Disappointingly, despite excellent graft patency and limb salvage rates, only 14.3% of their infrainguinal bypass patients achieved the *ideal* result at 6 months (Allie et al., 2009). Avoidance of incisional wound creation and subsequent common healing problems have been strongly considered an advantage in favor of endovascular intervention versus infrainguinal bypass in our practice (Allie et al., 2009; Chung et al., 2006).

Meanwhile, in patients expected to live more than two years and who were fit, the apparent improved durability and reduced re-intervention rate of surgery might outweigh the short-term considerations of increased morbidity and cost (Adam et al., 2005).

4.2 Endovascular approach

The endoluminal therapy for lower extremity occlusive disease has extraordinary evolved in the last decade and the armamentarium now available for the vascular interventionist is quite considerable (DeRubertis et al., 2007). This has allowed an impressive expansion of the endovascular approach in complex, formerly considered unachievable, infra-inguinal lesions (Allie et al., 2009). As a result, the endoluminal intervention is now considered the first-line treatment in CLI patients for a majority of authors.

In addition, the understanding of CLI patients had improved considerably (Allie et al., 2009). The so called *limb salvage-graft patency gap* has been consistently identified in all infrainguinal bypass surgery reports regardless of conduits (Allie et al., 2009). Even after an occlusion of an infrainguinal bypass graft following limb salvage, the limb will oftentimes remain viable and not regress back to CLI since the blood flow and metabolic needs to achieve wound healing in CLI are much greater than to keep viability (Allie et al., 2009). This paradigm shift has opened the door to a potential change of the goals in the post procedural follow-up of the CLI patients from vessel patency to limb salvage. This has become the cornerstone in treating CLI patients, allowing an impressive expansion of endovascular therapy indications (Allie et al., 2009).

In fact, scrutinizing the data of endovascular approach for CLI treatment from the last decade shows very encouraging results in regard to limb salvage.

Dorros et al. used percutaneous transluminal angioplasty (PTA) as the first treatment in 235 CLI patients with a 91% 5-year limb salvage rate and a small number of complications (Dorros et al., 2001).

Faglia et al. reported tibial PTA as primary treatment in 993 CLI diabetic patients. During a 26±15 months follow-up, only 1.7% underwent major amputation. Limb salvage was achieved in more than 98% of patients and an 88% 5-year primary clinical patency rate was described (Faglia et al., 2005).

Kudo et al. also published a 10-year PTA experience in 111 CLI patients. A 0.9% procedural mortality and a 96.4% technical success rate were described. The 5-year limb salvage rate was 89.1% (Kudo et al., 2005). The same authors published their 12-year experience of tibial PTA versus bypass surgery in 192 CLI patients. They further concluded that PTA was safe and effective, pointing it as the primary treatment for CLI (Kudo et al., 2006).

A meta-analysis of 30 articles from Romiti et al. looked at immediate technical success, primary and secondary patency, limb salvage, and survival after infrapopliteal PTA in CLI patients. The results were compared with a meta-analysis of popliteal-to-distal vein bypass graft that the authors had previously published (Albers et al., 2006). Even if there was a significant difference in favor of vein bypass concerning durability, the limb salvage rates were equivalent between both techniques (Albers et al., 2006; Romiti et al., 2008).
From the data presented, it results that endovascular approach is currently considered as the first-line treatment for CLI patients with below-the-knee arteries involvement.

5. Below-the-knee intervention – Technical issues

5.1 Access

The access for below the knee (BTK) vessels can be granted either by antegrade ipsilateral approach or by retrograde contralateral approach.

5.1.1 Antegrade ipsilateral approach

As it allows a nearer distance to the tibial arteries, the antegrade technique permits the utilization of shorter devices, which leads to an improvement of the guidewires and catheters' characteristics like pushability, torqueability, crossability or trackability. As a result, it may become easier to treat complex lesions as long occlusions, distal lesions as in foot vessels or use complex techniques like the pedal-plantar loop technique. However, the antegrade puncture implies that the iliac arteries and the proximal superficial femoral artery are free of significant disease. Even if the pattern of arterial involvement in diabetic, CLI patients is mostly at BTK level, the presence of palpable femoral and popliteal pulses should not be considered as synonym of absence of an upstream significant lesion. As so, an arterial ultrasound of the iliac and femoral arteries should be previously performed to insure that an adequate inflow is available. Moreover, the antegrade approach can be difficult in obese patients. In those patients, some tricks can help in turning the puncture easier: (1) wrap the abdominal pannus with tape in cranial and contralateral directions; (2) put a folded sheet under the ipsilateral hip; (3) place the patient in Trendelenburg position; (4) consider longer needles; (5) consider reinforced sheaths (e.g. SuperArrow® Flex). The antegrade technique is also more prone to local complications and should be performed using a single wall needle to avoid a double puncture and its consequent additional potential problems. It should also be completed under fluoroscopy to localize the femoral head and puncture the common femoral artery (Dotter et al., 1978; Grier and Hartnell, 1990). In hostile heavily scarred groins or in very obese patients, ultrasound guided puncture of either the common femoral or the superficial femoral arteries may reduce radiation doses, screen times and complications (Biondi-Zoccai et al., 2006; Marcus et al., 2007; Yeow et al., 2002).

5.1.2 Retrograde contralateral approach

Contralateral puncture is technically easier to achieve and safer in regard to local complications (Nice et al., 2003). It permits performing a strategic arteriography and the correction of proximal iliac and femoral lesions. It allows a more secure utilization of closure devices and maintains the puncture site remote from the treated segment. The utilization of long sheaths especially designed for BTK intervention (e.g. Cook® Shuttle Tibial) may provide additional external support, allowing intervention in more demanding cases, but

potentially increasing total costs. Meanwhile, distal lesions are still difficult to reach and unfavorable aortic bifurcations or aortic grafts may preclude its utilization.
Table 1 summarizes the advantages and disadvantages of each approach.

	Antegrade access	Contralateral access
More complex and distal lesion	√	
Iliac and proximal SFA lesions		√
More technically demanding	√	
More frequent local complications	√	
Remote access from treated segment		√
Safer closure devices utilization		√

Table 1. Antegrade and contralateral retrograde access

5.2 Tibial vessel selection for intervention – The key step

Perhaps the most critical decision in revascularizing CLI patients with predominant BTK arteries involvement is to decide which vessel(s) should be approached to achieve successful limb salvage. In spite of arbitrarily recanalize a tibial artery only based on arteriography, one should consider some basic and prevailing principles.

5.2.1 Angiosome model

The angiosome concept was initially described in plastic and reconstructive surgery papers and was intended to provide the basis for a logical planning of incisions and flaps (Taylor and Palmer, 1987; Taylor and Pan, 1998). These anatomical studies delineated three-dimensional anatomic units of tissue (from skin to bone) fed by a given source artery, defined as angiosomes. In foot it has been described six angiosomes, arising from the posterior tibial artery (n=3), the anterior tibial artery (n=1), and the peroneal artery (n=2) (figure 1). The posterior tibial artery gives rise to a calcaneal branch that supplies the medial ankle and plantar heel, a medial plantar artery that feeds the medial plantar instep and a lateral plantar artery that supplies the lateral forefoot, plantar midfoot and entire plantar forefoot. The anterior tibial artery continues as the *dorsalis pedis* artery feeding the dorsum of the foot. The peroneal artery supplies the lateral ankle and plantar heel via the calcaneal branch and the lateral anterior upper ankle via an anterior perforating branch. Alexandrescu et al. applied more recently this angiosome model to guide endovascular procedures in diabetic CLI patients with remarkable results (Alexandrescu et al., 2008). This rational approach for the revascularization of the foot was followed by several authors who confirmed its relevance for ulcer healing and consequent limb salvage (Alexandrescu et al., 2011; Iida et al., 2010; Neville et al., 2009). In fact, Iida et al. analyzed 203 limbs in 177 patients and separated them into direct and indirect groups depending on whether feeding artery flow to the site of ulceration was successfully acquired or not based on the angiosome concept. They found that limb salvage rate was significantly higher in the direct group (86%) than in the indirect group (69%) for up to 4 years after the procedure (Iida et al., 2010).

Lately, Alexandrescu et al. compared 213 CLI limbs revascularized prior (n=89) and after (n=134) the introduction of the angiosome model. They also concluded that angiosome-targeted revascularization was associated with significantly higher limb preservation (89% vs. 79% at 36 months) (Alexandrescu et al., 2011). To simply allow pulsatile flow to the correct portion of the foot is the contemporary paramount for ulcer healing.

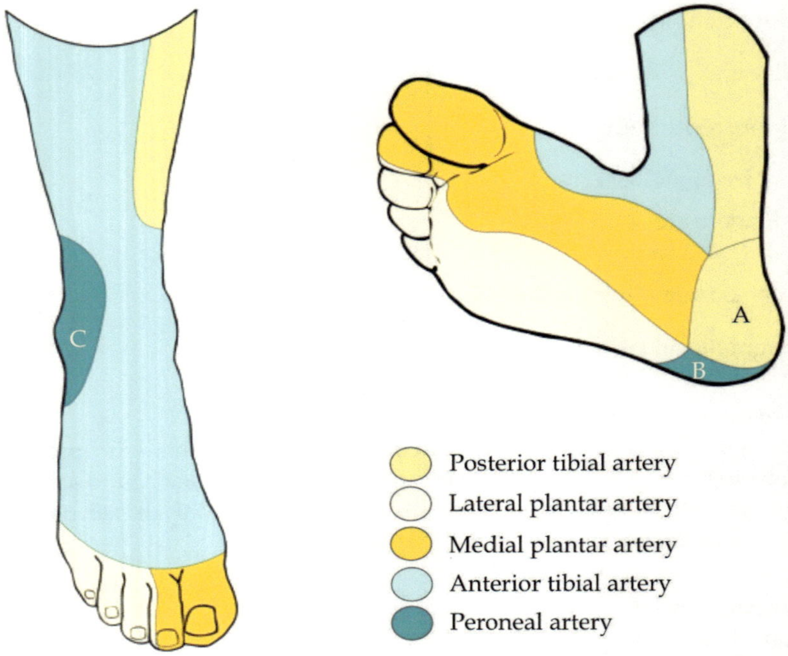

Fig. 1. Angiosome model. A – Calcaneal branch of the posterior tibial artery. B - Calcaneal branch of the peroneal artery. C – Anterior perforating branch of the peroneal artery.

5.2.2 Additional concepts

Adjacent angiosomes are bordered by reduced caliber (choke) or artery-similar caliber (true) anastomoses, which link neighboring angiosomes to one another and demarcate the border of each angiosome (Attinger et al., 2006; Taylor and Pan, 1998). In addition, these vessels are important safety conduits that allow a given angiosome to provide blood flow to an adjacent angiosome if the latter's source artery is damaged.

This concept should be taken into account in CLI limb revascularization. In fact, after having revascularized the key artery according to the angiosome concept, one may consider revascularizing other tibial vessels. The rationale to do so can be based on: (1) limited permeability rates with current angioplasty techniques may compromise the feeding artery before complete lesion healing; (2) trophic lesion may include more than one angiosome. Nevertheless, this attempt should never place the recanalized feeding artery at risk.

Meanwhile, some technical issues, as the lack of visible run-off, the presence of heavy calcification precluding transluminal or subintimal occlusion crossing, an occlusion at an arterial bifurcation (like the anterior tibial artery origin) or the presence of an important collateral at the beginning of an occlusion may restrict or prevent revascularization according to the angiosome model. In those circumstances, approaching an alternative tibial vessel considering the anastomoses between angiosomes may be the only option available in trying to preserve a CLI limb.

5.3 BTK Recanalization

In the past, the BTK interventional techniques were performed with large caliber, non-specific instruments, which resulted in poor results and skepticism upon its applicability in this specific sector. The relative similarity between BTK and coronary vessels led vascular interventionists to employ low profiling coronary devices, which improved outcomes. Additional developments brought specifically designed devices, achieving results that changed the paradigm of CLI patients treatment approach.

5.3.1 Imaging

Fluoroscopy is supposed to have high resolution (less than 0.3 mm), should allow roadmapping and overlay techniques and must permit a high range of angulation. In fact, the last point is highly relevant since some significant lesions can be occulted or underestimated by standard posterior-anterior view. Moreover, oblique incidences allow clear observation of tibial vessels avoiding superposed bone and potentially revealing useful calcifications that can be used as *natural roadmapping*.

5.3.2 Guidewires

One may start with a 0.035" regular angled glidewire™ to cross simple stenoses. However, more complex lesions must be addressed with specific guidewires.

Vascular specialists began BTK treatment with some scarcity of options in regard to guidewires, but currently there has been an increasing choice in this particular matter (Table 2).

Tip load, tip stiffness, hydrophilic/hydrophobic coating of the tip and body, guidewire flexibility, ability to shape, shaping memory, shaft support, torque transmission, trackability, and pushability are all critical components for a BTK intervention guidewire, especially for chronic total occlusions (CTOs) (Godino et al., 2009) (see tables 2 & 3).

The selection should consider some specificities of the lesion: (1) the localization (some authors prefer 0.018" guidewires for tibial arteries, leaving 0.014" guidewires for pedal arteries); (2) CTO or stenosis (occlusions may require specifically designed tip); (3) length (long lesions, especially CTOs, usually demand additional support to allow the passage of other interventional devices).

Non-hydrophilic guidewires allow a better tactile feel and a more controlled torque response when compared with hydrophilic wires. They are less likely to cause dissection of a vessel but have a higher resistance within the lesion, which may decrease the chances of successful crossing, particularly in CTOs. To counterweigh this, some uncoated, spring-coil wires have a specifically designed tapered-tip which confers more penetrating power to the tip. On the other hand, some guidewires may have, rather than increased sharpness, greater tip stiffness due to weights addition, which increases their penetration ability.

Hydrophilic wires typically advance with minimal resistance, providing good maneuverability in tortuous and long vessels but at a cost of reduced tactile feel. They are also more prone in penetrating beneath plaque inducing a dissection of the vessel.

0.014″ Guidewires	Hydrophilic		Tapered tip	Tip stiffness (g)	Remarks
	tip	body			
Abbott HT Winn™ 40, 80, 200	Y	HF	Y (0.012-0.009″)	4.8, 9.7, 13	BTK GW
Abbott Pilot™ 50, 150, 200	Y	Y	N	2,4,6	Coronary GW
Abbott Wisper LS, MS, ES	Y	N	N	1	Coronary GW
Asahi Confianza™	N	N	Y (0.009″)	9	Coronary GW
Asahi Intecc Miracle ™	N	N	N	3, 4.5, 6, 9, 12	Coronary GW
Biotronik Cruiser® Hydro MS, ES	Y	N	N	0.27	Coronary GW
Biotronik Cruiser® MS, ES	HF	N	N	0.27	Coronary GW
Biotronik XT-14	Y	N	N	NA	BTK GW
BS PT Graphix™; Grafix P2™ LS, MS	Y	Y	N	3-4	Coronary GW
Cook Approach® Hydro ST	Y	N	N	NA	BTK GW
Cook Approach® CTO	N	N	N	6, 12, 18, 25	BTK GW
Cordis Shinobi™	Y	N	N	2	Coronary GW
Medtronic Provia™	N	Y/N	Y (0.009″)*1	3, 6, 9, 12, 15	BTK GW

Table 2. Possible 0.014″ guidewires for BTK purposes. BS – Boston Scientific. LS, MS, ES (light, medium, and extra support). Y/N – Both versions are available. *1 – Only in the 9, 12 and 15 g tips. GW – Guidewire; HF hydrophobic; NA – Not Available.

0.018″ Guidewires	Hydrophilic		Tapered tip	Tip stiffness (g)	Remarks
	tip	body			
Abbott SteelCore 18 LT	N	N	N	NA	
Biotronik Cruiser® 18	Y	N	N	NA	Increased body stiffness
BS V-18™ Control Wire®	Y	N	N	3-4	Increased body stiffness
Cook Roadrunner® ES	N	N	N	NA	Increased body stiffness

Table 3. Possible 0.018″ guidewires for BTK purposes. BS – Boston Scientific; NA – Not Available.

5.3.3 Chronic Total Occlusions (CTOs)

CTOs are generally defined as occluded arteries of three months duration or longer (Stone et al., 2005). CTOs are characterized by proximal and distal fibrous caps, a mix of luminal *soft* and *hard* plaque, thrombin, fibrin, inflammatory cells (in the intima, media, and adventitia), and neovascularization. The plaque is composed of a collagen rich extracellular matrix, intra, and extracellular lipids, smooth muscle cells, and calcium (Katsuragawa et al., 1993; Srivatsa et al., 1997). The proximal and distal caps have higher concentrations of collagen and calcium (fibrocalcific), even if the distal cap is frequently softer than the proximal cap (Fefer et al.,

2010). This may explain, at least partially, the relative ease in crossing tibial CTOs by retrograde pedal approach. The composition of the core correlates with CTO age. Older CTOs have higher concentrations of fibrocalcific material ("*hard plaque*"), while CTOs present for less than one year have more cholesterol clefts and foam cells among less fibrous material ("*soft plaque*"). This may, in part, explain the greater simplicity in crossing these younger CTOs.
Neovascularization starts early, as part of the organization of the CTO, and increases with time. As it has been demonstrated in coronary arteries, many CTOs are not completely occluded when examined under the microscope (Srivatsa et al., 1997). In fact, the new sprouting vessels, in contrast with *vasa vasorum* that run in radial directions, proceed within and parallel to the occluded parent vessel (Strauss et al., 2005). As a result they may originate microchannels throughout the CTO which diameter can vary between 100 and 500 μm (Srivatsa et al., 1997; Stone et al., 2005). Those can be used to engage the tip of the guidewire, which can further help in crossing CTOs. In this particular matter, tapered tips increase the ability to insert the guidewire in those microchannels, while hydrophilic tips are more prone to progress inside them.

5.3.3.1 Crossing CTOs

According to the lesion and the guidewire, different techniques to penetrate CTOs fibrous caps may be applied.

5.3.3.1.1 Antegrade techniques

In the *drilling technique*, the tip is bended in a short extension and clockwise and counter-clockwise rotations of the guidewire are performed while the tip is pushed modestly against the CTO lesion (figure 2). The important issue in this technique is that one does not push the guidewire very hard. If the tip of the guidewire does not advance any more with gentle pushing, it is by far better to exchange for a stiffer wire, rather than continue pushing. If one pushes the wire hard, it will easily go into the subintimal space. Yet, when a stiff guidewire is used, it may be difficult to perceive whether the tip has been engaged in the true or in a false lumen inside the CTO. The movement of the tip may help in distinguishing one from the other. Typically, when the guidewire is in the subadventitial space, the tip budges markedly. Additionally, the extension of the tip curve may look exaggerated, especially when using floppy tip guidewires. Tactile feel from the guidewire during pullback can also aid as true lumen usually offers higher resistance. This technique has an increased risk of perforation, especially when using stiff tips guidewires and is not usually recommended for complex lesions (Godino et al., 2009; Kim, 2010).

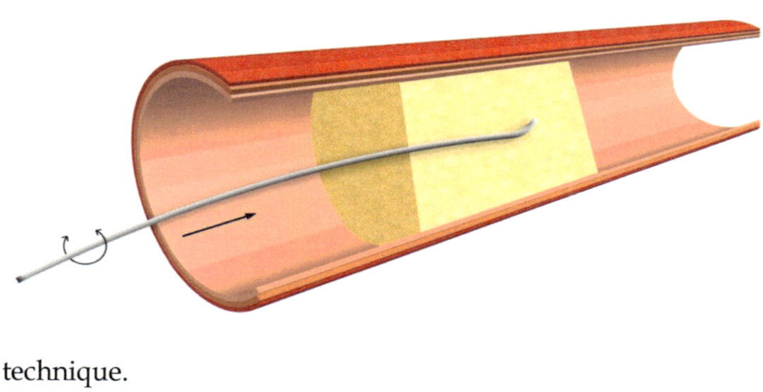

Fig. 2. Drilling technique.

In the *penetration technique*, the tip shape is usually straighter than in the drilling technique and a less rotational tip motion and a more direct forward probing is used (figure 3). Some heavily calcified CTO caps may require the use of very aggressive guidewires to achieve passage using the described technique (tapered stiff tips and increased body support guidewires, like the Abbott HT Winn 200™). Additionally, the target has to be clearly identified and careful monitoring of the progressive guidewire advancement should be done. Only experienced interventionists should make use of this technique in difficult CTOs, due to the particularly augmented risk of complications.

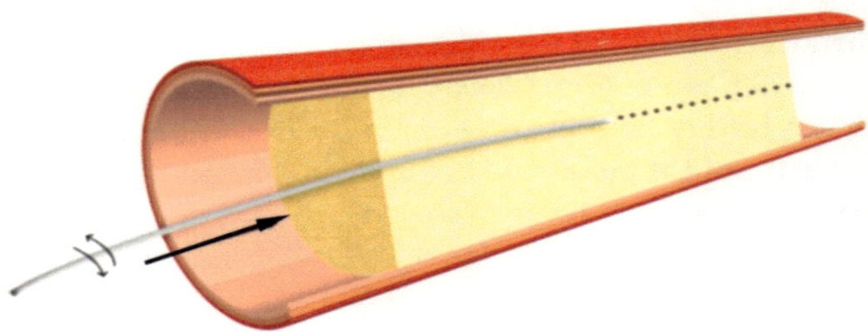

Fig. 3. Penetration technique.

The *sliding technique* utilizes hydrophilic guidewires. Reduced surface friction enhances passage through the CTO core. It is recommended that the tip is initially shaped with a single, long shallow bend and movement consists of simultaneous smooth tip rotation and gentle probing. The guidewire typically advances with minimal resistance and tactile feel, resulting frequently in inadvertent entry to the subintimal space.
This technique is particularly indicated for engaging softer CTOs with microchannels, subtotal occlusions or angulated lesions (Godino et al., 2009).
The *subintimal dissection technique* is usually performed when transluminal crossing has been unsuccessful. A hydrophilic guidewire with a floppy tip and an intermediate or stiff body is generally preferred. The loop is made with the floppy tip of the guidewire and should be relatively small to reduce the risk of perforation (figure 4).

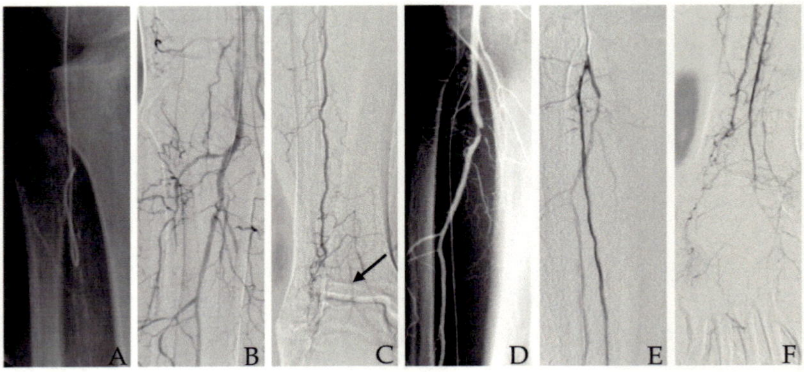

Fig. 4. A – Loop of the guidewire tip for *subintimal dissection* technique (BS V-18™ Control Wire®); B, C – Case of a long anterior tibial artery (ATA) occlusion (arrow pointing to distal ATA); D – Guidewire advanced subintimally all the way through ATA. E, F – Final result.

Highly calcified lesions may add some resistance to the guidewire progression, making pre-dilatation necessary, and can, in addition, make difficult or impede re-entry in true lumen. Recoil is more common and care should be especially taken to avoid damaging collaterals. As subintimal space is larger than true lumen, the balloon should be slightly oversized (0.5 mm).

In the *parallel wire technique*, when the initial wire passes into a dissection plane, it is left there using it as a reference point to assist in passing a second wire through the true lumen (figure 5. This technique has two main purposes: re-directing a wire inside the CTO and puncturing distal CTO fibrous cap.

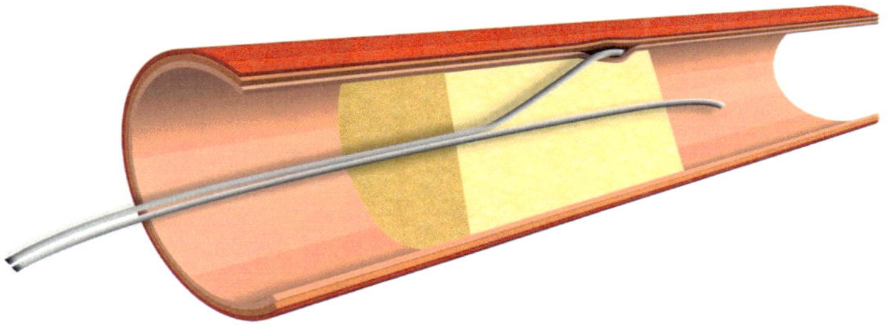

Fig. 5. Parallel wire technique.

5.3.3.1.2 Subintimal Arterial Flossing with Antegrade–Retrograde Intervention (SAFARI)

During antegrade recanalization, reentry into the distal true lumen can be difficult or impossible for several reasons. In those circumstances retrograde puncture has to be considered. This technique should also be envisaged when the proximal occlusion stump cannot be determined, which occurs most frequently with the anterior tibial artery (figure 6, case 1). It can be performed in all three leg arteries at the calf, ankle or foot levels. The puncture is performed under fluoroscopic guidance. Vessel calcification can be very useful. At the ankle or foot level, a 21 G, 4 cm long, needle can be used (the same needle used in a radial artery line placement). Crural level puncture implies a longer needle (21 G, 7 cm long, from a micropuncture kit). When the needle is in the artery lumen, a weak back-bleeding of arterial blood is observed. At that point, a 300 cm, 0.014", hydrophilic, intermediate or stiff shaft guidewire is engaged in the true lumen of the target vessel, subsequently assisted by a low profile support catheter or balloon catheter, without sheath placement. Subsequently, retrograde subintimal recanalization is carried out and continued until entry in the proximal true lumen or in the subintimal space from the antegrade approach is achieved. Sometimes, neither are obtained after several attempts. At that moment, the *rendez-vous technique* should be performed to break the membrane that separates the retrograde and antegrade subintimal spaces and, consequently, get continuity between them (figures 6-F and 7). At that time, the guidewire is typically snared or directed into the antegrade catheter or sheath to create a *flossing*-type guidewire which provides reliable access and adequate support (as it is fixed at both ends) for antegrade balloon angioplasty or stent placement (Figure 6) (Spinosa et al., 2003). When adequate flow has been reestablished into the target vessel, a catheter (diagnostic catheter, low profile support catheter or balloon catheter) is advanced distally to the lesion. The guidewire is then retrieved proximally, inverted and re-inserted (if not damaged). Hemostasis of the retrograde puncture site in foot and ankle is achieved by gentle local compression. At the calf level, hemostasis is performed by inflating a short balloon in the artery at the puncture site, usually for two minutes and at low pressure.

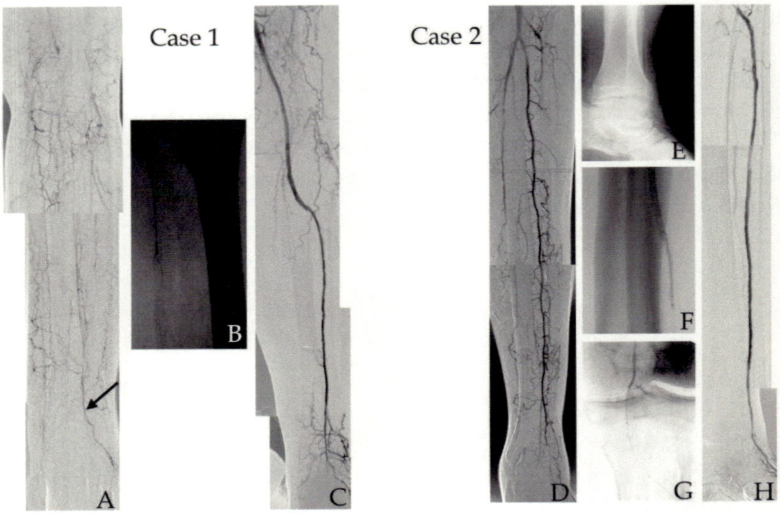

Fig. 6. SAFARI interventions. *Case 1.* A – Initial arteriography; occlusion of popliteal and all three tibial arteries (black arrow: patent *dorsalis pedis* artery). B – Snaring of the retrograde guidewire. C – Final result. / *Case 2.* D – Initial arteriography; patent peroneal artery, but ending in unsatisfactory collaterals (black arrow head: proximal anterior tibial artery). E – X-Ray showing percutaneous retrograde guidewire. F – *Rendez-vous technique.* G – Retrograde guidewire introduced inside 4F Bernstein catheter (the catheter should be turned to the arterial wall; the angled tip of the guidewire have to be engaged inside catheter lumen through simultaneous smooth tip rotation and gentle probing). H – Final result (guidewire can still be seen in the foot in a percutaneous position).

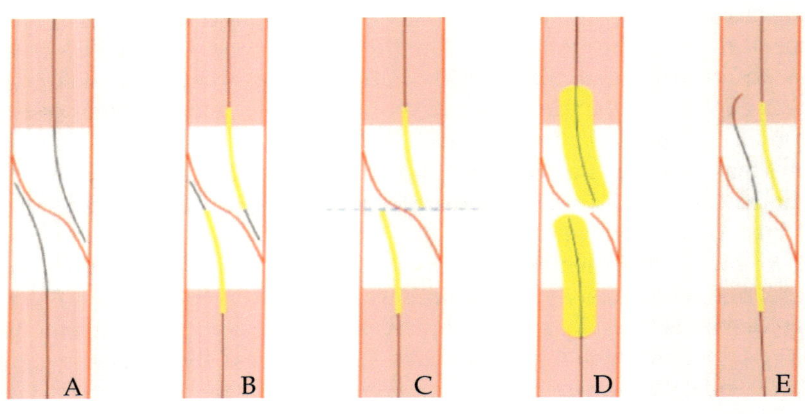

Fig. 7. *Rendez-vous technique.* A – Antegrade and retrograde guidewires in their respective subintimal space. B – A balloon catheter is advanced over each guidewire. C – The tip of the balloons are placed at the same level and guidewires tips are retrieved inside the balloon catheter. D – Balloons are inflated and the separating membrane broken. E – Retrograde guidewire is thoroughly advanced to proximal true lumen.

Meanwhile, there are several limitations to this technique. As so, an occluded or severely diseased artery may impede the puncture. Additionally, one should be extremely careful when the working artery is the only one patent in the leg, as a dissection, perforation or rupture may preclude a possible rescue surgery bypass.

5.3.3.1.3 Pedal-plantar loop technique

This technique consists in creating a loop with the guidewire from the anterior tibial artery to the posterior tibial artery, or the inverse, through the foot vessels (Fusaro et al., 2007; Manzi et al., 2009). The most common pathway is through *dorsalis pedis* artery, deep plantar artery, deep plantar arterial arch, lateral plantar artery and posterior tibial artery. Indications for this technique are similar to the SAFARI technique. However, unlike the SAFARI technique, it can be performed when no distal vessel is available for puncture, being also less invasive. Moreover, this technique can provide a better outflow for tibial arteries.

On the other hand, complications related to foot vessels manipulations can precipitate a serious worsening of the ischemic condition.

Additional information in regard to this technique is provided in the chapter from the present book written by Manzi et al.

5.3.3.1.4 Revascularization through peroneal artery collaterals

If neither the anterior nor the posterior tibial artery can be treated despite several intraluminal and subintimal crossing attempts, the alternative treatment may consist of providing direct flow along the peroneal artery. The distal peroneal artery has several collateral branches that connect with foot arteries. In particular, the communicating branch connects the peroneal with the posterior tibial artery, whereas the perforating branch goes through the interosseous membrane and links the peroneal to the *dorsalis pedis* artery. This technique aims at creating an effective pathway from the peroneal to tibial vessels by means of guidewire tracking through the referred collaterals (figure 8).

The *transcollateral* technique may be of value specifically when a proximal occlusion stump is not evident, when a dissection flap or a perforation in the proximal tract of the target vessel impairs guidewire advancement, or when distal disease makes retrograde percutaneous puncture impossible.

The major limitation of this technique is the absence of collaterals suitable for wiring (Fusaro et al., 2008; Graziani et al., 2008).

In all the above described techniques, a low-profile supportive catheter (Cook CXI™, Spectranetics® Quickcross®, Medtronic/Invatec Diver) or a low-profile balloon catheter can be used to provide additional support to the advancement of the guidewire. They also allow wire exchange without sacrificing the progress made through the lesion. Additionally, their lumen can be used to inject contrast and verify position and distal outflow. In this circumstances, diluted contrast, with diminished viscosity, may be preferable as the very low profile of catheter lumen is associated with high flow resistance.

5.3.4 Balloons

Specific low-profile balloons (less than 4F) have been recently designed for BTK purposes. They are made to work on a 0.014" or a 0.018" platform. The catheters of those balloons should provide increased shaft strength to allow adequate pushability, particularly in complex CTOs. In those circumstances, the over-the-wire technique should be preferred as it

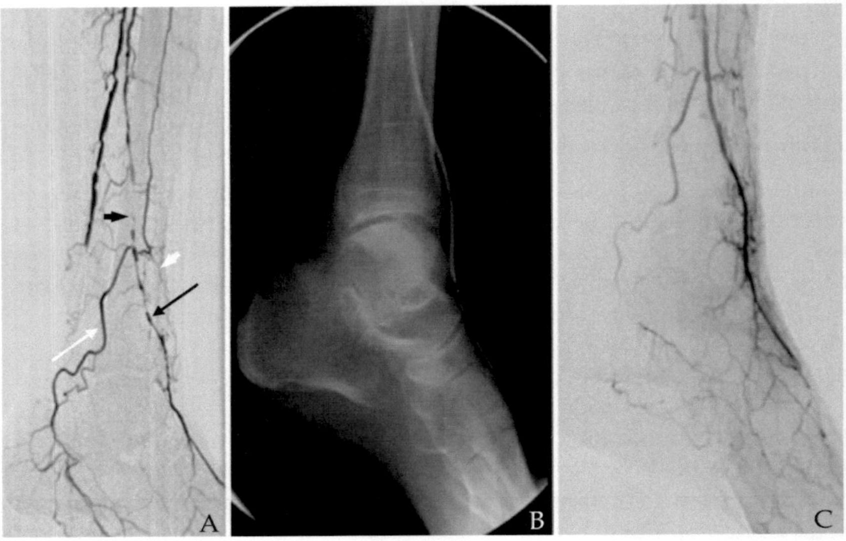

Fig. 8. *Transcollateral* technique. A – Black arrow head: peroneal artery; white arrow head: occlusion of the distal anterior tibial artery; white arrow head: occlusion of the distal anterior tibial artery; white arrow: communicating branch of peroneal artery anastomosing with posterior tibial artery; black arrow: perforating branch anastomosing with *dorsalis pedis* artery. B – Inflated balloon throughout distal peroneal artery, perforating branch and *dorsalis pedis* artery. Notice the posterior to anterior transition. C - Final result.

promotes better support when compared to the rapid-exchange monorail technique. The transition between the guidewire and the tip of the catheter should be as smooth as possible to avoid the catheter getting stuck in the lesion, optimizing its crossability. Hydrophilic coating of the catheter is particularly relevant in long complex lesions. Long catheters should be considered when the contralateral approach is performed.

In regard to the balloon itself, its compliance should be kept at minimum, as diameter accuracy is crucial for BTK interventions. In this particular matter, even conical balloons have been recently released. Long sizes are now available allowing angioplasty of an almost entire tibial vessel. The shoulders should be reduced to keep precision on the extension of the vessel to be treated. Segmental pre-dilatation with smaller diameter balloons may be required to allow the passage of the definitive balloon.

Although there is no consensus on insufflation time, most of the authors recommend a period longer than 3 minutes.

5.3.5 Bare-metal stents

The tibial arteries are small diameter vessels and have a limited flow. As so, they are particularly prone to neointimal hyperplasia and re-stenosis after balloon-expandable bare-metal stent (BMS) placement (Siablis et al., 2005). In fact, reocclusion occurs in up to 50% of the cases by one year (Scheinert et al., 2006; Siablis et al., 2007; Siablis et al., 2005). Additionally, balloon-expandable stents are available in only small lengths as they are originally coronary stents. There is only one long balloon-expandable stent device (up to 8 cm) dedicated to the infrapopliteal segment (Medtronic Invatec Chromis Deep). However, data regarding its behavior is lacking (Karnabatidis et al., 2009a). Meanwhile, balloon expandable stents in tibial vessels seem to be surprisingly less vulnerable to compressions and fracture than in the femoro-popliteal sector, except if placed distally (Karnabatidis et al., 2009b).

Long, thin-strut, low-profile, self-expanding nitinol stents designed and engineered specifically for the infrapopliteal arteries are now commercially accessible. Yet, data concerning their efficacy is still scarce. More concrete and solid evidence will arise when the results from the Expand-Trial (Astron Pulsar Stent versus PTA in patients with symptomatic critical limb ischemia or Severe intermittent claudication) and the XXS-Trial (Balloon Angioplasty Versus Xpert Stent in CLI Patients) will become available.

Though, considering the existing data, bare metal stents should be reserved to bailout situations after balloon angioplasty. As so, they should be inserted in the following situations: flow-limiting dissection resistant to prolonged balloon angioplasty, significant elastic recoil, and relevant residual stenosis (higher than 30%). Still, they have also been advocated to correct challenging lesions in bifurcations using the *crush technique* originally described in coronary arteries (Colombo et al., 2003; Schwarzmaier-D'Assie et al., 2007).

5.4 Complications

Systemic and access complications are common to all endovascular procedures. Additional considerations should be made in regard to some direct local complications.

A perforation or an arteriovenous fistula that occurs while attempting to cross a tibial CTO is rarely of any clinical significance as it will almost constantly closes within few minutes when only a guidewire or a low-profile catheter has passed extraluminally (Lyden, 2009) (figure 9). Thus, one should be sure to be inside the vessel before inflating a balloon. Removing the devices to above the proximal extremity of the CTO and reattempting to cross the lesion from the top, may allow successful passage and aid in solving the perforation or the arteriovenous fistula. When those complications do not auto-resolve, external compression guided by angiography or temporary vessel occlusion with a balloon can be attempted. In very rare situations, coiling must be envisaged.

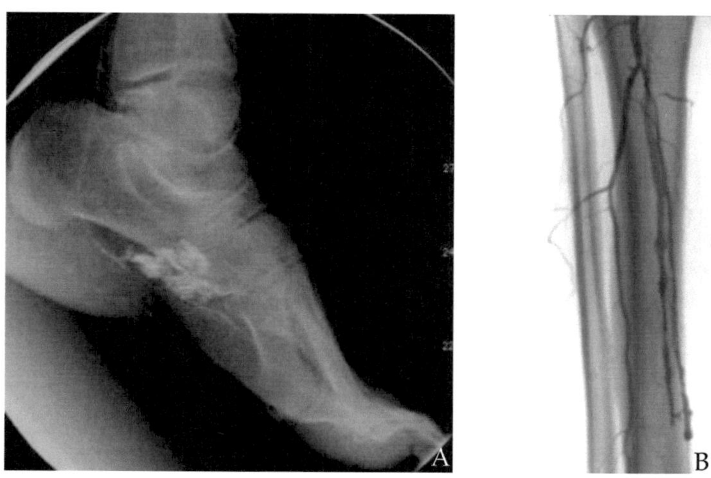

Fig. 9. A – Perforation; extraluminal contrast is easily noticed. B – Peroneal arteriovenous fistula.

5.5 Adjunctive medication

All patients should be placed on intravenous heparin when the sheath is introduced. The dose should be adjusted to keep an activated clotting time between 250 and 300. Other anticoagulants, such as bivalirudin, have been shown to be equally effective (Patel et al., 2010).

All patients should already be on a chronic aspirin regimen. Clopidogrel should be started 5 days before the procedure. Alternatively, a 300 mg load can be administrated peri-procedure. Although adequate evidence is lacking, aspirin plus clopidogrel should be kept for six months.

Tibial arteries are particularly prone to vasospasm. As so, arterial vasodilators should be available at all times. There are mostly four that can be used in: nitroglycerin, papaverine, tansolusine and verapamil, although nitroglycerin is most commonly used (Cronenwett et al., 2005). Besides their use in treating catheterization-associated vasospasm, they may be administrated prophylactically before balloon insufflation or guidewire manipulation of tortuous vessels, especially foot vessels.

Thrombolytics should also be accessible, as dissection, spasm or elastic recoil may precipitate an acute thrombosis.

5.6 Emergent techniques and alternatives

5.6.1 Drug-eluting stents

Driven by the encouraging results of the trials on drug-eluting stents in coronary arteries, some vascular interventionists have applied them in the infrapopliteal arteries to overcome restenosis and prolong amputation- and reintervention-free survival of CLI patients (Schofer et al., 2003). Several single-center series have demonstrated that drug-eluting stents effectively seem to be associated with a higher primary patency and a reduced need for reintervention in comparison to bare metal stents (Scheinert et al., 2006; Siablis et al., 2009).

Meanwhile, considering that bare metal stents have currently restricted indications, most of CLI patients have long complex infrapopliteal lesions, only short coronary drug-eluting balloon-expandable stents are currently available, and taking into account the so called *limb salvage-graft patency gap*, one could consider that the potential role for drug-eluting stents in BTK vessels is still to be determined.

5.6.2 Drug-coated balloons

The concept of delivering a local antiproliferative drug to the vessel surface utilizing drug-coated balloons to prevent restenosis without placing a permanent foreign material seems very appealing. Moreover, in opposition to current drug-eluting stents, drug-coated balloons can treat long lesions.

Nevertheless, more solid evidence is required to clarify the utility of drug-coated balloons in infrapopliteal arteries. The PICOLLO and PADI ongoing trials may provide the needed additional data (Hawkins and Hennebry, 2011).

5.6.3 Atherectomy devices

The OASIS trial proved that orbital atherectomy in infrapopliteal vessels may provide predictable and safe lumen enlargement. Short-term data demonstrated substantial symptomatic improvement and infrequent need for further revascularization or amputation (Korabathina et al., 2010). Specific directional atherectomy devices are also available for tibial vessels. Nevertheless, more consistent data is needed to determinate the precise role of these tools in BTK intervention.

5.6.4 Additional technology

There are additional devices, some already available, other still in the pipeline of manufacturers, which may become relevant in near future. Bioabsorbable stents (drug-eluting or not), cryoplasty, and laser atherectomy are among them.

6. Conclusions

Endoluminal therapy for BTK arteries is now a key part of the vascular specialist armamentarium. Tibial arteries endovascular approach has demonstrated to lead to high limb salvage rates with low morbidity and mortality. As a result, the paradigm for treatment of CLI patients has changed. One should now consider endovascular intervention as the first line treatment in the majority of CLI patients, especially in those with significant medical comorbidities. To do so, the vascular specialist should have a consistent knowledge of the BTK endovascular techniques and devices. The first step decision in tibial endovascular therapy is the access. In this context, antegrade ipsilateral approach is generally preferred. The next critical decision is the choice of the vessel(s) to be approached in order to reach successful limb salvage. Allowing pulsatile flow to the correct portion of the foot is the contemporary paramount for ulcer healing. As so, an adequate understanding of the current angiosome model should enhance clinical results. However, this concept does not preclude the recanalization of the other tibial vessels as trophic lesion may include more than one angiosome and the limited long-term permeability rate of angioplasty may compromise the feeding artery before complete lesion healing. The selection of the devices should be judicious. The choice of the guidewire is extremely relevant and should be based on the characteristics of the lesion (location, length, and stenosis/occlusion) as well as on the characteristics of the guidewire itself (tip load, stiffness, hydrophilic/hydrophobic coating, flexibility, torque transmission, trackability, and pushability). Going through chronic total occlusions may be quite challenging. Therefore, the vascular interventionist should master the techniques that have been recently described: antegrade techniques, including the drilling technique, the penetrating technique, the subintimal technique and the parallel technique; subintimal arterial flossing with antegrade-retrograde intervention (SAFARI); pedal-plantar loop technique and revascularization through peroneal artery collaterals. The specifically designed, low-profile, increased shaft strength, balloons catheters were conceived for a 0.0.014" or a 0.018" platform. The balloons should have minimal compliance and be available in long sizes. Bare metal stents should be available, even though their use is presently reserved for bailout situations.
Meanwhile, the continuous arising of new technologies will possibly convulse the currently accepted BTK endovascular techniques. In fact, drug-eluting stents, drug-coated balloons, atherectomy devices, bioabsorbable stents among others may play a relevant role in BTK intervention in the near future.

7. Acknowledgements

The authors would like to thank the staff of the Angiology and Vascular Surgery Department, the Radiology Technicians, the Radiology Nurses and the Staff of Diabetic Foot

Outpatient Clinic of the Vila Nova de Gaia/Espinho Hospital Center for their tireless efforts in providing the best possible conditions for the success of the endovascular procedures and the achievement of limb salvage.

8. References

Abou-Zamzam, A.M., Jr., Lee, R.W., Moneta, G.L., Taylor, L.M., Jr. & Porter, J.M. (1997). Functional outcome after infrainguinal bypass for limb salvage. *J Vasc Surg* 25, 287-295.

Adam, D.J., Beard, J.D., Cleveland, T., Bell, J., Bradbury, A.W., Forbes, J.F., Fowkes, F.G., Gillepsie, I., Ruckley, C.V., Raab, G., et al. (2005). Bypass versus angioplasty in severe ischaemia of the leg (BASIL): multicentre, randomised controlled trial. *Lancet* 366, 1925-1934.

Albers, M., Romiti, M., Brochado-Neto, F.C., De Luccia, N. & Pereira, C.A. (2006). Meta-analysis of popliteal-to-distal vein bypass grafts for critical ischemia. *J Vasc Surg* 43, 498-503.

Alexandrescu, V., Vincent, G., Azdad, K., Hubermont, G., Ledent, G., Ngongang, C.& Filimon, A.M. (2011). A Reliable Approach to Diabetic Neuroischemic Foot Wounds: Below-the-Knee Angiosome-Oriented Angioplasty. *J Endovasc Ther* 18, 376-387.

Alexandrescu, V.A., Hubermont, G., Philips, Y., Guillaumie, B., Ngongang, C., Vandenbossche, P., Azdad, K., Ledent, G.& Horion, J. (2008). Selective primary angioplasty following an angiosome model of reperfusion in the treatment of Wagner 1-4 diabetic foot lesions: practice in a multidisciplinary diabetic limb service. *J Endovasc Ther* 15, 580-593.

Allie, D.E., Hebert, C.J., Ingraldi, A., Patlola, R.R.& Walker, C.M. (2009). 24-carat gold, 14-carat gold, or platinum standards in the treatment of critical limb ischemia: bypass surgery or endovascular intervention? *J Endovasc Ther* 16 Suppl 1, I134-146.

Attinger, C.E., Evans, K.K., Bulan, E., Blume, P.& Cooper, P. (2006). Angiosomes of the foot and ankle and clinical implications for limb salvage: reconstruction, incisions& revascularization. *Plast Reconstr Surg* 117, 261S-293S.

Biondi-Zoccai, G.G., Agostoni, P., Sangiorgi, G., Dalla Paola, L., Armano, F., Nicolini, S., Alek, J.& Fusaro, M. (2006). Mastering the antegrade femoral artery access in patients with symptomatic lower limb ischemia: learning curve, complications& technical tips and tricks. *Catheter Cardiovasc Interv* 68, 835-842.

Blevins, W.A., Jr.& Schneider, P.A. (2010). Endovascular management of critical limb ischemia. Eur J Vasc Endovasc Surg 39, 756-761.

Brosi, P., Dick, F., Do, D.D., Schmidli, J., Baumgartner, I.& Diehm, N. (2007). Revascularization for chronic critical lower limb ischemia in octogenarians is worthwhile. *J Vasc Surg* 46, 1198-1207.

Chung, J., Bartelson, B.B., Hiatt, W.R., Peyton, B.D., McLafferty, R.B., Hopley, C.W., Salter, K.D.& Nehler, M.R. (2006). Wound healing and functional outcomes after infrainguinal bypass with reversed saphenous vein for critical limb ischemia. *J Vasc Surg* 43, 1183-1190.

Colombo, A., Stankovic, G., Orlic, D., Corvaja, N., Liistro, F., Airoldi, F., Chieffo, A., Spanos, V., Montorfano, M.& Di Mario, C. (2003). Modified T-stenting technique with crushing for bifurcation lesions: immediate results and 30-day outcome. *Catheter Cardiovasc Interv* 60, 145-151.

Cronenwett, J.L., Johnston, K.W.& Rutherford, R.B. (2005). *Rutherford's vascular surgery*, 6th ed. / [edited by] Jack L. Cronenwett, Peter Gloviczki. edn (Philadelphia, Pa., Saunders).

DeRubertis, B.G., Pierce, M., Chaer, R.A., Rhee, S.J., Benjeloun, R., Ryer, E.J., Kent, C.& Faries, P.L. (2007). Lesion severity and treatment complexity are associated with outcome after percutaneous infra-inguinal intervention. *J Vasc Surg* 46, 709-716.

Dorros, G., Jaff, M.R., Dorros, A.M., Mathiak, L.M.& He, T. (2001). Tibioperoneal (outflow lesion) angioplasty can be used as primary treatment in 235 patients with critical limb ischemia: five-year follow-up. *Circulation* 104, 2057-2062.

Dotter, C.T., Rosch, J.& Robinson, M. (1978). Fluoroscopic guidance in femoral artery puncture. *Radiology* 127, 266-267.

Faglia, E., Dalla Paola, L., Clerici, G., Clerissi, J., Graziani, L., Fusaro, M., Gabrielli, L., Losa, S., Stella, A., Gargiulo, M., et al. (2005). Peripheral angioplasty as the first-choice revascularization procedure in diabetic patients with critical limb ischemia: prospective study of 993 consecutive patients hospitalized and followed between 1999 and 2003. *Eur J Vasc Endovasc Surg* 29, 620-627.

Fefer, P., Carlino, M.& Strauss, B.H. (2010). Intraplaque therapies for facilitating percutaneous recanalization of chronic total occlusions. *Can J Cardiol* 26 Suppl A, 32A-36A.

Fusaro, M., Agostoni, P.& Biondi-Zoccai, G. (2008). "Trans-collateral" angioplasty for a challenging chronic total occlusion of the tibial vessels: a novel approach to percutaneous revascularization in critical lower limb ischemia. *Catheter Cardiovasc Interv* 71, 268-272.

Fusaro, M., Dalla Paola, L.& Biondi-Zoccai, G. (2007). Pedal-plantar loop technique for a challenging below-the-knee chronic total occlusion: a novel approach to percutaneous revascularization in critical lower limb ischemia. *J Invasive Cardiol* 19, E34-37.

Godino, C., Sharp, A.S., Carlino, M.& Colombo, A. (2009). Crossing CTOs-the tips, tricks, and specialist kit that can mean the difference between success and failure. *Catheter Cardiovasc Interv* 74, 1019-1046.

Graziani, L., Silvestro, A., Bertone, V., Manara, E., Andreini, R., Sigala, A., Mingardi, R.& De Giglio, R. (2007). Vascular involvement in diabetic subjects with ischemic foot ulcer: a new morphologic categorization of disease severity. *Eur J Vasc Endovasc Surg* 33, 453-460.

Graziani, L., Silvestro, A., Monge, L., Boffano, G.M., Kokaly, F., Casadidio, I.& Giannini, F. (2008). Transluminal angioplasty of peroneal artery branches in diabetics: initial technical experience. *Cardiovasc Intervent Radiol* 31, 49-55.

Grier, D.& Hartnell, G. (1990). Percutaneous femoral artery puncture: practice and anatomy. *Br J Radiol* 63, 602-604.

Hawkins, B.M.& Hennebry, T.A. (2011). Local Paclitaxel delivery for treatment of peripheral arterial disease. *Circ Cardiovasc Interv* 4, 297-302.

Ihnat, D.M.& Mills, J.L., Sr. (2010). Current assessment of endovascular therapy for infrainguinal arterial occlusive disease in patients with diabetes. *J Vasc Surg* 52, 92S-95S.

Iida, O., Nanto, S., Uematsu, M., Ikeoka, K., Okamoto, S., Dohi, T., Fujita, M., Terashi, H.& Nagata, S. (2010). Importance of the angiosome concept for endovascular therapy in patients with critical limb ischemia. *Catheter Cardiovasc Interv* 75, 830-836.

Karnabatidis, D., Katsanos, K.& Siablis, D. (2009a). Infrapopliteal stents: overview and unresolved issues. *J Endovasc Ther* 16 Suppl 1, I153-162.

Karnabatidis, D., Katsanos, K., Spiliopoulos, S., Diamantopoulos, A., Kagadis, G.C.& Siablis, D. (2009b). Incidence, anatomical location, and clinical significance of compressions and fractures in infrapopliteal balloon-expandable metal stents. *J Endovasc Ther* 16, 15-22.

Katsuragawa, M., Fujiwara, H., Miyamae, M.& Sasayama, S. (1993). Histologic studies in percutaneous transluminal coronary angioplasty for chronic total occlusion: comparison of tapering and abrupt types of occlusion and short and long occluded segments. *J Am Coll Cardiol* 21, 604-611.

Kim, H.Y. (2010). Percutaneous recanalization of coronary chronic total occlusions: current devices and specialized wire crossing techniques. *Korean Circ J* 40, 209-215.

Korabathina, R., Mody, K.P., Yu, J., Han, S.Y., Patel, R.& Staniloae, C.S. (2010). Orbital atherectomy for symptomatic lower extremity disease. *Catheter Cardiovasc Interv* 76, 326-332.

Kroger, K., Stang, A., Kondratieva, J., Moebus, S., Beck, E., Schmermund, A., Mohlenkamp, S., Dragano, N., Siegrist, J., Jockel, K.H., et al. (2006). Prevalence of peripheral arterial disease - results of the Heinz Nixdorf recall study. *Eur J Epidemiol* 21, 279-285.

Kudo, T., Chandra, F.A.& Ahn, S.S. (2005). The effectiveness of percutaneous transluminal angioplasty for the treatment of critical limb ischemia: a 10-year experience. *J Vasc Surg* 41, 423-435; discussion 435.

Kudo, T., Chandra, F.A., Kwun, W.H., Haas, B.T.& Ahn, S.S. (2006). Changing pattern of surgical revascularization for critical limb ischemia over 12 years: endovascular vs. open bypass surgery. J Vasc Surg 44, 304-313.

Lyden, S.P. (2009). Techniques and outcomes for endovascular treatment in the tibial arteries. *J Vasc Surg* 50, 1219-1223.

Manzi, M., Fusaro, M., Ceccacci, T., Erente, G., Dalla Paola, L.& Brocco, E. (2009). Clinical results of below-the knee intervention using pedal-plantar loop technique for the revascularization of foot arteries. J *Cardiovasc Surg (Torino)* 50, 331-337.

Marcus, A.J., Lotzof, K.& Howard, A. (2007). Access to the superficial femoral artery in the presence of a "hostile groin": a prospective study. *Cardiovasc Intervent Radiol* 30, 351-354.

Neville, R.F., Attinger, C.E., Bulan, E.J., Ducic, I., Thomassen, M.& Sidawy, A.N. (2009). Revascularization of a specific angiosome for limb salvage: does the target artery matter? *Ann Vasc Surg* 23, 367-373.

Nice, C., Timmons, G., Bartholemew, P.& Uberoi, R. (2003). Retrograde vs. antegrade puncture for infra-inguinal angioplasty. Cardiovasc Intervent Radiol 26, 370-374.

Norgren, L., Hiatt, W.R., Dormandy, J.A., Nehler, M.R., Harris, K.A., Fowkes, F.G., Bell, K., Caporusso, J., Durand-Zaleski, I., Komori, K., et al. (2007). Inter-Society Consensus for the Management of Peripheral Arterial Disease (TASC II). *Eur J Vasc Endovasc Surg* 33 Suppl 1, S1-75.

Patel, P.J., Hieb, R.A.& Bhat, A.P. (2010). Percutaneous revascularization of chronic total occlusions. *Tech Vasc Interv Radiol* 13, 23-36.

Pomposelli, F.B., Kansal, N., Hamdan, A.D., Belfield, A., Sheahan, M., Campbell, D.R., Skillman, J.J.& Logerfo, F.W. (2003). A decade of experience with dorsalis pedis artery bypass: analysis of outcome in more than 1000 cases. *J Vasc Surg* 37, 307-315.

Romiti, M., Albers, M., Brochado-Neto, F.C., Durazzo, A.E., Pereira, C.A.& De Luccia, N. (2008). Meta-analysis of infrapopliteal angioplasty for chronic critical limb ischemia. *J Vasc Surg* 47, 975-981.

Scheinert, D., Ulrich, M., Scheinert, S., Sax, J., Braunlich, S.& Biamino, G. (2006). Comparison of sirolimus-eluting vs. bare-metal stents for the treatment of infrapopliteal obstructions. *EuroIntervention* 2, 169-174.

Schofer, J., Schluter, M., Gershlick, A.H., Wijns, W., Garcia, E., Schampaert, E.& Breithardt, G. (2003). Sirolimus-eluting stents for treatment of patients with long atherosclerotic lesions in small coronary arteries: double-blind, randomised controlled trial (E-SIRIUS). *Lancet* 362, 1093-1099.

Schwarzmaier-D'Assie, A., Karnik, R., Bonner, G., Vavrik, J.& Slany, J. (2007). Fracture of a drug-eluting stent in the tibioperoneal trunk following bifurcation stenting. *J Endovasc Ther* 14, 106-109.

Siablis, D., Karnabatidis, D., Katsanos, K., Diamantopoulos, A., Spiliopoulos, S., Kagadis, G.C.& Tsolakis, J. (2009). Infrapopliteal application of sirolimus-eluting versus bare metal stents for critical limb ischemia: analysis of long-term angiographic and clinical outcome. *J Vasc Interv Radiol* 20, 1141-1150.

Siablis, D., Karnabatidis, D., Katsanos, K., Kagadis, G.C., Kraniotis, P., Diamantopoulos, A.& Tsolakis, J. (2007). Sirolimus-eluting versus bare stents after suboptimal infrapopliteal angioplasty for critical limb ischemia: enduring 1-year angiographic and clinical benefit. *J Endovasc Ther* 14, 241-250.

Siablis, D., Kraniotis, P., Karnabatidis, D., Kagadis, G.C., Katsanos, K.& Tsolakis, J. (2005). Sirolimus-eluting versus bare stents for bailout after suboptimal infrapopliteal angioplasty for critical limb ischemia: 6-month angiographic results from a nonrandomized prospective single-center study. *J Endovasc Ther* 12, 685-695.

Spinosa, D.J., Leung, D.A., Harthun, N.L., Cage, D.L., Fritz Angle, J., Hagspiel, K.D.& Matsumoto, A.H. (2003). Simultaneous antegrade and retrograde access for subintimal recanalization of peripheral arterial occlusion. *J Vasc Interv Radiol* 14, 1449-1454.

Srivatsa, S.S., Edwards, W.D., Boos, C.M., Grill, D.E., Sangiorgi, G.M., Garratt, K.N., Schwartz, R.S.& Holmes, D.R., Jr. (1997). Histologic correlates of angiographic chronic total coronary artery occlusions: influence of occlusion duration on neovascular channel patterns and intimal plaque composition. *J Am Coll Cardiol* 29, 955-963.

Stone, G.W., Kandzari, D.E., Mehran, R., Colombo, A., Schwartz, R.S., Bailey, S., Moussa, I., Teirstein, P.S., Dangas, G., Baim, D.S., et al. (2005). Percutaneous recanalization of chronically occluded coronary arteries: a consensus document: part I. *Circulation* 112, 2364-2372.

Strauss, B.H., Segev, A., Wright, G.A., Qiang, B., Munce, N., Anderson, K.J., Leung, G., Dick, A.J., Virmani, R.& Butany, J. (2005). Microvessels in chronic total occlusions: pathways for successful guidewire crossing. *J Interv Cardiol* 18, 425-436.

Taylor, G.I.& Palmer, J.H. (1987). The vascular territories (angiosomes) of the body: experimental study and clinical applications. *Br J Plast Surg* 40, 113-141.

Taylor, G.I.& Pan, W.R. (1998). Angiosomes of the leg: anatomic study and clinical implications. *Plast Reconstr Surg* 102, 599-616.

Van Dieren, S., Beulens, J.W., van der Schouw, Y.T., Grobbee, D.E.& Neal, B. (2010). The global burden of diabetes and its complications: an emerging pandemic. *Eur J Cardiovasc Prev Rehabil* 17 Suppl 1, S3-8.

Varu, V.N., Hogg, M.E.& Kibbe, M.R. (2010). Critical limb ischemia. *J Vasc Surg* 51, 230-241.

Yeow, K.M., Toh, C.H., Wu, C.H., Lee, R.Y., Hsieh, H.C., Liau, C.T.& Li, H.J. (2002). Sonographically guided antegrade common femoral artery access. *J Ultrasound Med* 21, 1413-1416.

4

Investigation of the Oxidative Stress, the Altered Function of Platelets and Neutrophils, in the Patients with Peripheral Arterial Disease

Maria Kurthy et al*

Department of Surgical Research and Techniques, Pecs University Medical School, Pecs Hungary

1. Introduction

Ischemia reperfusion injury (I/R) is a relevant problem in case of myocardial infarction (Moens AL, Claeys MJ et al. 2005.), stroke, (Kato H and Kogure K 1999), coronary bypass surgery, (Bakkaloglu C, and Soyagir B, 2006), under thrombolysis, (Krumholz HM and Goldberger 2006), revascularization surgery of lower limb (Arato et al 2006., Laird IR 2003), balloon angioplasty (Weissand A.G. and Zahger AT 1999) and in every cases, when the physiological blood flow in the occluded vessels are restored (Falkensammer J and Oldenburg WA 2006), (Ferencz A et al 2004). Vessel closure and hypoxia can be caused by embolism (thrombus, tumour, fat, foreign body) stenotic arteriopathy, arterial spasm, compression, arterial thrombus, trauma, etc. During the exclusion of a segment of the vessels from the circulation, ischemia and acidosis appeared in the surrounding tissues. In case of the heart, when oxygen supply is inadequate, the respiration shift from aerobic fatty acid consumption and metabolism to anaerobic glycolysis, resulting in a reduced ATP production. The results of hypoxia in the metabolically active tissues (cardiac, skeletal muscle and neuronal tissues) are more profound than in other cell types. The cells are exposed to hypoxia try to adapt to the absence of oxygen, by switching their metabolism from aerobic to anaerobic. Finally this strategy leads to tissue damages and loss of cells too, as it can be seen in acute or chronic occlusive diseases, as well. The measures of the tissue injuries depend on the duration of hypoxia, the mass of tissues are involved, the ATP requirement of the cell types and the blood pressure of the patients. Under hypoxic condition the generations of reactive oxygen species (ROS), such as $O^{2.-}$, H_2O_2, are increased. During normoxyc, physiological condition mitochondria generate low level of ROS by the respiratory chain. These are managed by natural antioxidants, such as manganese superoxid dismutase (SOD) in the mitochondria, or copper-zinc SOD in the inter-membrane space in the mitochondria, and in the cytosol, making the dismutation of superoxide anion

*Gabor Jancso[2], Endre Arato[2], Laszlo Sinay[2], Janos Lantos[1], Zsanett Miklos[1], Borbala Balatonyi[1], Szaniszlo Javor[1], Sandor Ferencz[1], Eszter Rantzinger[1], Dora Kovacs, Viktoria Kovacs, Zsofia Verzar[2], Gyorgy Weber[1], Balazs Borsiczky[1] and Erzsebet Roth[1]

[1]*Department of Surgical Research and Techniques, Pecs University Medical School, Pecs*

[2]*Department of General and Vascular Surgery of Baranya County Hospital, Pécs, Hungary*

generation to H_2O_2, which transformed further by catalase, glutathion plus glutathion peroxydase. Under hypoxic condition several sources of free radicals activated, e.g. the NADPH oxydase, xanthin oxidase, and others. ROS generated by hypoxia disrupts respiratory chain, causing a vicious cycle, manifested in modification in permeability transmission, loss of membrane potential, altering the function of mitochondrial complex I, III, and generating ubisemiquinon radical, which donates its electron to oxygen resulting in superoxyde anion. In reduced oxygen tension complex II switches its activity from succinate dehydrogenase to fumarate reductase (Henrich M et al, 2004.), Kolamunne RT et al 2011). Chronic sever hypoxia induces ATP depletion, and cell death. In the course of hypoxia, ATP generation decrees, exhausting the ATP sources, which responsible for the overflow of hypoxanthine, an ATP metabolite. Hypoxanthine in normoxyc condition metabolized further by xanthine dehydrogenase to xanthine (by means of nicotinamide adenine dinucleotide (NAD) as cofactor), but during hypoxia xanthin dehydrogenase converted to xanthin oxidase, which is unable to catalyse this conversion, but in the presence of high oxygen level in reoxygenation phase it continuously generates toxic ROS, because it uses oxygen as cofactor. ROS are effective oxidizing and reducing agents that directly damage cellular membranes, leading to impairment of membrane ion channels, disturbing cellular ionic balance resulting in cell swelling. ROS can activate leucocytes as well, and induce chemotaxis, cytokine release, leukocyte infiltration into the injured tissues, and due to endothelium dysfunction, a systemic reperfusion inflammatory response occurs. The most serious consequences of IR are the development of remote organ injuries in non-ischemic organs and can induce systemic inflammatory response injury (SIRS) or multiorgan failure syndrome (MOFS) which are responsible for of 20-40% of death in intensive care units (Levy JH, and Tanaka KA 2003). Tough reconstruction of the flow in the occluded vessels is not without risk, because of the generated volume, pressure and metabolic load, accompanied by further tissue damages resulting in the so-called reperfusion injury.

The main components of the molecular pathophysiological cascades are the activated circulating cells, first of all the white blood cells (WBC), mainly the neutrophils, due to their intensive free radical production, but, thrombocytes (PLT), red blood cells (RBC), and the cells of the vessel wall (endothelial cells and smooth muscle cells) also participate in the free radical production and the tissue damage (Roth and Hejjel 2003). In the early reperfusion the release of inflammatory cytokines, such as tumor necrosis factor alpha (TNF) increase too. These events together with the elevated Ca^{2+} levels inside the attached cells threat the integrity of the whole organism, destroying the crucial macromolecules, proteins, lipids and nucleic acids (Arato et al. 2005), (Blaisdell FW 1989).

Reactive oxygen species are Janus-faced agents. They have important role in eliminating pathogen microorganisms from the body, and can regulate cell growth and differentiation. ROS can act as important signalling molecules, in the circulation and participate in the maintenance of intra- and extracellular milieu. They can induce redox sensitive transcription factors, regulate redox sensitive signalization cascades and can act as secondary messengers (Kathy K et al 2000), (Dröge W, 2002). Oxygen free radicals can act as second messengers and they are able to influence the function of enzymes, and transcription factors, leading to the induction of genes are sensitive to them (Li W et al 2008). Their intra- and extracellular levels are regulated by SOD and catalase (the enzymes are present in almost all living organisms are exposed to oxygen) and other antioxidant, respectively. On the other hand they can cause endothelial dysfunction due to eliminating vital nitrogenous monoxides

(NO), which are absolutely necessary for the endothelium dependent relaxation of the vessels (Moncada et al 1991), for the proper function of cardiomyocytes (Umar S, van der Laarse A. 2010), and for the physiological function of circulating cells, such as thrombocytes (Massberg S 1998) and leukocytes, and red blood cells. It can be stated that free radicals are both our friends and enemy at the same time (Downey JM, and Cohen MV 2008).

It is very difficult to monitor the cellular processes which influence the outcome of the surgical interventions, or serves as a marker of the postoperative events. A huge amount of data emerged for the characterization of ischemia reperfusion injury, but function of platelets and other circulating cells or their interaction with each other or with endothelial cells has been hardly investigated (Buchholz AM, Bruch L 2003.). Limitation of reperfusion injury is inevitably important to prevent tissue damages, manifested in apoptosis, necrosis or both, and frequently occurred after restoration of circulation after stroke, myocardial infarction, organ transplantations, and in all types of revascularization surgeries. There are pharmacologic tools, and protective processes, which can reduce IR injury. Antioxidants, such as N-acetylcysteine, vitamin E, mannitol, thiols, alkaloids and endogenous antioxidants, such as superoxide dismutase, reduced glutathion, glutathione reductase, catalase, or ion chelators functions due to inactivation of free radicals, which are key element in IR induced tissue damages (Arato et al 2010), (Peto K, et al 2007), but leukocyte depletion, anti-cytokine or leukocyte adhesion molecule monoclonal antibody therapies ended with conflicting results (Arato et al 2010) (Loberg AG et al ,2011). Among other effective possibilities, ischemic postconditioning is one of the most effective processes in reducing IR caused damages, which was first introduced by Vinten-Johansen's group in 2003. The main essence of application of short (some seconds) repetitive interruption of early reperfusion by brief ischemic episodes resulting in reduced infarct size in the heart, diminished tissue edema, reduced infiltration of leukocytes into the area of injury, as they were improved in animal studies (Vinten-Johansen J 2007).

Angioplasty with or without vascular stenting is an effective method, was developed by Dotter and Judkins (Misty M et al 2001) to reconstruct the proper flow within the narrowed or occluded vessels. The procedure is carried out mainly in the coronary arteries, but it is frequently applied in other parts of the circulation. The procedure itself is a typical example of I/R injury was characterized above, with main risks of endothelium dysfunction and reocclusion due to thrombus formation and/or smooth muscle proliferation. The potential role of the circulating cells, such as PLT, WBC, and RBC in the vessel closure is intensively studied, and their interactions with the components of vessel wall, mainly with the smooth muscle cells and the endothelial linage have special attention (Ming Wei Liu et al 1989). Platelet leukocyte interaction is also investigated, because of their unique role in reocclusion (Szabo S. et al 2005).

In the present study we aimed to investigate the function of circulating cells in the course of acute (emergency) and elective revascularization surgery in lower limb of patients with Peripheral arterial disease (PAD). In our studies thrombocyte function, antioxidant and prooxidant status were investigated in two groups of patients, who were scheduled to elective revascularization surgery (Elective) and were compared to the patients with acute vessel closure and were undergone revascularization surgery in emergency, 4-6 hours after of vessel closure (Acute). Data obtained in the two patients groups were compared to the same parameters of healthy veterinary blood donors (Control). Patients of the two groups (Acute and Elective) have other chronic diseases too, such as diabetes mellitus. Diabetes is a disease when patients have high blood sugar concentration due to the inadequate production: DM1, or inadequate effects on the tissues of otherwise physiological or high level of circulating insulin: DM2. In the second series of experiments, thrombocyte function and prooxidant/antioxidant status of DM1 and DM2 patients with PAD were also investigated. In vitro effects of exogenous insulin (Actrapid Insulin (Novo-Nordisk) In 0, 40, 80, 160 μU/ml) were also investigated on collagen induced platelet aggregation and phorbol - 12 myristate-13 acetate (PMA) induced reactive oxygen species (ROS) production in whole blood.

2. Materials and methods

Patients selection and investigation in this randomized, open, prospective studies was carried out according to the Helsinki declaration (1996), considering the statute of Hungarian Ministry of Health (32/2005. (VIII:26), with the permission of the local ethical board of the Pecs University, Medical School. (Permission No.: 2498).

2.1 The first series of experiments

The aim of this study was to investigate the effect of the duration of hypoxia on the thrombocyte function, free radical production and antioxidant/prooxidant statuses of the patients who were undergone revascularization surgery of lower limb.

Patients: Two groups of patients were investigated:

1. Acute group: n=12; 9 males and 3 female, age: 58.1±7.3 years, suffered from ischemia 4-6 hours before revascularization surgery of lower limb because of seriously ischemic extremities due to embolism, acute arterial thrombosis or rupture of infrarenal artery before the surgery. They were undergone revascularization surgery in emergency.
2. Elective group n=10, (6 male 4 female) were scheduled to elective revascularization surgery because of chronic obliterative arterial stenosis. Ischemia was diagnosed by angiography, and Doppler test.

Other chronic diseases accompanied by PAD in our patients are summarized in Table 1.

Surgical interventions were carried out in General and Vascular Surgery Department of Baranya County Hospital (Pecs; Hungary), and were performed in spinal anaesthesia, with 43.8±17 min ischemic time. Patients of both groups received similar anticoagulant and antiplatelet therapy (at least 75 mg Aspirin) and low molecular weight heparin was also prescribed in the perioperative period. Medication of the patients is summarized in Table 2.

Disease	Acute group	Elective group
Hypertension	6/12	8/10
Ischemic heart disease	3/12	4/10
Diabetes mellitus	4/12	5/10
Lung complications	4/12	4/10
Smooking	5/12	4/10

Table 1. Chronic diseases accompanied with PAD in the first series of the study

Blood sampling: Venous blood samples were obtained by venipuncture. Samples of 10 healthy blood donors (Blood Donation Center of Pecs, Hungary) served as Control. Venous blood samples of the two patients groups were obtained before and 2 and 24 hours and one week after the surgery. Blood samples were collected into three Vacutainer tubes containing trisodium citrate (3.8%) or K3-EDTA (7.5 %) (Becton Dickinson, UK). Informed consents were obtained from all patients and volunteers participated in the study.

Groups of medicine	Acute	Elective
PLT aggregation inhibitors (Aspirin protect or Astrix)	12/12	10/10
Anticoagulant (perioperative)	12/12	10/12
Antihypertensive	6/12	8/10
Antidiabetic	4/12	5/10
Others	12/12	10/10

Table 2. Medication of patients with PAD in the 1st series of the study

Laboratory measurements: were carried out in Department of Surgical Research and Techniques of Pecs University Medical School, Hungary. **Hematologic measurement:** red and white blood cell numbers, haemoglobin concentration, platelet numbers were measured by Minitron automatic analysator (Diatron LTD Budapest, Hungary). **Platelet aggregation measurements:**

1. in platelet rich plasma (PRP), according to Born's turbidimetric method (Born 1965a), Born et al 1965b), by means of Carat aggregometer (Carat Diagnostic ltd, Budapest, Hungary), using ADP (5 μM; and 10 μM) and collagen (2 μg/ml) as inductors. Aggregation was followed for 8 minutes after its induction and expressed in %.
2. **in whole blood** was measured by the method of Ingerman-Wojenski and Silver by Chrono-log lumino-aggregometer (type 560VS, USA), according to the user's manual of the instrument (Ingerman-Wojenski CM and Silver MJ), using the same inductors as was used in PRP. In whole blood platelet aggregation was measured by impedance, and expressed in Ohm, and was followed for six minutes from its induction.

Measurement of main antioxidants: *SOD* is an ancient antioxidant enzyme of pro- and eukaryotic organisms, containing metal (Cu, Zn, Fe, Mn Ni, respectively) in its active centre, and it has several isoforms, which can be found intra- and extracellularly, in almost all living creature, as well. Measurement of SOD activity was carried out by the method of Misra and Fridovich (Misra and Fridovich 1972). Reduced glutathione *(GSH)* levels were determined in plasma were obtained after centrifugation of anticoagulated whole blood, using Ellman's reagent (Sedlak and Lindsday 1968). GSH cystein is able to neutralize free radicals by donating one electron and stabilizes them. In the course of this reaction it became reactive, as well, but an other GSH can neutralize it, forming GSSG, which will be regenerated to GSH by glutathione reductase. Plasma proteins (such as albumin) contain sulphydril groups, as well and exert remarkable antioxidant capacity though its -SH groups, was measured also.

Measurement of prooxidants: Reactive oxygen species *(ROS)* was measured in the mixture of whole blood (20 μl) and phosphate buffered saline (1400 μl) by chemiluminometric, kinetic method, by means of Chrono-Log lumino-aggregometer. The main sources of ROS in the blood are leukocytes. ROS production was induced in whole blood by phorbol -12-miristate-13-acetate (PMA) and was made detectable by luminol (Arato et al 2010b).) Malondialdehyde *(MDA),* the main lipid peroxidation marker, which signs the polyunsaturated fatty acid peroxidation of the biological membranes. It was measured in anticoagulated whole blood and in plasma (Ohkawa H (1979). Myeloperoxidase *(MPO)* produces hypochlorous acid (HOCl) from hydrogen peroxide (H_2O_2) and chloride anion (Cl^-) (or the equivalent from a non-chlorine halide) during the neutrophil's respiratory burst.

It requires hem as a cofactor. Furthermore, it oxidizes tyrosine to tyrosyl radical using hydrogen peroxide as an oxidizing agent. MPO level was measured in plasma, according to the method of (Xia and Zweier 1997).

2.2 The second series of experiments

The aim of this study

Insulin resistance and diabetes mellitus are causal or worsening factors in the peripheral arterial diseases (Jude EB 2001). In the second part of the study we intended to investigate thrombocyte function parallel with antioxidant prooxidant status of ambulant diabetic (DM1 and DM2) patients with PAD were under the care of General and Vascular Surgery Department of Baranya County Hospital (Pecs; Hungary). Eleven healthy volunteers of Blood Donation Centre of Pecs served as controls

Methods

This study involved 24 patients with DM1 (18 male and 6 female; age: 62 ± 2.3 year), and 22 with DM2 (18 male and 4 female; age: 65,7 ±3.7) with PAD. Healthy blood donors served as control (8 male and 2 female; age: 33 ± 6.7 years). Anticoagulated whole blood of ambulant patients and volunteers were used. Informed consents were obtained from all participants. Regular medication of the two patients group is summarized in **Table 3.**

Medication	**DM1**	**DM2**
Platelet aggregation inhibitors (Aspirinprotect or Astrix)	24/24	22/22
Anticoagulant (Syncumar)	4/24	4/22
Anticoagulant (LMWH)	12/24	10/22
Antihypertensive	18/24	18/22
Insulin	24/24	2/22
Oral antidiabetic	0/24	20/22
Other	24/24	22/22

Table 3. Medication of the DM1 and DM2 patients.

Parameters to be measured

Clinical chemistry data: Glucose triglyceride, cholesterol was measured by commercial kits (Diagnosticum Ltd Budapest) by photometric method. Platelet aggregation was measured in whole blood and in PRP. PMA induced ROS production; endogenous antioxidant and prooxidant status of these patients were measured as it was described above. *Platelet aggregation*: Platelet aggregation was measured in PRP and in whole blood as it was described above. In the latter case area under the aggregation curves were calculated as well, using Origin 6.0 data analyzing and graphing software. Collagen induced platelet aggregation, and PMA induced ROS production were measured in the presence of 0, 40, 80, 160 μU/ml insulin (Actrapid), too. **Statistical analyses:** Student's paired and unpaired t-test and one way analysis of variance were used. Differences were considered significant, when p was less than 0.05. The results were expressed as mean ± SD or in percentage.

3. Results

3.1 Results of the first series of experiment

3.1.1 Results of clinical chemistry measurements

Red blood cell numbers were similar in the three groups, but haemoglobin concentration was significantly lower and leukocyte number was higher in Acute group, compared to the **Elective** and **Control** ones, in the course of the study

3.1.2 Platelet aggregation in platelet-rich plasma

ADP and Collagen were selected as aggregation inductors. These agents were used to control the efficacy of the two most frequently used groups of antiplatelet drugs, the cyclooxygenase (COX) inhibitors and adenosine diphosphate (ADP) receptor antagonists.

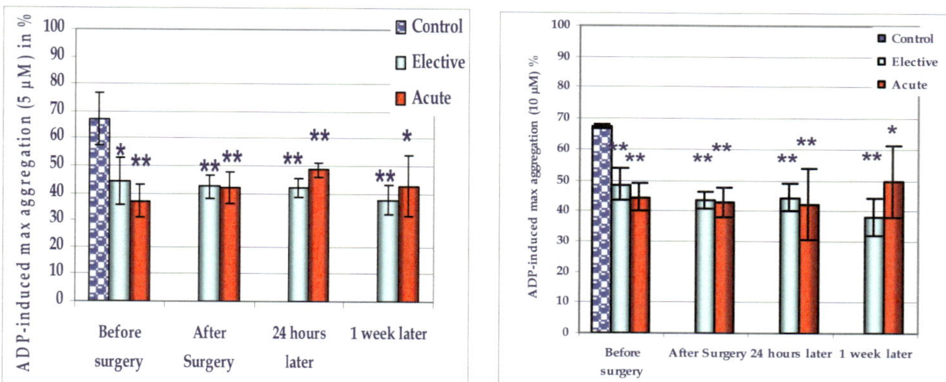

Fig. 1. ADP (5 and 10 µM) induced aggregation in platelet rich plasma. Antiplatelet therapy seemed to be effective in both patients groups using 5 and 10 µM ADP, as inductor in PRP.*= p<0.05 vs. Control, **= p<0.01 vs. control.

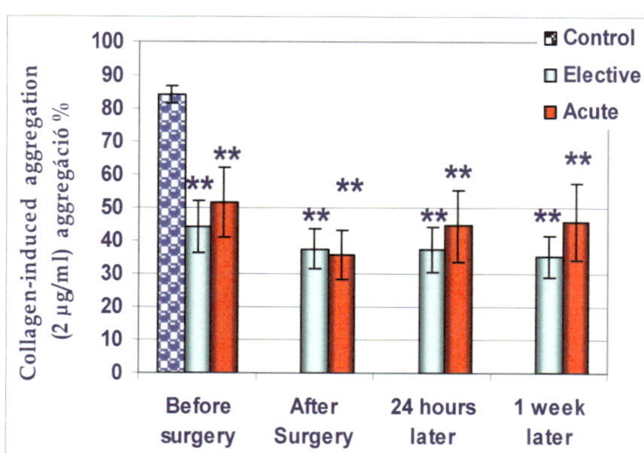

Fig. 2. Maximum values of collagen (2 µg / ml) induced platelet aggregation in PRP, compared to Control. *= p<0,05, **=p<0.01 compared to controls.

In figure 1 and 2 the ADP- and in figure 3 the collagen induced aggregation maximums were summarized, and compared to the values of healthy subjects. According to our data antiplatelet therapy received by both patients groups were effective on the level of isolated thrombocytes in the whole observation time. Platelet aggregation in Control group was within the normal range either ADP or collagen was used as inductors (61-91% of ADP, and 64-92 of collagen), contrarily in both groups of patients a significantly reduced response to ADP and Collagen were measured, signing an effective anti-platelet therapy.

3.1.3 Investigation of platelet aggregation in whole blood

3.1.3.1 ADP induced platelet aggregation in acute and elective groups

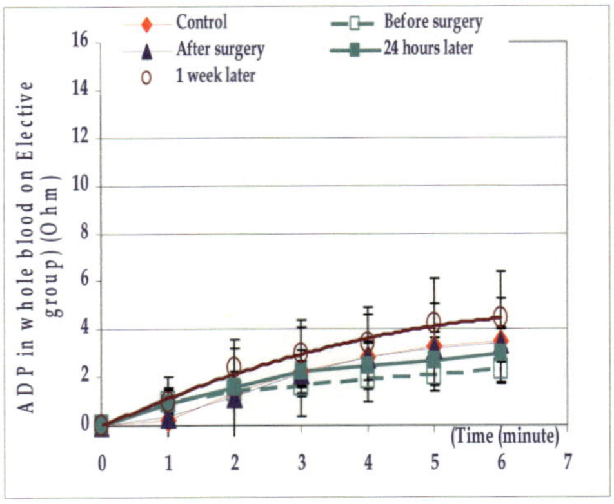

Fig. 3. ADP induced platelet aggregation in Elective group, compared to Control (red line)

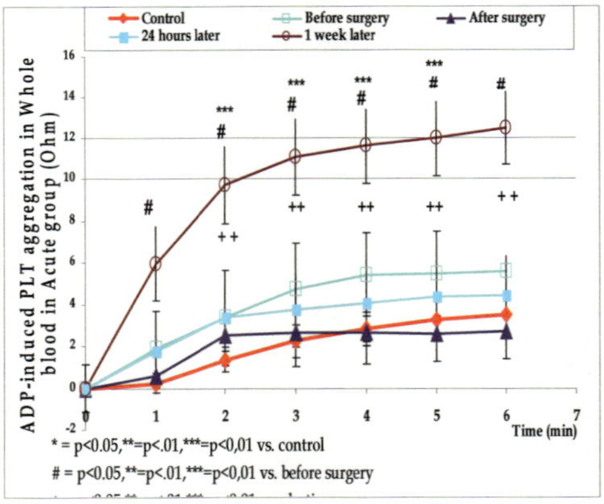

Fig. 4. ADP induced aggregation in Acute group, compared to Control (red line).

ADP induced platelet aggregation in whole blood was similar in Acute and Elective and Control groups before the surgery. In the Elective group ADP induced platelet aggregation did not changed significantly in the course of the study. In the Acute group a significant gradual increase was observed in the function of time, with a four times increase at the end of the week (Figure 4).

3.1.3.2 Collagen induced aggregation in whole blood

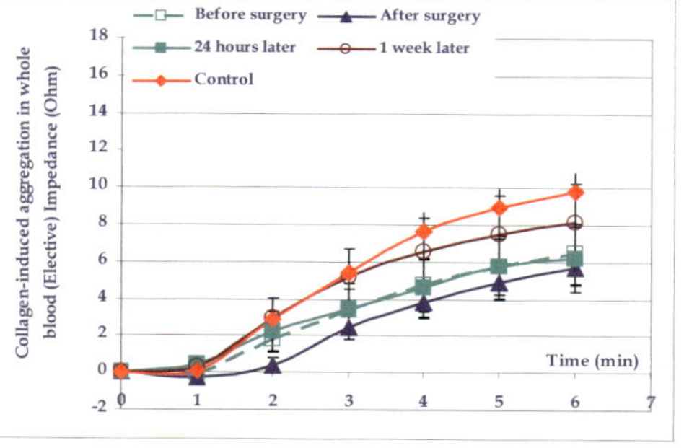

Fig. 5. Collagen induced platelet aggregation in Elective group.

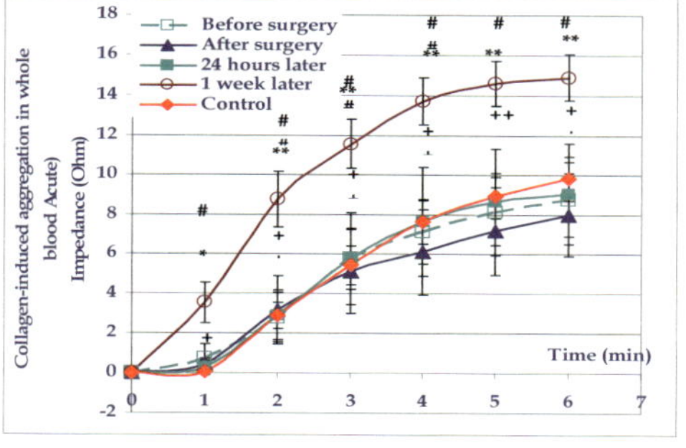

Fig. 6. Collagen induced aggregation in whole blood in Acute group.

In whole blood of healthy subjects, the collagen induced platelet aggregation started with one minute delay. In the patient groups, collagen induced aggregation started without delay, mainly in Acute group, one week after the surgery. Application of the inductor in this case resulted in an immediate induction of platelet aggregation. The effect of antiplatelet therapy was detected in platelet- rich plasma was missed in whole blood.

3.1.4 Investigation of antioxidants

3.1.4.1 GSH level

Before surgery GSH levels were similar in the three groups. In patients groups a transient reduction occurred 2 hours after and one day after the surgery, but returned to the baseline level one week after the surgery.

3.1.4.2 Plasma thiol groups

Before the surgery the plasma SH-group concentration of the patient groups did not differed from each other or the healthy controls, but a transient, significant reduction was measured 2 hours and 24 hours after surgery in both patients groups, which returned to the normal level 1 week later.

3.1.4.3 SOD activity

Before surgery SOD activity was lower in both patients groups, compared to Control, however SOD activity in Elective group was higher than in Acute group, and remained unchanged during the study. In Acute group SOD level decreased further 24 hours after the surgery. SOD levels of patients groups remained below the normal range in the course of the whole study (Figure 7.)

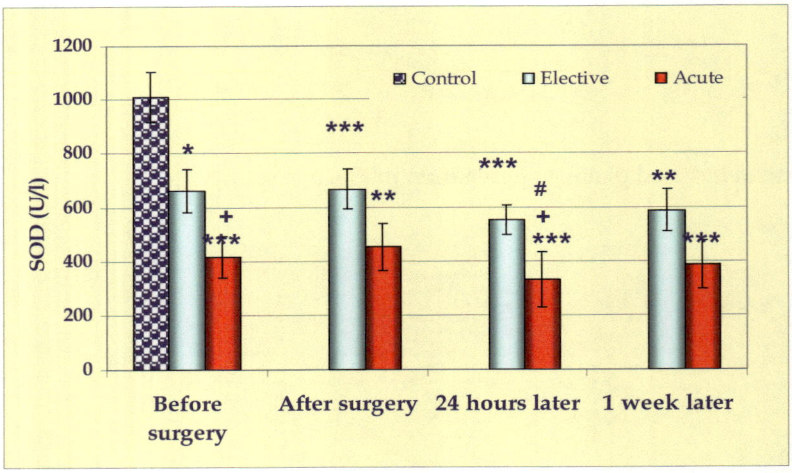

Fig. 7. **Changes in SOD activity.** *= p<0.05, **=p<0.01, **=p<0.005, +=p<0.05 vs. elective, #=p<0,05 vs. before surgery

Before surgery SOD activity in both patients groups were lower compared to healthy volunteers. This low level decreased further significantly n Acute group until the 24th hour of reperfusion and remained in this low level during the study. In elective group SOD level was on a constant low-level during the study. I/R injury was described almost 50 years ago, but the correct mediation, the way of prevention or treatment is under investigation in nowadays, as well. The inflammatory responses can be detected following reperfusion varies greatly and depends on the time and severity of ischemia, as it was measured in our cases too. Restoration of blood flow of ischemic tissues initiates a chain reaction of complications which can categorize into two main groups: regional and systemic. In our case restoration of blood flow in lower limb, generated a systemic response, which had been detected in blood samples (in serum, haemolysate, plasma) obtained in a great distance from the intervention.

3.1.5 Investigation of prooxidants

3.1.5.1 PMA induced free radical production

Before surgery PMA induced ROS production was higher in Acute than in Elective and Control groups. This value elevated further in the course of the study. Free radical generation was characterized with four parameters: 1. the lag-time: the time elapsed between the induction and the beginning of the free radical production, 2. maximum of free radical production corrected to the WBC numbers, 3. the Slope: the rate of rise of the ascending part of the free radical generation curves and the WBC numbers (Figure 8.).

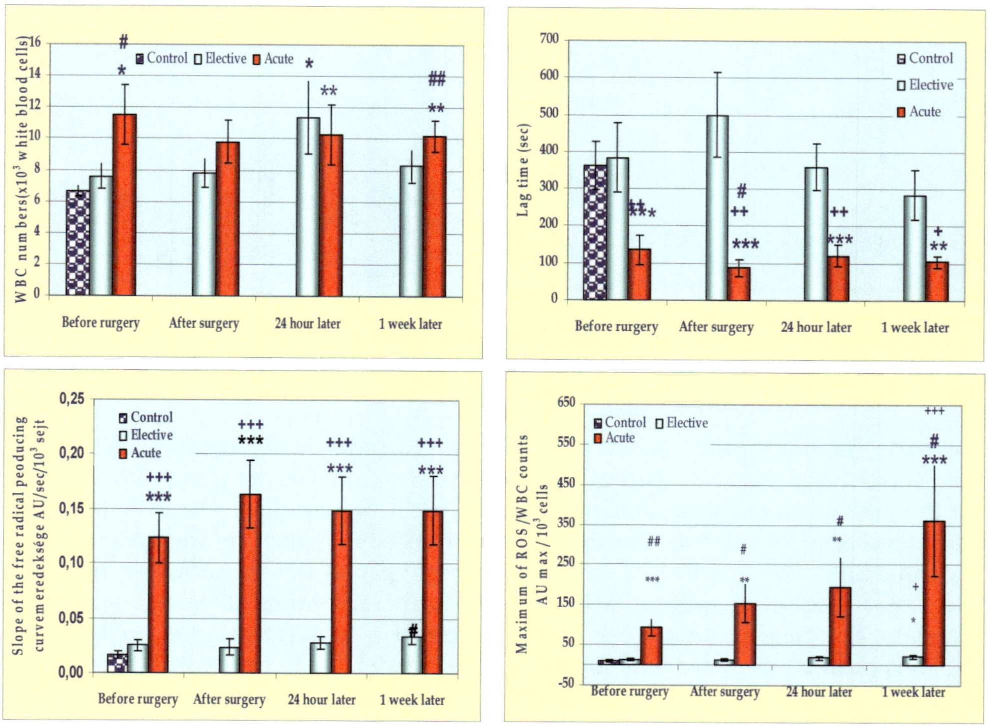

Fig. 8. Upper left panel: white blood cell numbers, upper right panel: lag time, bottom left panel: slope of free radical curve, bottom right panel: maximal free radical production. ***=<0.001 vs. control, +++=p<0.001 vs. elective, #= p< 0.01 vs. before surgery).

In Acute group WBC numbers were significantly higher (upper left panel) and Lag time was significantly shorter (upper right panel) before and one week after the surgery, than the similar values in Elective and Control Groups (*=p<0.05 vs. Control, # = p<0.05 vs. Elective groups). Slope of the free radical producing curves became steeper in acute and elective groups, signing that more and more active WBC are present before and one week after the surgery, but in Acute group this free radical generation was significantly higher, than in the other two groups. The maximum of free radical production continuously elevated both in acute and in elective groups, but these elevation in acute group was several times higher than it was measured in elective group (figure 8.).

3.1.5.2 Investigation of lipid peroxidation due to measurement of MDA in plasma and in red blood cell haemolysate

It is a well known fact, that one of the main consequence of long-lasting atherosclerosis is the significant decrease in the polyunsaturated fatty acid (PUFA) content of the membranes, due to saturation of the membrane lipids which responsible for the rigidity of the membranes. MDA is one of the lipid peroxydation end products, generated in the course of free radical induced peroxydation of PUFA. MDA is frequently used as a lipid peroxydation marker in biological tissues.

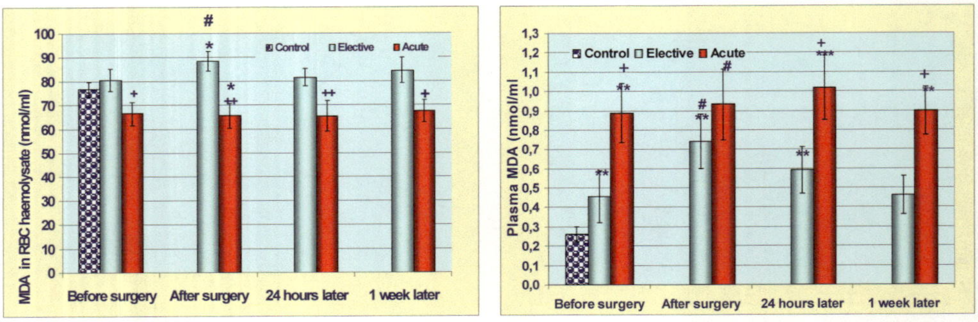

Fig. 9. MDA level in red blood cell (RBC) hemolysate (left panel) and in plasma (right panel), *= $p<0.05$ vs. Control, **= $p<0.01$ vs. Control, ***= $p<0.0051$ vs. Control +=$p<0.05$ vs. Elective, #=$p<0.05$ vs. before surgery

Surprisingly, in our case MDA concentration of erythrocyte membrane remained in a standard, relatively low level during the whole study, in the Acute group. We speculated about the background of this phenomenon, and finally we concluded that the long-lasting hypoxia preceeded the surgery may exhausted of the PUFA contents of the lipidmembranes. At the same time, plasma MDA of Acute group (right panel) were significantly higher than in Elective and Control groups, and elevated further 24 hours after the surgery, and returned to the baseline one week after the surgery. In Elective group a bell-shaped elevation appeared which peaked 2 hours after surgery (Figure 9. right panel).

3.1.5.3 Changes in MPO

In spite of MPO have not been evaluated in routine clinical chemistry studies, according to a recent study of Brevetti and coworkers its elevated level, but not C-reactive protein, predicts cardiovascular risk in peripheral arterial disease (Brevetti G , 2008). According to an other study it is a marker of myocardial infarction too. The base-line myeloperoxidase level independently predicts the risk of major adverse coronary events within 30 days.

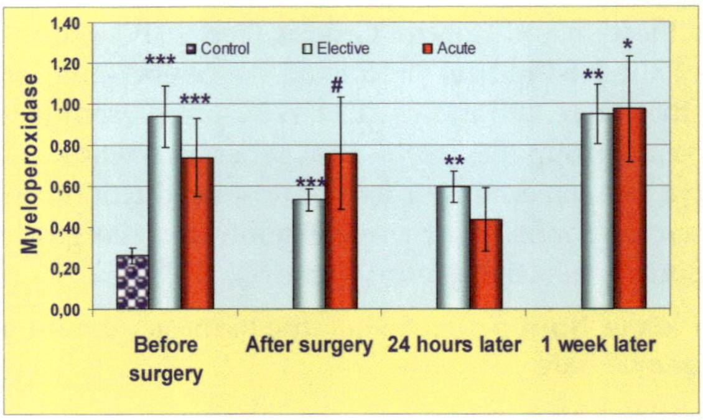

Fig. 10. **Myeloperoxidase level in Control, Elective and Acute groups.** MPO level both in Elective and Acute groups were significantly higher than in Control before surgery, than after a transient decrease in the postoperative period returned to the preoperative level.

(Brennan ML et al 2003). MPO is a hydrogen peroxide oxidoreductase, specifically found on mammalian polymorphonuclear leukocytes (PMN), responsible for the bactericidal capability of these cells. PMN activation and mediator release are partially responsible for the morbidity and mortality of revascularization of ischemic lower limb, regardless of the mode of intervention, surgery or application of thrombolytics.

3.1.5.4 Conclusion of the first series of the experiments

Ischemia/reperfusion injury, accompanied by revascularization surgeries of lower limb, was in the focus of the present study. This problem has great importance in the clinical practice because of its poor outcome (postoperative mortality is 15-60%). Tissue injury appears not only under ischemia, but after restoration of the blood flow in the formerly ischemic areas, due to the reperfusion injury, as well (Yasin) NM et al. 2002), (Arato et al 2009). Ischemia reperfusion injury of lower limb is accompanied by muscle changes with progressive micro-vascular damage, and affects all circulating cells (RBC, WBC, and PLT), as well. These cells are in connection with each other and with cells of the vessel walls, too. Inflammatory response following reperfusion varies greatly, and depends on the time and severity of ischemia. According to our results in accordance with several other studies, the duration and severity of ischemia is proportional to the damage occurred after it. Studying thrombocyte function and antioxidant prooxidant status of our unique patient groups, several new aspects of ischemia reperfusion injury were revealed. Peripheral arterial disease is a common progressive disorder that attaches the circulation of the legs, particularly in people over 55 years, strengthening in these patients the greatly increased risk of heart attack or stroke, and of dying within a decade. Several aspects of the problem were intensively studied, but platelet function during the restoration of the circulation of ischemic lower limb was hardly investigated before. It was revealed in this study that an effective antiaggregating therapy was applied in these patients, and effectively reduced the aggregation induced by ADP and collagen in PRP, but this reduction in whole blood was completely disappeared, both in ADP and collagen induced aggregation in Acute and Elective groups too. Above this a highly significant increase in platelet aggregation was measured in whole blood, in response to both types of inductors, one week after the surgery in Acute group. We concluded on the basis of our result that the long-lasting hypoxia is responsible for the increased PLT aggregation in whole blood, as the consequence of the shift of the antioxidant-prooxidant balance to the prooxidant direction lead to the increased response to aggregation inductors.

3.2 Results of the second series of experiments

3.2.1 Clinical chemistry data

Monitoring thrombocyte function and antioxidant prooxidant status of diabetic patients with peripheral arterial disease is inevitably important, because of the increased risk of complication. Patients suffering from both diabetes and PAD are at risk of developing critical limb ischemia, ulceration and potentially requiring limb amputation. In addition, diabetes complicates surgical treatment of PAD and impairs vascular functions. The presence of diabetes increases the frequency of intermittent claudication. The relative risk of amputation in diabetic population is 12,4-fold higher compared to the non diabetic patients (95%, 10,9-14,9), and this value doubles above 65 years. Diabetes increases the sensing of shear stress and the response to vasoconstrictor stimuli, reducing the recruitment and dilatation of collateral arteries (Brennan ML et al 2010).

Group of patients	Glucose	Triglyceride	Cholesterol
DM1	11.4 ±1.6	1.9 ± 0.3	4.3±0.6
DM2	7.3 ±0.7	4.3 ±1.4	5.2 ±0.7
Healty	4.82 ±0.27	1.1±0.15	4.2 ±0.5
Normal values	4.2-6.1 mmol/l	0.4-1.7 mmol/l	3.7-5.2 mmol/l

Table 4. Clinical Chemistry of Control subjects and DM1 and DM2 patients.

Glucose and triglyceride levels of diabetic patients were higher than the normal values. The mean value of cholesterol level was within the normal range, but individually high values were measured, as well.

3.2.2 Investigation of platelet aggregation

3.2.2.1 Investigation of PLT function in platelet rich plasma

Investigation of platelet function by turbidimetric method in PRP is a more frequently used method, than impedance measurement in whole blood. Our own investigations focused our attention on the usefulness of the parallel measurements. There are several advantages using both methods parallel, e.g. in PRP platelet function can be measured independently from other circulating cells. It is very advantageous if we investigate the effect of antiplatelet drug in a specific direction. Contrary, in whole blood the effects of the other components of circulating cells of blood (leukocytes, red blood cells) can be studied together.

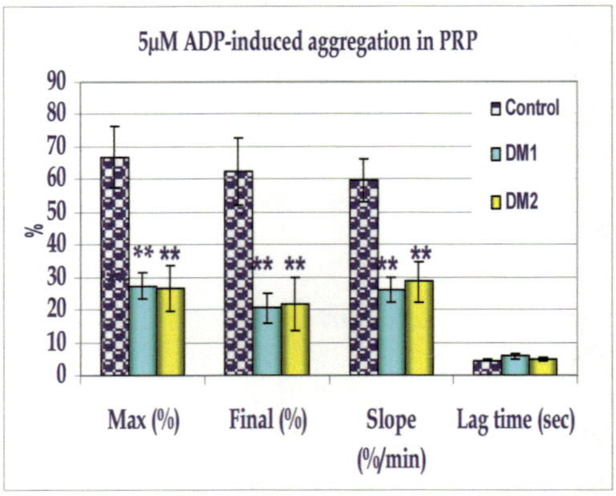

Fig. 11. ADP induced platelet aggregation in PRP of diabetic patients with PAD.

All parameter were measured in DM1 and DM2 Patients were reduced, compared to Control. In DM2 patients Slope of the aggregation curve was significantly higher compared to Elective groups.

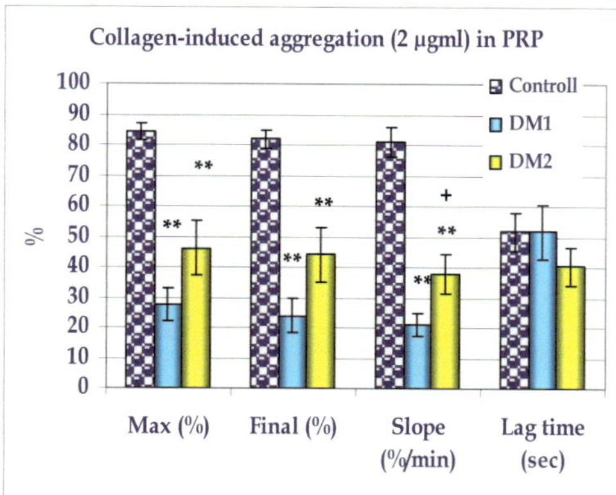

Fig. 12. Collagen induced platelet aggregation in PRP of diabetic patients with PAD.

3.2.2.2 Investigation of ADP induce platelet aggregation in whole blood in control and diabetic patients with PAD

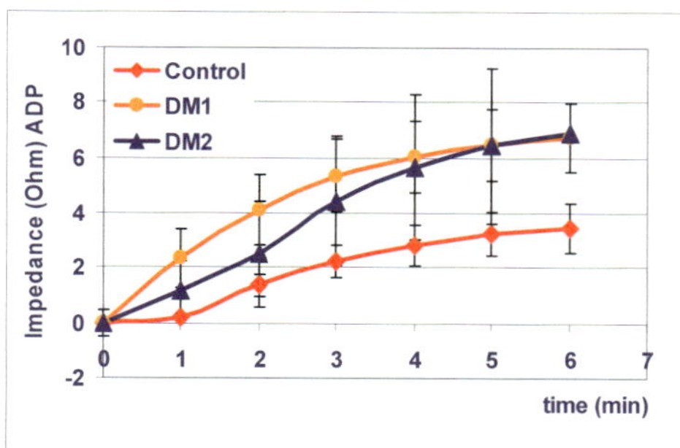

Fig. 13. ADP induced platelet aggregation of healthy and diabetic patients with PAD in the function of time. However patient's data were higher in every time points compared to Control, significant difference can't be detected.

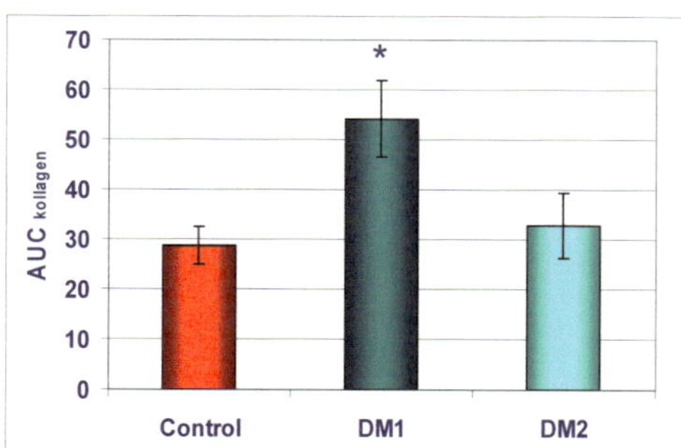

Fig. 14. Area under the ADP induced platelet aggregation curves (AUC). AUC of patients with PAD were significantly higher ($p<0.05$), than that of Control

3.2.2.3 Investigation of PLT function in whole blood in control and diabetic patients collagen induce platelet aggregation in whole blood

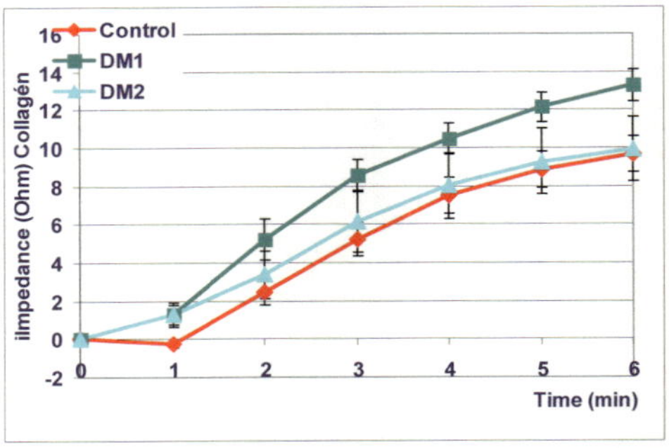

Fig. 15. Collagen induced platelet aggregation in whole blood of healthy and diabetic subjects with PAD in the function of time. Platelet aggregation of diabetic patients was higher in each point of times, but significant difference has not been observed among the groups.

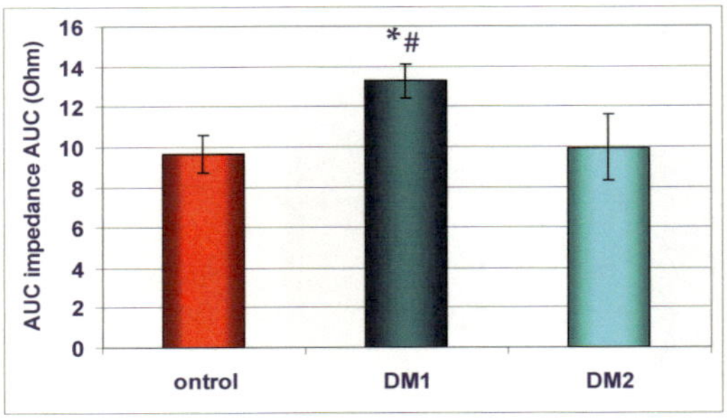

Fig. 16. AUC of the platelet aggregation curves of healthy and diabetic patients. Significant differences were measured among DM1 and DM2 groups, compared to each other (#)., and between DM1 and Control.

3.2.3 Antioxidant and prooxidant levels

Plasma GHS levels were similar in the three groups, however SOD activity was significantly lower in both patients groups, compared to Control (Figure 17). WBC numbers in the DM1 group was the double and ROS production/10^3 WBC was 20 times higher in DM1 group than in Control and was double of the DM2 (Fig.18)

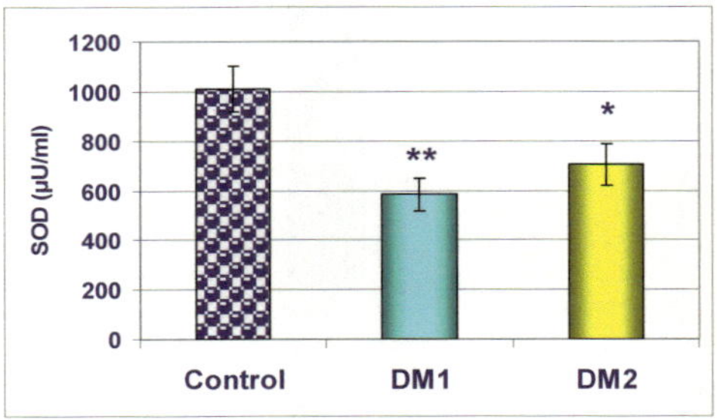

Fig. 17. SOD activity was significantly lower in patients groups than in Control.

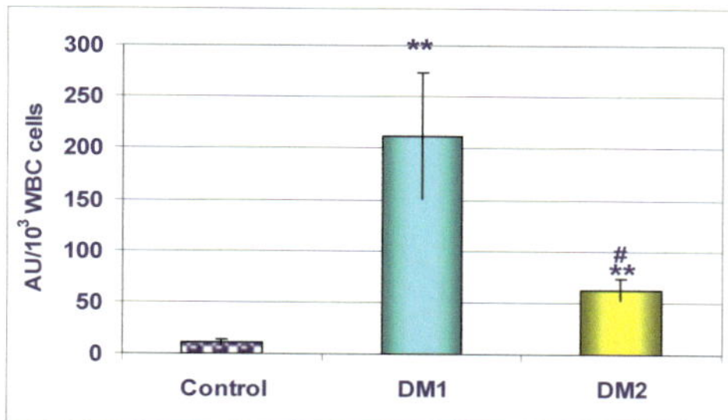

Fig. 18. PMA induced ROS production was higher in patients then in Control

3.2.4 In vitro effects on insulin on platelet aggregation in whole blood

3.2.4.1 In vitro effect of actrapid insulin on collagen induced platelet aggregation in whole blood of healthy volunteers, DM1 and DM2 patients with PAD was investigated

Actrapid insulin exerts its effect within a short time in patients too, that was the reason why we chose this. Platelet aggregation was expressed in Ohm, and area under the curves was calculated as well, and we expressed in %. AUC without insulin was considered as 100%.

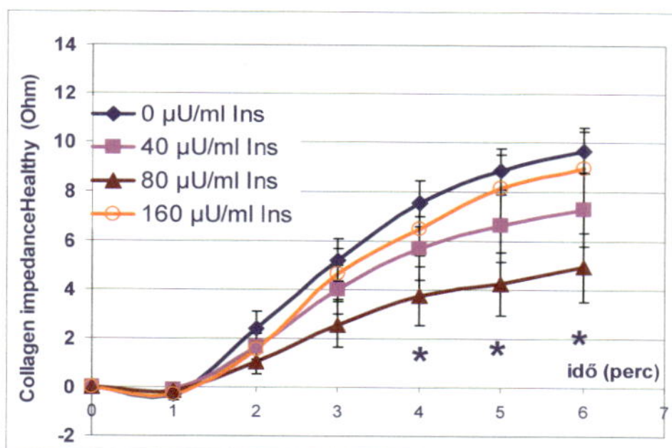

Fig. 19. Collagen induced aggregation in healthy volunteer's whole blood in the function of time, in the presence or absence of Actrapid insulin. A significant decrease occurred in the presence of 80 μU/ml of insulin

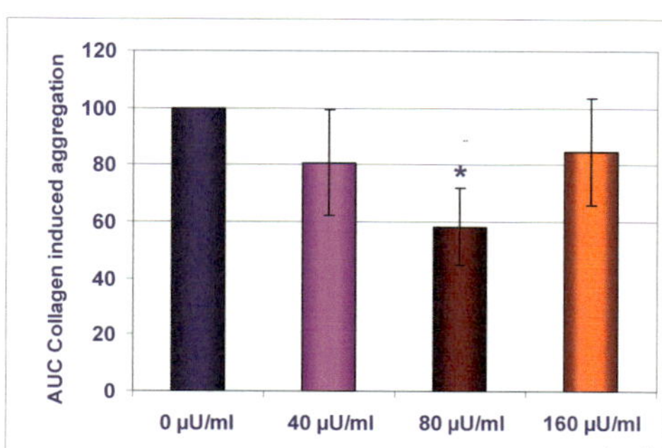

Fig. 20. AUC in healthy subjects. Significant decrease was detected in the presence of 80 μU/ml of insulin, considering 100% of AUC without insulin

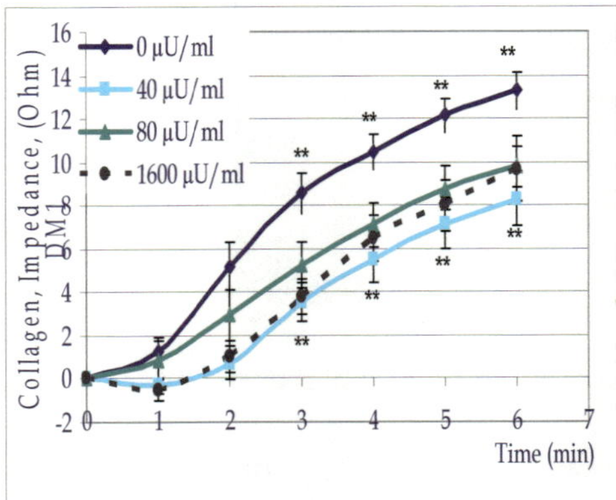

Fig. 21. Collagen induced platelet aggregation in the function of time on whole blood in DM1 patients. DM1 patient's blood was sensitive to each concentration of insulin, without any significant difference among the groups.

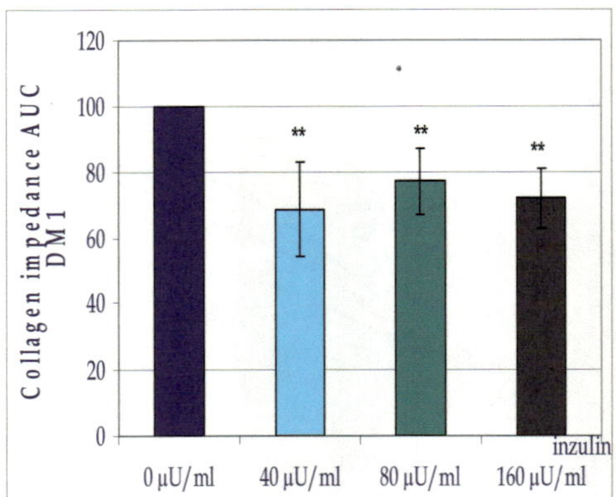

Fig. 22. AUC of collagen induced platelet aggregation curves in DM1. The three insulin concentration caused similar, but significant decrease in the aggregation.

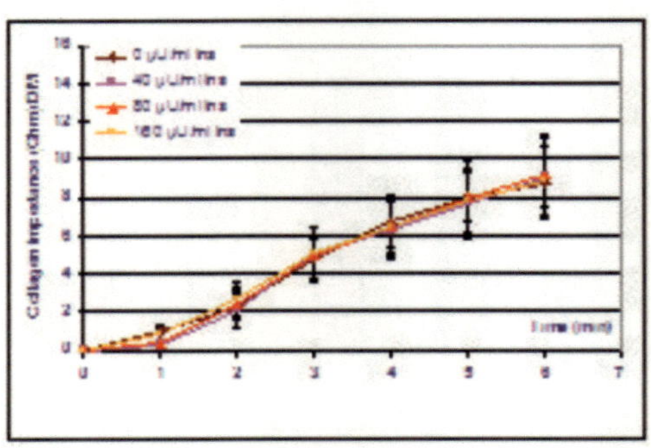

Fig. 23. Collagen induced platelet aggregation in DM2 patients. Insulin was ineffective on collagen induced platelet aggregation.

3.2.5 Effect of exogenous insulin on PMA induced ROS production in whole blood

Insulin effect on the maximum of PMA induced ROS production was investigated, as well. The presence of insulin in whole blood was able to reduce PMA induced ROS production in whole blood in healthy subjects and that of DM1 patients' blood too, but not in DM 2 patients (Figure 24.)

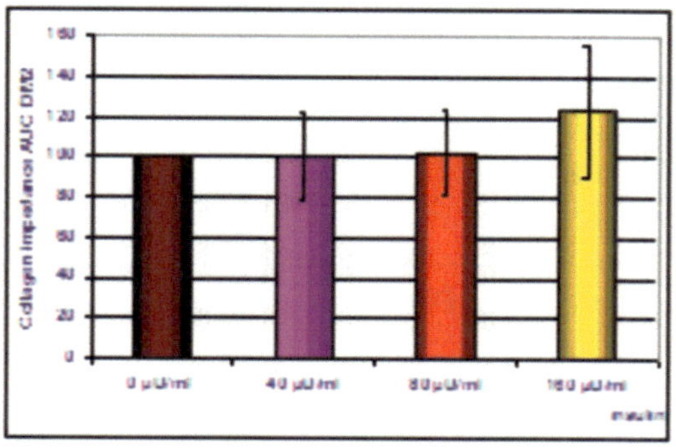

Fig. 24. Insulin was not able to reduce area under platelet aggregation curve in blood samples of patients with DM2.

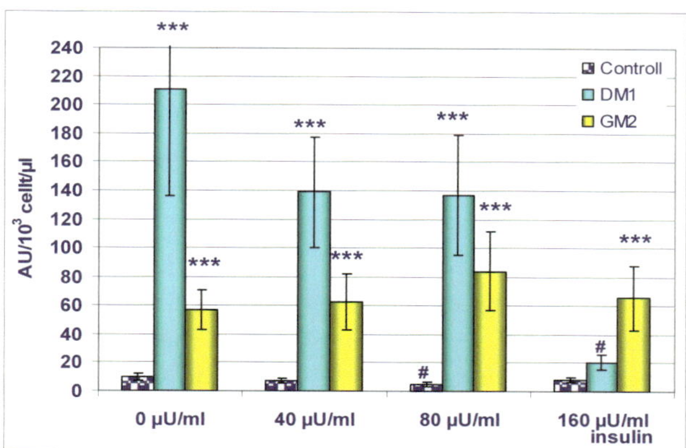

Fig. 25. Effect of insulin on PMA induced ROS production on whole blood of Control, DM1 and CM2 patients' whole blood, in vitro.

3.3 Summary of data obtained from investigation of diabetic patients blood

The presence of DM1 or DM2 diabetes differently influenced the thrombocyte function and antioxidant status of PAD patients, and the in vitro effects of insulin on collagen induced platelet aggregation and PMA induced ROS generation.

Investigating platelet aggregation in whole blood of patients neither in ADP, nor in collagen induced aggregation curves differed significantly from each other or the control. Calculating area under curves (AUC), significant differences were revealed, showing that platelets of DM1 patients was more sensitive to both inductors than that of in other two groups (Figure 13-16). This increased sensitivity was accompanied by lower SOD activity (Figure 17.) and highly significant increase in PMA induced ROS generation (Figure 18.).

In vitro effects of insulin on collagen induced platelet aggregation, and PMA induced ROS generation were also investigated in the presence of 0, 40, 80, 160 μU/ml insulin in the whole blood. A U-shaped inhibition in collagen induced aggregation was detected in healthy subjects, a constant decrease in DM1 patients, without dose dependence, but insulin was ineffective in DM2 patients blood (figure 19-25). The maximum values of PMA induced ROS generation was significantly higher than in other two groups, but insulin pre-treatment was able to reduce it. Insulin was able to reduce the low ROS levels were induced by PMA in the blood donor's blood, but not in DM2 patient's blood.

4. Conclusion

Reconstruction of blood flow in the formerly ischemic tissues induces chain reactions, which affect not only the tissues are involved, but threats the integrity of the whole organism, causing multiorgan failure and death. The irreversible muscle cell damage begins 3 hour after ischemia and completed about within 6 hours (Blaisdell W. 2002). Tissue damage induced by the revascularization surgery of lower limbs had been in the focus of our studies. Our main aims were to study and characterize the role of the duration of the hypoxia on the thrombocyte function, and on the other circulating cells, especially on the leukocytes. ADP and collagen were used as platelet aggregation inductors. ADP is able to potentate the effects of other inductors, such as thrombin, due to stimulate and stabilize the thrombus. Collagen appears in the blood steam in the course of the injury of endothelial lineage. Collagen directly acts due to GPIIbIIIa receptors, and indirectly by Von-Willebrand factor, induces platelet aggregation and increases the adherence of platelet to the vessel wall, too.

Our studies can be considered new, in the respects of the parallel measurement of aggregation in platelet rich plasma and in whole blood within the same samples, at the same time. We revealed significant differences using the two methods. In isolated thrombocyte the effectiveness of antiplatelet therapy can be tested directly on the thrombocyte itself, during the hospitalization. In whole blood, the modulating effects of other cellular and non cellular components of blood can be studied. The disturbances in antioxidant/prooxidant balance are in the background of this phenomenon. The most surprising results were in our studies, that in PRP a satisfactory aggregation inhibition was detected in both the Acute and Elective groups (Figure1 and 3), but in whole blood (Figure 3., 4.,5., 6.) a highly significant elevation in ADP and collagen induced aggregation were revealed in the Acute group, compared to the Elective and Control ones. We concluded that the increased leukocyte numbers, the elevated free radical production of the individual leukocytes, and the exhausted antioxidant capacity, mainly the significant reduction in SOD activity, had important role (Figure 7. and 8). We pointed out the importance of the increase of prooxidants, while antioxidant capacity decreases especially in Acute group and in a less extensive way in Elective group too.

It has to be mentioned that SOD deficiency is a highly important determinant of the increased ROS production and the increase in platelet aggregation one week after the surgery. Pipinos and co-workers published that, the SOD enzyme mutation of gastrocnemius muscle of rats is a risk factor of PAD, (Pipinos II and Swanson SA 2008). Intracellular GSH and the plasma -SH groups possess remarkable antioxidant capacities. Before the surgery their levels were almost equal in the three groups, but after surgery a small but significant transient reduction was measured in their levels, mainly in the Acute group. Conflicting results are published about the effects of volatile anaesthetics on oxidative stress, and some local anaesthetics can cause transient decrease in GSH level in skeletal muscles (Jia-Li Luo, et al 1996). It can be supposed that transient decrease in GSH level is partially caused by the surgical intervention. Further alterations are caused by the disease itself, due to the sclerotic vessels, and/or the presence of hypertension, and other disturbances. These states also complicated by increased free radical generation, which usually increased further by the surgical intervention. Activated platelets play definitive role in the development of atherosclerosis and increase of the risk of surgical interventions. In spite of these there are only few data which can highlight the background of the poor prognosis of PAD and the role of thrombocytes in these processes. Other risk-factors which have definitive role, the activated complement system (Beinrohr L), leukocyte-thrombocyte interaction, and the increased endothelin release. The consequences of IR affect not only the great conduit vessels, but microcirculation is also affected (Kaszaki et al 2006). In the course of the animal studies they improved the protective effects of endothelin-A receptor antagonists and preconditioning against IR induced micro-vascular alterations.

Diabetes is also a well defined risk factor which worsens the outcome the surgical intervention. In the second series of our study thrombocyte function and antioxidant prooxidant status of diabetic patients with peripheral arterial disease were investigated and effects of exogenous insulin were tested. Platelet aggregation of PRP in diabetic patients was reduced compared to healthy blood donors signing the efficacy of their antiplatelet treatment. This difference failed to appear in whole blood. Free radical productions were significantly higher and SOD enzyme activities were significantly lower in diabetic patients compared to control. Low concentrations of insulin reduced the aggregation and free radical production in healthy and Type 1 diabetic patient's blood but failed to induce such effects in Type 2 diabetic ones. Insulin resistance is developed against not only the metabolic effects of insulin, but against other activities of this important hormone, as well. Revealing the alterations caused by surgical intervention in the function of circulating cells is inevitably important to improve the outcome of these procedures and reduce the complication of surgical intervention and facilitate recovery. Insulin is a vital hormone which essential for the glucose uptake of skeletal muscle and the heart. Insulin resistance increases the harmful effect of IR. Insulin effect can be improved and free radical production can be decreased by antioxidant, signing the important roles of free radicals in the pathogenesis of IR. Mice overexpressing extracellular SOD are less sensitive to IR (Sheng H et al 1999), signing that endogenous antioxidants have important role in tissue protection.

Present study support the importance of antioxidant prooxidant equilibrium and the role of endogenous antioxidants.

5. References

Adiseshiah M, Round JM, Jones DA. Reperfusion injury in skeletal muscle: a prospective study in patients with acute limb ischaemia and claudicants treated by revascularization. Br J Surg. 1992. 79. (10) 1026-10269.

Alsousou J, Thompson M, Hulley P, Noble A, Willett K. The biology of platelet-rich plasma and its application in trauma and orthopaedic surgery: a review of the literature. J Bone Joint Surg Br. 91(8):987-96.2009.

Arato E, Kurthy M, Jancso G, Sinay L, Kasza G, Verzar Z, Benko L, Cserepes B, Kollar L, Roth E. [Oxidative stress and leukocyte activation after lower limb revascularization surgery] Magy Seb. 59. (1):50-57.2006.

Arató E, Kürthy M, Sínay L, Kasza G, Menyhei G, Hardi P, Masoud S, Ripp K, Szilágyi K, Takács I, Miklós Z, Bátor A, Lantos J, Kollár L, Roth E, Jancsó G. Effect of vitamin E on reperfusion injuries during reconstructive vascular operations on lower limbs Clin Hemorheol Microcirc. 44. (2):125-36.2010.

Arató E., Kürthy M., Jancsó G., Kasza G., Sinay L., Rozsos I., Kollár L., Rõth E.: [Role of oxidative stress in revascularization surgery in lower limb] Az oxidatív stressz szerepe az alsóvégtagi revaszkularizációs szindrómában. Érbetegségek, S2; 39. 2005.

Arató E, Kürthy M, Sínay L, Kasza G, Menyhei G, Masoud S, Bertalan A, Verzár Z, Kollár L, Roth E, Jancsó G. Pathology and diagnostic options of lower limb compartment syndrome. Clin Hemorheol Microcirc. 41.(1):1-8.2009.

Arató E, Kürthy M, Sínay L, Kasza G, Menyhei G, Hardi P, Masoud S, Ripp K, Szilágyi K, Takács I, Miklós Z, Bátor A, Lantos J, Kollár L, Roth E, Jancsó G. Effect of vitamin E on reperfusion injuries during reconstructive vascular operations on lower limbs. Clin Hemorheol Microcirc. 44(2):125-36.2010a.

Arató et al 2010b E, Kürthy M, Sínay L, Kasza G, Menyhei G, Hardi P, Masoud S, Ripp K, Szilágyi K, Takács I, Miklós Z, Bátor A, Lantos J, Kollár L, Roth E, Jancsó G. Effect of vitamin E on reperfusion injuries during reconstructive vascular operations on lower limbs. Clin Hemorheol Microcirc. 44(2):125-36.2010b

Bakkaloglu C, Soyagir B, Torun M, Karagoz H, Simsek B. Oxidative stress is decreased in off-pump versus on-pump coronary artery surgery. J Biochem Mol Biol. 31;39(4):377-82. 2006.

Beinrohr L, Dobó J, Závodszky P, Gál P. C1, MBL-MASPs and C1-inhibitor: novel approaches for targeting complement-mediated inflammation. Trends Mol Med. 14(12):511-21. 2008.

Blaisdell W. The pathophysiology of skeletal muscle ischemia and the reperfusion syndrome: a review Cardiovascular Surgery, 10, (6). 620–630, 2002.

Born G.V.Haslam RJ, Goldman M. Nature. 13;205:678-80. 1965.

Born, G.V.R. Platelets in thrombogenesis: mechanism and Inhibition of platelet aggregation Ann R Coll Surg Engl. 36:200-6 1965.

Brennan ML, Penn MS, Van Lente F, Nambi V, Shishehbor MH, Aviles RJ, Goormastic M, Pepoy ML, McErlean ES, Topol EJ, Nissen SE, Hazen SL. Prognostic value of myeloperoxidase in patients with chest pain. N Engl J Med. 349(17):1595-604.2003.

Brevetti G, Schiano V, Laurenzano E, Giugliano G, Petretta M, Scopacasa F, and Chiariello M. Myeloperoxidase, but not C-reactive protein, predicts cardiovascular risk in peripheral arterial disease Eur Heart J. 29: 224-230. 2008.

Buchholz AM, Bruch L, Schulte KL. Activation of circulating platelets in patients with peripheral arterial disease during digital subtraction angiography and percutaneous transluminal angioplasty. Thromb Res. 109(1):13-22. 2003.

Claesson K, Kölbel T, Acosta S. Role of endovascular intervention in patients with diabetic foot ulcer and concomitant peripheral arterial disease. Int Angiol. 30 (4):349-58. 2011.

Combined thrombolysis with abciximab favourably influences platelet-leukocyte interactions and platelet activation in acute myocardial infarction. J Thromb Thrombolysis. 20(3):155-61.2005.

Comparative effectiveness of adenosine analogues as inhibitors of blood-platelet aggregation and as vasodilators in man. Nature. 13;205:678-80. 1965

Downey JM, and Cohen MV. Free radicals in the heart: friend or foe? Expert Rev Cardiovasc Ther. 6(5):589-91.2008.

Dröge W, Free Radicals in the Physiological Control of Cell Function Physiological Review 82 47-95. 2002.

Falkensammer J, Oldenburg WA. Surgical and medical management of mesenteric ischemia. Curr Treat Options Cardiovasc Med. 8(2): 137-143.2006.

Ferencz A, Szanto Z, Kalmar-Nagy K, Horvath OP, Roth E. Mitigation of oxidative injury by classic and delayed ischemic preconditioning prior to small bowel autotransplantation. Transplant Proc. 2004. 36. (2) 286-288. 2004.

Foo F, Oldroyd KG. Clinical value of antiplatelet therapy in patients with acute coronary syndromes and in percutaneous coronary intervention. Biomark Med. 5(1):9-30.2011.

Henrich M, Paddenberg R, Haberberger RV, Scholz A, Gruss M, Hempelmann G, Kummer W. Hypoxic increase in nitric oxide generation of rat Sensory neurons requires activation of mitochondrialComplex ii and voltage-gated calcium channels Neuroscience.;128(2):337-45.2004.

Ingerman-Wojenski CM, Silver MJ. A quick method for screening platelet dysfunctions using the whole blood lumi-aggregometer. Thromb Haemost. 51(2):154-6. 1984.

J Interv Cardiol. 14(5):539-546. 2001.

Jia-Li Luo, Folke Hammarqvist, Kerstin Andersson, Jan Wernerman Skeletal Muscle Glutathione After Surgical trauma Annals of Surgery 223, (4) 420-427. 1996.

Jude EB, Oyibo SO, Chalmers N, Boulton AJPeripheral arterial disease in diabetic and nondiabetic patients: a comparison of severity and outcome. Diabetes Care. 24(8):1433-7.2001.

Kathy K. Griendling; Dan Sorescu; Bernard Lassègue; Masuko Ushio-Fukai Modulation of Protein Kinase Activity and Gene Expression by Reactive Oxygen Species and Their Role in Vascular Physiology and Pathophysiology Arteriosclerosis, Thrombosis, and Vascular Biology.20:2175-2183. 2000.

Kaszaki J, Wolfárd A, Szalay L, Boros M. Pathophysiology of ischemia-reperfusion injury. Transplant Proc. 2006 Apr;38(3):826-8.

Kato H, Kogure K.: Biochemical and molecular characteristics of the brain with developing cerebral infarction. Cell Mol Neurobiol. 19. (1):93-108. 1999

Kolamunne RT, Clare M, Griffiths HR. Mitochondrial superoxide anion radicals mediate induction of apoptosis in cardiac myoblasts exposed to chronic hypoxia. Arch Biochem Biophys.505(2):256-65. 2011.

Krumholz HM, Goldberger AL. Reperfusion arrhythmias after thrombolysis. Electrophysiologic tempest, or much ado about nothing. Chest. 99 (4 Suppl):135S-140S.1991.

Laird JR. The management of acute limb ischemia: techniques for dealing with thrombus.

Levy JH, Tanaka KA. Inflammatory response to cardiopulmonary bypass. Ann Thoracic Surgery. 75.(2):S715-20.2003.

Li W, Khor TO, Xu C, Shen G, Jeong WS, Yu S, Kong AN. Activation of Nrf2-antioxidant signaling attenuates NFkappaB-inflammatory response and elicits apoptosis. Biochem Pharmacol. 76(11):1485-9. 2008.

Lin JK, Shih CA. Inhibitory effect of curcumin on xanthine dehydrogenase/oxidase induced by phorbol-12-myristate-13-acetate in NIH3T3 cells. Carcinogenesis. 15.:1717-71.1994

Loberg AG, Stallard J, Dunning J, Dark J. Can leukocyte depletion reduce reperfusion injury following cardiopulmonary bypass? Interact Cardiovasc Thorac Surg. 12(2):232-7. 2011.

Massberg S., Enders G, Leiderer R, Eisenmenger S, Vestweber D, Krombach K, Messmer K. Platelet-Endothelial Cell Interactions During Ischemia/Reperfusion: The Role of P-Selectin Blood 92. (2) 507-515. 1998.

Mhairi J. Maxwell, Erik Westein, Warwick S. Nesbitt, Simon Giuliano, Sacha M. Dopheide P. Jackson Identification of a 2-stage platelet aggregation process mediating shear-dependent thrombus formation Blood 109. 566-576. 2007.

Ming Wei Liu, Gary S. Roubin and Spencer B. King III Restenosis After Coronary Angioplasty Potential Biologic Determinants and Role of Intimal Hyperplasia Circulation 79:1374-1387.1989.

Misra HP, Fridovich I. The role of superoxide anion in the autoxidation of epinephrine and a simple assay for superoxide dismutase. J Biol Chem. 247(10):3170-5. 1972.

Misty M. Payne Charles, Theodore Dotter The Father of Intervention Tex Heart Inst J. 28(1): 28–38.2001.

Moens AL, Claeys MJ, Timmermans JP, Vrints CJ. Myocardial ischemia/reperfusion-injury, a clinical view on a complex pathophysiological process. Int J Cardiol. 2005 Apr 20;100(2):179-190.

Moncada S, Palmer RM, Higgs EA. Nitric oxide: physiology, pathophysiology, and pharmacology. Pharmacol Rev. (2):109-42. 1991.

Ohkawa H, Ohishi N, Yagi K. Assay for lipid peroxides in animal tissues by thiobarbituric acid reaction. Anal Biochem 95(2):351-8. 1979.

Peto K, Nemeth N, Brath E, Takacs IE, Baskurt OK, Meiselman HJ, Furka I, Miko I. The effects of renal ischemia-reperfusion on hemorheological factors: preventive role of allopurinol. Clin Hemorheol Microcirc. 37(4):347-58.2007.

Pipinos II, Swanson SA, Zhu Z, Nella AA, Weiss DJ, Gutti TL, McComb RD, Baxter BT, Lynch TG, Casale GP. Chronically ischemic mouse skeletal muscle exhibits myopathy in association with mitochondrial dysfunction and oxidative damage. Am J Physiol Regul Integr Comp Physiol.;295(1):R 290-296. 2008

R Hille and T Nishino Flavoprotein structure and mechanism. 4. Xanthine oxidase and xanthine dehydrogenase The FASEB Journal, 9, 995-1003.

Röth E, Hejjel L: Oxygen free radicals in the heart disease, In:Cardiac Drug Development Guide. ED. M.K. Pugsley. Human Press Inc. Totowa NJ. 47-66. 2003.

Ruiter MS, van Golde JM, Schaper NC, Stehouwer CD, Huijberts MS. Diabetes impairs arteriogenesis in the peripheral circulation: review of molecular mechanisms. Clin Sci 8;119(6):225-38.2010.

Sedlak J, Lindsay RH. Estimation of total, protein-bound, and nonprotein sulfhydryl groups in tissue with Ellman's reagent. Anal Biochem. 24;25(1):192-205. 1968.

Sinay L, Kürthy M, Horváth S, Arató E, Shafiei M, Lantos J, Ferencz S, Bátor A, Balatonyi B, Verzár Z, Süto B, Kollár L, Wéber G, Roth E, Jancsó G. Ischaemic postconditioning reduces peroxide formation, cytokine expression and leukocyte activation in reperfusion injury after abdominal aortic surgery in rat model. Clin Hemorheol Microcirc. 40(2):133-42.2008.

Smyth SS, McEver RP, Weyrich AS, Morrell CN, Hoffman MR, Arepally GM, French PA, Dauerman HL, Becker RC; 2009. Platelet Colloquium Participants. Platelet functions beyond hemostasis. J Thromb Haemost. 7. (11):1759-66. 2009.

Szabo S, Etzel D, Ehlers R, Walter T, Kazmaier S, Helber U, Hoffmeister HM.

Umar S, van der Laarse A. Nitric oxide and nitric oxide synthase isoforms in the normal, hypertrophic, and failing heart. Mol Cell Biochem. 333 .(1-2):191-201. 2010.

Vinten-Johansen J, Zhao ZQ, Jiang R, Zatta AJ, Dobson GP. Preconditioning and postconditioning: innate cardioprotection from ischemia-reperfusion injury.Journal of Applied Physiology 103. 1441-1448. 2007.

Virchow R. Gesammelte Abhandlungen zur Wissenschaftlichen Medicin. Frankfurt, Germany: Medinger Sohn & Co.; 219-732.1856.

Weiss A.G and Zahger AT: Coronary angioplasty or intravenous thrombolysis: the dilemma of optimal reperfusion in acute myocardial infarction: A critical review of the literature. J Thromb. Thrombolysis 8(2):113-21. 1999.

Xia Y and Zeier J.L. Analytical Biochemistry 245, 1, 93-96, 1997.

Yassin MM, Harkin DW, Barros D'Sa AA, Halliday MI, Rowlands BJ. Lower limb ischemia-reperfusion injury triggers a systemic inflammatory response and multiple organ dysfunction. World J Surg. 6(1):115-21.2002.

Sheng H, Bart RD, Oury TD, Pearlstein RD, Crapo JD, Warner DS. Mice overexpressing extracellular superoxide dismutase have increased resistance to focal cerebral ischemia. Neuroscience. 88. (1): 185-91.199

5

Antithrombotic Therapy After Peripheral Angioplasty

Beniamino Zalunardo[1], Diego Tonello[1], Fabio Busato[1], Laura Zotta[1], Sandro Irsara[2] and Adriana Visonà[1]
[1]*Angiology Unit, San Giacomo Hospital, Castelfranco Veneto (TV)*
[2]*Vascular Surgery, San Giacomo Hospital, Castelfranco Veneto (TV)*
Italy

1. Introduction

Peripheral arterial disease affects approximately 12% of adults and 20% of adults over 70 years (Hiatt et al., 1995). This disease results from one or more lesions in the arterial system of the lower extremity that restrict blood flow. The restriction of blood flow during ambulation may cause intermittent claudication, i.e. muscular pain due to lack of blood supply. About one fifth of people with peripheral arterial disease have intermittent claudication. About half of people with peripheral arterial disease are asymptomatic. A small part of people with peripheral arterial disease (< 10%) have critical limb ischemia, i.e. rest muscular pain and/or ischemic ulceration or gangrene of toes. Based on the severity of symptoms, the stages of the disease are classified as Fontaine stages I-IV, where stage I is asymptomatic, stage IIa is the occurrence of intermittent claudication after a pain-free walking distance of more than 200 m, stage IIb is intermittent claudication after less than 200 m, stage III is rest pain, and stage IV is the presence of ischemic ulcers.

Patients with peripheral arterial disease, which is an expression of systemic atherosclerosis, have an increased risk of cardiovascular events (Hankey et al., 2006).

Medical therapy should include modification or elimination of atherosclerotic risk factors (cigarette smoking, diabetes mellitus, hypertension, hyperlipidemia), and antiplatelet therapies to decrease the risk of cardiovascular events and to improve survival. Moreover, the initial approach to the treatment of limb symptoms should focus to relieve discomfort, to improve exercise performance, and daily functional abilities by means of structured exercise and, in selected patients, pharmacotherapies to treat the exercise limitation of claudication (Norgren et al, 2007). Lower extremity revascularization is indicated for patients with a lifestyle-limiting disability due to intermittens claudication or with chronic critical limb ischemia (Hirsch et al., 2006; Norgren et al., 2007).

There are two types of revascularization procedure: endovascular or surgical. Percutaneous transluminal angioplasty with or without stenting is an endovascular technique for revascularizing obstructed arteries. It was first introduced by Dotter and Judkins (Dotter & Judkins, 1964), and subsequently improved by Grüntzig (Grüntzig & Hopff, 1974).

In peripheral transluminal angioplasty the recanalization of obstructed arteries is obtained by dilatation of a stenosis (i.e. a narrowing of the vessel diameter) or recanalization of a total occlusion, using a wire-guided inflatable balloon catheter. Usually the femoral artery in the groin is cannulated and a deflated balloon catheter is inserted and pushed forward along the guide-wire to the sites of obstruction. Stenting is usually added to reduce the risk of reocclusion, especially if there is a major endothelial damage, arterial dissection or non-satisfactory dilatation with relevant residual stenosis. Self-expanding metallic stents are mainly applied at the aortic bifurcation or iliac segments, whereas the femoropopliteal level, until recently, was associated with a higher risk for reocclusion due to smaller vessel diameters in distal arteries (Do et al., 1992; Mahler et al., 1999; Palmaz et al., 1985; Strecker et al., 1988).

The implantation of drug-eluting stents, nitinol stents, paclitaxel-coated angioplasty balloons, or treatment by intravascular brachytherapy following peripheral angioplasty of the femoropopliteal arteries have been considered as interventions with the capacity of reducing the occurrence of restenosis/reocclusion (Schillinger et al., 2006; Gray et al., 2008).

In patients with peripheral arterial disease endovascular procedures are generally the treatment of choice for short-segment iliac or femoral-popliteal artery lesions (TASC-A, single stenosis less than 3 cm long). Longer segment iliac or femoral-popliteal artery lesions (TASC-B, single iliac stenosis 5-10 cm long, two iliac lesions 3-5 cm long, single occlusion of an iliac artery, tandem femoral-popliteal stenoses less than 3 cm long, single femoral-popliteal lesion 3-5 cm in length) are frequently treated by endovascular techniques (Norgren et al., 2007).

Restenosis (or reocclusion) is the main complication of peripheral transluminal angioplasty. Balloon angioplasty has been shown to induce endothelial injury and oxidative stress with subsequent endothelial dysfunction, platelet aggregation, macrophage activation, and smooth muscle cell proliferation (McBride et al., 1988; Taniyama & Griendling, 2003). Peripheral transluminal angioplasty induces a prothrombotic condition: atherosclerotic plaques are disrupted and platelets aggregate at the site of the damaged arterial wall (Fuster et al., 1995). Thus, as a result of platelet aggregation, activated blood clotting in the damaged atheromatous artery and low shear stress, restenosis (or reocclusion) is frequent (Schwartz, 1998; Wentzel et al., 2003).

In particular, the effects of balloon angioplasty on the platelet activation have been studied previously in vitro and in vivo. Peripheral transluminal angioplasty has been shown to result in significant imbalance between the production of prostacyclin, an effective vasodilatator and platelet antiaggregator produced in endothelial cells, and thromboxane A2, a potent smooth muscle constrictor and platelet aggregator formed in platelets, with shift more toward increased thromboxane A2 production. This finding is suggestive of significant platelet activation and may have implication for future failure of peripheral angioplasty (Parmar et al., 2010). An increased formation of thromboxane A2 was also seen in other two studies, one in patients undergoing peripheral angioplasty and one in patients after coronary angioplasty (Rossi et al., 1997; Peterson et al., 1986).

In addition, in the initial phase after balloon and stent procedures, coagulation system is activated, as demonstrated by increased serum levels of thrombin-antithrombin complexes, D-dimer and fibrinopeptide A. This condition favours early thrombotic occlusion, where 'early' is usually defined as a period covering the first 4 weeks after the intervention (Tsakiris et al., 1999; Tschöpl et al., 1997). Subsequently, intimal hyperplasia, a redundant healing of the arterial wall, which is responsible for restenosis and reocclusion in the mid- and long-term, may follow. Intimal hyperplasia occurs as a result of denudation (tearing off of the inner lining) of the endothelium caused by damage to the vessel wall with the catheter. Smooth muscle cells in the medial layer are stimulated to grow and migrate into the intimal layer (Haudenschild, 1995; Jørgensen et al., 1990).

Risk factors for restenosis/reocclusion include severity of atherosclerosis in run-off arteries, length of diseased segments, number of treated lesions, stage of disease, and presence of cardiovascular risk factors (Norgren et al., 2007). Female gender may be an independent predictor of decreased primary patency of external iliac artery stents (Timaran et al., 2001). Inflammation, revealed by an elevated C-reactive protein, was also considered as a risk factor for restenosis at six months after successful femoropopliteal angioplasty (Schillinger et al., 2002).

The rate of restenosis/reocclusion of suprainguinal (iliac) arteries after peripheral transluminal angioplasty ranges from 14% after one year to 29% after 5 years, while the rate of restenosis/reocclusion of infrainguinal (femoropopliteal) arteries after peripheral transluminal angioplasty with or without stenting ranges from 23-35% after one year to 45-58% after 5 years (Norgren et al., 2007). Patients with stenoses or occlusions of infrainguinal arteries of less than 3 cm had a favourable long-term patency rate of 74% (Gallino et al., 1984).

Patients subjected to local thrombolysis show higher incidences of restenosis/reocclusion (Decrinis et al., 1993).

It is important to define the lesion suitable for balloon angioplasty in both the suprainguinal and infrainguinal districts.

Inter-Society Consensus for the Management of Peripheral Arterial Disease (TASC II) redefined the indications for endovascular or surgical revascularization on the basis of anatomical characteristics of the lesions. Endovascular interventions are recommended for: i) unilateral or bilateral stenosis of common iliac artery; unilateral or bilateral single short (≤ 3 cm) stenosis of external iliac artery; ii) single stenosis ≤ 10 cm in length of femoropopliteal arteries; single occlusion ≤ 5 cm in length of femoropopliteal arteries (TASC Type A lesions) (Norgren et al., 2007).

Endovascular interventions are the preferred treatments for: i) short (≤ 3 cm) stenosis of infrarenal aorta; unilateral common iliac artery occlusion; single or multiple stenosis totaling 3-10 cm involving the external iliac artery not extending into the common femoral artery; unilateral external iliac artery occlusion not involving the origin of internal iliac or common femoral artery; ii) multiple lesions (stenoses or occlusions), each ≤ 5 cm of femoropopliteal segment; single stenosis or occlusion ≤ 15 cm not involving the infra geniculate popliteal artery; single or multiple lesions in the absence of continuous tibial vessels to improve inflow for a distal bypass; heavily calcified occlusion ≤ 5 cm in length; single popliteal stenosis (TASC Type B lesions) (Norgren et al., 2007).

Provisional stent placement is indicated for iliac arteries as salvage therapy for a suboptimal or failed result from balloon dilatation (persistent translesional gradient, residual stenosis greater than 50%, flow-limiting dissection). Stenting is effective as primary therapy for common and external iliac artery stenoses and occlusions. Moreover, stents can be useful in the femoral, popliteal and tibial arteries as a salvage therapy for suboptimal or failed results from balloon dilatation (Hirsch et al., 2006).

As mentioned above, the implantation of drug-eluting stents, nitinol stents, paclitaxel-coated angioplasty balloons, or treatment by intravascular brachytherapy following peripheral angioplasty have been considered as interventions with the capacity of reducing the occurrence of restenosis/reocclusion. A study by Schillinger et al. showed better results at one year with self-expanding nitinol stent in femoropopliteal segments (Schillinger et al., 2006). Use of paclitaxel-coated angioplasty balloons during percutaneous treatment of femoropopliteal disease has been shown to be associated with significant reductions in late lumen loss (Tepe et al., 2008). Endovascular brachytherapy has been proposed as a promising treatment modality to reduce restenosis after angioplasty (Minar et al., 2000). However, the phenomenon of late acute thrombotic occlusion in patients receiving endovascular brachytherapy after stenting of the femoropopliteal arteries may compromise the benefits of endovascular radiation. The fact that late acute thrombotic occlusions occurs concomitantly with stopping clopidogrel in patients treated with a double antiplatelet regimen (aspirin 100 mg / day and clopidogrel 75 mg / day) suggests an intensive and prolonged antithrombotic prevention in these patients (Bonvini et al., 2003).

There are much few data concerning antithrombotic therapy after peripheral arterial revascularization, and patients with peripheral arterial disease are often treated on the basis of experiences extrapolated from coronary arteries (Visonà et al., 2009).

Antithrombotic therapy has been shown to lower the incidence of associated cardiovascular events (Sobel & Verhaeghe, 2008). A meta-analysis of 42 trials has shown a statistically significant 23% reduction of vascular events (vascular death, nonfatal myocardial infarction or stroke) in 9,214 patients with peripheral arterial disease treated with antiplatelet therapy. Even patients having peripheral angioplasty benefited to a similar degree (Antithrombotic Trialists' Collaboration, 2002). Clopidogrel seems to be superior to aspirin in reducing cardiovascular events, particularly in patients with peripheral arterial disease (relative risk reduction of 23%) (CAPRIE Steering Committee, 1996), but this advantage is minimal. Life-long antiplatelet therapy is usually recommended for all patients with peripheral arterial disease to prevent death and disability from stroke and myocardial infarction.

Antithrombotic drugs to prevent restenosis would make an important contribution to the sustained success of endovascular treatment. The main questions concern the most effective and safe antithrombotic therapy and its duration.

2. Methods

We performed a Medline search of English language studies published between 1976 and 2010 with the keywords "antithrombotic therapy, peripheral angioplasty". We also considered the reviews and meta-analyses. We selected two meta-analyses, two reviews, and fifteen original articles.

3. Results

Two meta-analyses and two reviews evaluated the efficacy and safety of antithrombotic agents for the prevention of restenosis after balloon angioplasty in patients with peripheral arterial disease (Girolami et al., 2000; Dörffler-Melly et al., 2005; Watson & Bergqvist, 2000; Visonà et al. 2009).

The first meta-analysis evaluated the efficacy of conservative adjuvant therapy after endovascular or surgical revascularization procedures. The meta-analysis, including thirty-two studies, showed that, compared to non-active control, aspirin (100-300 mg daily) with dipyridamole (225-450 mg daily) improves patency (odds ratio 0.69) and mortality (odds ratio 0.57). Similarly, ticlopidine has been shown to improve patency and amputation rates (odds ratio 0.53 and 1.01, respectively), and therefore may be used when aspirin is contraindicated. Data on the effectiveness of vitamin K inhibitors were not conclusive (Girolami et al., 2000).

The second meta-analysis is a Cochrane review of 14 randomized trials comparing different antithrombotic drugs (anticoagulants, antiplatelet agents and others) with no treatment or placebo to prevent restenosis/reocclusion following peripheral vascular treatment. The trials included patients with symptomatic peripheral arterial disease treated by endovascular revascularization of the iliac or femoropopliteal arteries. Various pharmacological interventions were analysed: anticoagulants, antiplatelet agents and other vasoactive drugs were compared with no treatment, placebo, or any other vasoactive drug. Clinical endpoints were reocclusion, amputation, death, myocardial infarction, stroke and major bleeding. The efficacy and safety of acetylsalcylic acid and low molecular weight heparins have been shown. Aspirin (50-300 mg daily) started prior to femoropopliteal peripheral transluminal angioplasty has been shown to be the most effective prophylactic treatment. Low molecular weight heparins seem to be more effective in preventing restenosis or reocclusion than unfractionated heparin (Dörffler-Melly et al., 2005).

Watson and Bergqvist identified eleven randomized trials with antithrombotic agents, but they didn't clarify their usefulness in reducing the likelihood of restenosis or reocclusion after balloon angioplasty of femoropopliteal lesions (Watson & Bergqvist, 2000).

Our group recently conducted a review on antithrombotic therapy after peripheral angioplasty (Visonà et al., 2009).

We analyse the studies identified in the following paragraphs (Table 1).

3.1 Aspirin with or without dipyridamole

Two studies compared aspirin combined with dipyridamole to placebo (Heiss et al., 1990; Study Group, 1994).

In a single-center trial 199 patients undergoing balloon angioplasty of femoropopliteal arteries were randomized to high dose aspirin (990 mg) combined with dipyridamole (225 mg), low dose aspirin (300 mg) plus dipyridamole (225 mg), or placebo. Clinical and angiographic improvement was observed in both treatment groups in comparison with placebo, but this was statistically significant only in the high-dose aspirin group (Heiss et al., 1990).

A multicenter study randomized 223 patients undergoing balloon angioplasty of iliac or femoropopliteal arteries to receive either placebo or aspirin (50 mg) plus dipyridamole (400 mg). No difference was observed between the two groups. A possible explanation of this result may be a higher percentage of patients with more favourable iliac lesions in the placebo group (65% versus 51%). Moreover, use of metallic stents was not performed (Study Group, 1994).

According the conclusions of the Cochrane review, a 60% reduction of restenosis/ reocclusion was found with aspirin 330 mg combined with dipyridamole as compared to placebo up to 12 months after angioplasty of femoropopliteal arteries. A similar positive effect on patency was found with aspirin 50 to 100 mg combined with dipyridamole as compared to placebo at 6 months, but this was not significant (Dörffler-Melly et al., 2005).

Aspirin/dipyridamole showed a superior effect on patency after femoropopliteal angioplasty compared to vitamin K antagonists at 3, 6, and 12 months, but even this effect was not significant (Do & Mahler, 1994; Pilger et al. 1991).

Aspirin 50 to 330 mg, with or without dipyridamole, started before femoropopliteal endovascular treatment, appeared to be the most effective and safest strategy, and reduced the incidence of restenosis/reocclusion at 6 and 12 months when compared with no therapy or vitamin K antagonists. Three trials compared the efficacy and safety of different doses of aspirin after peripheral angioplasty. The doses tested ranged from 50 mg / day to 1000 mg / day. The three studies showed that higher doses of aspirin had no advantage on early reocclusion (within one month) and were more likely to cause gastrointestinal side effects including peptic ulcer (Weichert et al., 1994; Minar et al., 1995; Ranke et al., 1994).

3.2 Oral anticoagulants

Anticoagulation is frequently combined with antiplatelet therapy after femoropopliteal or tibial artery balloon angioplasty, although the results of three randomized controlled trials do not support this practice (Schneider et al., 1987, as cited in Sobel & Verhaeghe, 2008; Pilger et al., 1991; Do & Mahler, 1994). In fact, in all three studies no significant difference was observed in arterial patency rate between the anticoagulation groups and the antiplatelet therapy groups (only slightly lower patency rate and more bleeding complications in the anticoagulation groups).

3.3 Low molecular weight heparins

Intimal hyperplasia is responsible for restenosis and reocclusion after angioplasty in the mid- and long-term. Low molecular weight heparins have been shown in experimental studies to have antiproliferative effects in addition to their antithrombotic properties (Wilson et al., 1991). Their potential to reduce restenosis remains to be established. The hypothesis that low molecular weight heparins plus aspirin are more effective than aspirin alone in reducing incidence of restenosis after peripheral transluminal angioplasty was tested in two trials. Nadroparin, administered at a dose adjusted to weight for 7 days after femoropopliteal angioplasty, has been shown to be more effective to prevent reocclusion at 6 months than unfractionated heparin, without causing increased bleeding (Schweizer et al., 2001). Despite this interesting result, dalteparin 2500 UI, administered for 3 months after femoropopliteal angioplasty plus aspirin 100 mg/day versus aspirin alone, failed to reduce incidence of restenosis/reocclusion at 12 months. However, dalteparin appeared to be beneficial at the 12-month follow-up in the subgroup of patients with critical limb ischemia (Koppensteiner et al., 2006).

3.4 New antiplatelet drugs (abciximab, thienopyridines)

There are few studies available on potent new antiplatelet drugs such as abciximab and thienopyridines.

3.4.1 Abciximab

In one study in high-risk patients with long segmental femoropopliteal interventions adjunctive administration of abciximab had a favorable effect on patency and clinical outcome in patients undergoing complex femoropopliteal catheter interventions not hampered by serious bleeding. Treatment effect of abciximab observed at 30 days was maintained at 6 months (Dörffler-Melly et al., 2005).

In another study adjunctive abciximab after nitinol stenting of the superficial femoral artery did not appear to demonstrate any identifiable effect on functional outcomes at 9 months (Ansel et al., 2006).

3.4.2 Thienopyridines

The thienopyridines, ticlopidine and clopidogrel, interfere with the adenosine diphosphate (ADP) pathway. They might represent a useful alternative to aspirin, when it is not

tolerated, and might be combined with aspirin, when increased risk factors for restenosis/reocclusion are detected, although specific data are lacking.
In one study ticlopidine was compared to vitamin K inhibitors. No significant difference in efficacy was found between the two drugs (Schneider et al., 1987, as cited in Sobel & Verhaeghe, 2008).
The administration of clopidogrel and aspirin leads to a potent platelet inhibition, whose benefits have been demonstrated for patients with acute coronary syndrome, symptomatic vascular disease, and presence of multiple cardiovascular risk factors. A randomized double-blind trial showed that the administration of clopidogrel and aspirin significantly suppresses platelet function up to 30 days after lower limb angioplasty, compared to aspirin and placebo (Cassar et al., 2005a). On the other hand, addition of clopidogrel to the standard antithrombotic therapy with aspirin had no effect on the levels of markers of coagulation activation, such as D-dimer and thrombin-antithrombin III, in patients with intermittent claudication before or after endovascular intervention (Cassar et al., 2005b). Moreover, therapy with clopidogrel and aspirin had no significant effect on markers of vascular smooth muscle cell proliferation before and after peripheral angioplasty (Wilson et al., 2009).

3.4.3 Dual antiplatelet therapy

Dual antiplatelet therapy (clopidogrel plus aspirin), leading to a potent platelet inhibition, has been shown to be more effective than aspirin alone in reducing cardiovascular events in patients with acute non-ST coronary syndrome. This finding has not been confirmed in patients at high cardiovascular risk but not in the acute phase, where risk-benefit ratio is less favourable (Keller et al., 2007). A potential benefit of clopidogrel and aspirin versus aspirin alone in patients with symptomatic vascular disease has been suggested by the CHARISMA trial, which enrolled more than 15,000 patients with either evident clinical cardiovascular disease or multiple risk factors (Bhatt et al., 2006).
The benefit of more potent platelet inhibition with dual therapy, aspirin and clopidogrel, has been shown in a trial on acute coronary syndromes (CURE) (Fox et al., 2004). However, the efficacy and safety of this dual antiplatelet therapy after peripheral angioplasty have not been evaluated in a randomized controlled trial. The Clopidogrel and Aspirin in the Management of Peripheral Endovascular Revascularization study (CAMPER) was designed to evaluate this outcome after femoropopliteal angioplasty, but it was stopped, due to difficulties of randomization, perhaps because many patients were already treated off-label with clopidogrel and aspirin (Patrono et al., 2004).
The administration of ticlopidine and acetylsalicylic acid has been shown to improve neurological outcome after carotid stenting without an additional increase in bleeding complications in patients undergoing carotid stenting, compared to acetylsalicylic acid alone (Dalainas et al., 2006).
Aspirin and clopidogrel were used as standard therapy in two major randomized controlled trials of carotid stenting (preprocedure and at least for 30 days) (SPACE Collaborative Group, 2006; Mas et al., 2006).
Although it is questionable to extrapolate experience from one anatomic region to another, in the absence of data on peripheral interventions, dual antiplatelet therapy seems to be a reasonable approach to reduce thrombotic complications after lower extremity balloon angioplasty and stenting, especially in the femoropopliteal and tibial districts. In fact, many physicians in the world use dual antiplatelet therapy with aspirin (100 mg / day) and clopidogrel (75 mg / day) before and after peripheral transluminal angioplasty and stenting of peripheral arteries. Dual antiplatelet therapy is continued for 4 weeks after the intervention.

Then aspirin is continued indefinitely (Visonà et al., 2009). Treatment with a loading dose of clopidogrel 6-24 hours before angioplasty seems to improve the clinical outcome (Verheugt et al., 2007), and a 600 mg loading dose versus 300 mg at least 12 hours before the procedure provides greater benefit in coronary syndromes (Cuisset et al., 2006). In addition, an intra-arterial bolus of heparin (3000 to 5000 U) is often administered at the time of the procedure.

Drugs	Author, year	Treatments	Pts	Design
ASA ± dipyridamole	Heiss, 1990	ASA 300 mg / dipyridamole 225 mg ASA 990 mg / dipyridamole 225 mg Placebo	47 51 47	R, DB, 1C
	Study Group, 1994	ASA 50 mg / dipyridamole 400 mg Placebo	105 110	R, DB, 12C
	Hess, 1978	ASA 990 mg ASA 990 mg / dipirydamole 225 mg	50 51	R, DB, 1C
	Ranke, 1992	ASA 50 mg ASA 900 mg	184 175	R, DB, 2C
	Weichert, 1994	ASA 300 mg ASA 1000 mg	106 105	R, DB, 2C
	Minar, 1995	ASA 100 mg ASA 1000 mg	105 102	R, O, 1C
Oral anticoagulants	Do, 1994	ASA 50 mg / dipyridamole 400 mg Anticoagulant	51 61	R, O, 1C
	Pilger, 1991	ASA 500 mg / dipirydamole 225 mg Anticoagulant	66 63	R, O, 1C
LMWHs	Schweizer, 2001	Weight adjusted nadroparin + ASA 100 mg Unfractionated heparin + ASA 100 mg	86 86	R, O, 1C
	Koppensteiner, 2006	Dalteparin 2500 IU + ASA 100 mg ASA 100 mg	137 138	R, O, 1C
Ticlopidine	Schneider, 1987	Ticlopidine Anticoagulant	103 94	R, O, 3C
Abciximab	Dörffler-Melly, 2005	Abciximab + ASA 100 mg Placebo + ASA 100 mg	47 51	R, DB, 1C
	Ansel, 2006	Abciximab Placebo	27 24	R, O, 1C
Iloprost	Horrocks, 1997	Iloprost 72 h + ASA 300 mg after 72 h ASA 300 mg None 72 h + ASA 300 mg after 72 h	11 13 14	R, O, 2C
Cilostazol	Iida, 2008	Cilostazol 200 mg Ticlopidine 200 mg	63 64	R, O, 1C

Pts= patients; ASA=acetylsalicylic acid; LMWHs=low molecular weight heparins; R=randomized; DB=double blind; O=open; nC=number of centres

Table 1. Drugs, studies published, patients analysed and study designs

Currently, for patients undergoing lower extremity balloon angioplasty (with or without stenting), the American College of Chest Physicians (ACCP) recommends long-term aspirin (75-100 mg / day) (grade 1C), and recommends against anticoagulation with heparin or vitamin K inhibitors (grade 1A) (Sobel & Verhaeghe, 2008).
Randomized, prospective studies with dual therapy are needed for resolving some issues, such as real efficacy of dual therapy in peripheral district, the optimal loading dose in patients undergoing endovascular revascularization, and the optimal duration of dual therapy following peripheral angioplasty and stenting (Plosker & Lyseng-Williamson, 2007).

3.5 Vasoactive drugs

Some drugs have interesting vasoactive properties, that may improve outcome after peripheral angioplasty. Iloprost, the prostacyclin analogue, and cilostazol, a phosphodiesterase type 3 inhibitor, have multiple effects, such as inhibition of platelet activation, vasodilation, antiproliferation of vascular smooth muscle cells, and improvement of endothelial cell function. These effects may lead to the inhibition of neointimal hyperplasia after stenting.
Iloprost was investigated in a small study in conjunction with aspirin. A 3-day periinterventional intravenous infusion of iloprost plus long-term aspirin didn't reduce incidence of restenosis, compared to aspirin alone (Horrocks et al., 1997).
Cilostazol after endovascular therapy for femoropopliteal lesions was more effective in reducing restenosis than ticlopidine (Iida et al., 2008).
Further studies are needed.

4. Conclusion

Patients with peripheral arterial disease benefit from receiving life-long aspirin at a daily dose of 75 mg to 100 mg or clopidogrel at a daily dose of 75 mg. Patients undergoing peripheral transluminal angioplasty should receive aspirin at a daily dose of 75 mg to 100 mg, started before the intervention and continued life-long. Thienopyridines, e.g. clopidogrel, might represent a useful alternative to aspirin in cases of intolerance to aspirin. Although randomized clinical trials are lacking, it is reasonable to consider short-term dual antiplatelet therapy with aspirin and thienopyridines for infrainguinal stenting, given the relatively high rate of restenosis/reocclusion after interventions. It is reasonable to administer a 300-600 mg loading dose 6-24 hours before angioplasty, and to continue dual therapy for 4 weeks. If a drug-eluting peripheral stent was placed, dual therapy is maintained for 6-12 months. Use of low molecular weight heparins may be reserved for patients with critical limb iischemia. Abciximab may be useful after extended femoropopliteal interventions in patients at high risk of restenosis/reocclusion.

5. References

Ansel, G.M.; Silver, M.J.; Botti, C.F. Jr; Rocha-Singh, K.; Bates, M.C.; Rosenfield, K.; Schainfeld, R.M.; Laster, S.B. & Zander, C. (2006). Functional and clinical outcomes of nitinol stenting with and without abciximab for complex superficial femoral artery disease: a randomized trial. *Catheter Cardiovasc Interv*, Vol.67, No.2, (February 2006), pp. 288-297, ISSN 1522-1946

Antithrombotic Trialists' Collaboration. (2002). Collaborative meta-analysis of randomised trials of antiplatelet therapy for prevention of death, myocardial infarction, and stroke in high risk patients. *BMJ*, Vol.324, No.7329, (January 2002), pp. 71–86, ISSN 0959-8138

Bhatt, D.L.; Fox, K.A.; Hacke, W.; Berger, P.B.; Black, H.R.; Boden, W.E.; Cacoub, P.; Cohen, E.A.; Creager, M.A.; Easton, J.D.; Flather, M.D.; Haffner, S.M.; Hamm, C.W.; Hankey, G.J.; Johnston, S.C.; Mak, K.H.; Mas, J.L.; Montalescot, G.; Pearson, T.A.; Steg, P.G.; Steinhubl, S.R.; Weber, M.A.; Brennan, D.M.; Fabry-Ribaudo, L.; Booth, J.; Topol, E.J. & CHARISMA Investigators. (2006). Clopidogrel and aspirin versus aspirin alone for the prevention of atherothrombotic events. *N Engl J Med*, Vol.354, No.16, (April 2006), pp. 1706-1717, ISSN 0028-4793

Bonvini, R.; Baumgartner, I.; Do, D.D.; Alerci, M.; Segatto, J.M.; Tutta, P.; Jäger, K.; Aschwanden, M.; Schneider, E.; Amann-Vesti, B.; Greiner, R.; Mahler, F. & Gallino, A. (2003). Late Acute Thrombotic Occlusion After Endovascular Brachytherapy and Stenting of Femoropopliteal Arteries. *J Am Coll Cardiol*, Vol.41, No.3, (February 2003), pp. 409–412, ISSN 0735-1097

CAPRIE Steering Committee. (1996). A randomised, blinded, trial of clopidogrel versus aspirin in patients at risk of ischaemic events (CAPRIE). *Lancet*, Vol.348, No.9038, (November 1996), pp. 1329-1339, ISSN 0140-6736

Cassar, K.; Ford, I.; Greaves, M.; Bachoo, P. & Brittenden, J. (2005). Randomized clinical trial of the antiplatelet effects of aspirin-clopidogrel combination versus aspirin alone after lower limb angioplasty. *Br J Surg*, Vol.92, No.2, (February 2005), pp. 159-165, ISSN 0007-1323

Cassar, K.; Bachoo, P.; Ford, I.; Greaves, M. & Brittenden, J. (2005). Clopidogrel has no effect on D-dimer and thrombin-antithrombin III levels in patients with peripheral percutaneous transluminal angioplasty. *J Vasc Surg*, Vol.42, No.2, (August 2005), pp. 252-258, ISSN 0741-5214

Cuisset, T.; Frere, C.; Quilici, J.; Morange, P.E.; Nait-Saidi, L.; Carvajal, J.; Lehmann, A.; Lambert, M.; Bonnet, J.L. & Alessi, M.C. (2006). Benefit of a 600-mg loading dose of clopidogrel on platelet reactivity and clinical outcomes in patients with non-ST-segment elevation acute coronary syndrome undergoing coronary stenting. *J Am Coll Cardiol*, Vol.48, No.7, (October 2006), pp. 1339-1345, ISSN 0735-1097

Dalainas, I.; Nano, G.; Bianchi, P.; Stegher, S.; Malacrida, G. & Tealdi, D.G. (2006). Dual antiplatelet regime versus acetyl-acetic acid for carotid artery stenting. *Cardiovasc Intervent Radiol*, Vol.29, No.4, (July-August 2006), pp. 519-521, ISSN 0174-1551

Decrinis, M.; Pilger, E.; Stark, G.; Lafer, M.; Obernosterer, A. & Lammer J. (1993). A simplified procedure for intra-arterial thrombolysis with tissue-type plasminogen activator in peripheral arterial occlusive disease: primary and long-term results. *European Heart Journal*, Vol.14, No.3, (March 1993), pp. 297–305, ISSN 0195-668X

Do, D.D.; Triller, J.; Walpoth, B.H.; Stirnemann, P. & Mahler, F. (1992). A comparison study of self-expandable stents vs balloon angioplasty alone in femoropopliteal artery occlusions. *Cardiovascular & Interventional Radiology*, Vol.15, No.5, (September 1992), pp. 306-312, ISSN 0174-1551

Do, D.D. & Mahler, F. (1994). Low-dose aspirin combined with dipyridamole versus anticoagulants after femoropopliteal percutaneous transluminal angioplasty. *Radiology*, Vol.193, No.2, (November 1994), pp. 567-571, ISSN 0033-8419

Dörffler-Melly, J.; Koopman, M.M.W.; Prins, M.H. & Büller, H.R. (2005). Antiplatelet and anticoagulant drugs for prevention of restenosis/reocclusion following peripheral endovascular treatment. *Cochrane Database of Syst Rev*, Vol.1., No. CD002071. (Jan 2005). DOI: 10.1002/14651858.CD002071.pub2, ISSN 1469-493X

Dörffler-Melly, J.; Mahler, F.; Do, D.D.; Triller, J. & Baumgartner, I. (2005). Adjunctive abciximab improves patency and functional outcome in endovascular treatment of femoropopliteal occlusions: initial experience. *Radiology*, Vol.237, No.3, (December 2005), pp. 1103-1109, ISSN 0033-8419

Dotter, C.T. & Judkins M.P. (1964). Transluminal treatment of arteriosclerotic obstruction. Description of a new technic and a preliminary report of its application. *Circulation*, Vol.30, No.5, (November 1964), pp. 654-670, ISSN 0009-7322

Faxon, D.P.; Spiro, T.E.; Minor, S.; Minor, S.; Coté, G.; Douglas, J.; Gottlieb, R.; Califf, R.; Dorosti, K.; Topol, E. & Gordon, J.B. (1994). Low molecular weight heparin in prevention of restenosis after angioplasty. Results of Enoxaparin Restenosis (ERA) Trial. *Circulation*, Vol.90, No.2, (August 1994), pp. 908-914, ISSN 0009-7322

Fox, K.A.; Mehta, S.R.; Peters, R.; Zhao, F.; Lakkis, N.; Gersh, B.J. & Yusuf S. (2004). Benefits and risks of the combination of clopidogrel and aspirin in patients undergoing surgical revascularization for non-ST-elevation acute coronary syndrome. The Clopidogrel in Unstable angina to prevent Recurrent ischemic Events (CURE) Trial. *Circulation*, Vol.110, No.10, (September 2004), pp. 1202-1208, ISSN 0009-7322

Fuster, V.; Falk, E.; Fallon, J.T.; Badimon, L.; Chesebro, J.H. & Badimon, J.J. (1995). The three processes leading to post PTCA restenosis: dependence on the lesion substrate. *Thrombosis and Haemostasis*, Vol.74, No.1, (July 1995), pp. 552–559, ISSN 0340-6245

Gallino, A.; Mahler, F.; Probst, P. & Nachbur, B. (1984). Percutaneous transluminal angioplasty of the arteries of the lower limbs: a 5 year follow-up. *Circulation*, Vol.70, No.4, (October 1984), pp. 619-623, ISSN 0009-7322

Girolami, B.; Bernardi, E.; Prins, M.H.; ten Cate, J.W.; Prandoni, P.; Simioni, P.; Andreozzi, G.M.; Girolami, A. & Büller, H.R. (2000). Antiplatelet therapy and other interventions after revascularisation procedures in patients with peripheral arterial disease: a meta-analysis. *Eur J Vasc Endovasc Surg*, Vol.19, No.4, (April 2000), pp. 370-380, ISSN 1078-5884

Gray, B.H.; Conte, M.S.; Dake, M.D.; Jaff, M.R.; Kandarpa, K.; Ramee S.R.; Rundback, J.; Waksman, R. and for the writing Group 7. (2008). Atherosclerotic Peripheral Vascular Disease Symposium II: Lower-Extremity Revascularization: State of the Art. *Circulation*, Vol.118, No.23, (December 2008), pp. 2864-2872, ISSN 0009-7322

Grüntzig, A. & Hopff, H. (1974). Percutaneous recanalization after chronic arterial occlusion with a new dilator-catheter (modification of the Dotter technique). *Deutsche Medizinische Wochenschrift*, Vol.99, No.49, (December 1974), pp. 2502–2011, ISSN 0012-0472

Hankey, G.J.; Norman, P.E. & Eikelboom, J.W. (2006). Medical treatment of peripheral arterial disease. *JAMA*, Vol.295, No.5, (February 2006), pp. 547-553, ISSN 0098-7484

Haudenschild, C.C. (1995). Pathophysiology of reocclusion and restenosis. *Fibrinolysis*, Vol.9, Suppl. 1, (April 1995), pp. 44–47, ISSN 0268-9499

Heiss, H.W.; Just, H.; Middleton, D. & Deichsel, G. (1990). Reocclusion prophylaxis with dipyridamole combined with acetylsalicylic acid following PTA. *Angiology*, Vol.41, No.4, (April 1990), pp. 263–269, ISSN 0003-3197

Hiatt, W.R.; Hoag, S. & Hamman, R.F. (1995). Effect of diagnostic criteria on the prevalence of peripheral arterial disease. The San Luis Valley Diabetes Study. *Circulation*, Vol.91, No.5, (March 1995), pp. 1472-1479, ISSN 0009-7322

Hirsch, A.T.; Haskal, Z.J.; Hertzer, N.R.; Bakal, C.W.; Creager, M.A.; Halperin, J.L.; Hiratzka, L.F.; Murphy, W.R.; Olin, J.W.; Puschett, J.B.; Rosenfield, K.A.; Sacks, D.; Stanley, J.C.; Taylor, L.M. Jr; White, C.J.; White, J.; White, R.A.; Antman, E.M.; Smith, S.C. Jr; Adams, C.D.; Anderson, J.L.; Faxon, D.P.; Fuster, V.; Gibbons, R.J.; Hunt, S.A.; Jacobs, A.K.; Nishimura, R.; Ornato, J.P.; Page, R.L. & Riegel, B.; American Association for Vascular Surgery; Society for Vascular Surgery; Society for Cardiovascular Angiography and Interventions; Society for Vascular Medicine and Biology; Society of Interventional Radiology; ACC/AHA Task Force on Practice Guidelines Writing Committee to Develop Guidelines for the Management of Patients With Peripheral Arterial Disease; American Association of Cardiovascular and Pulmonary Rehabilitation; National Heart, Lung, and Blood Institute; Society for Vascular Nursing; TransAtlantic Inter-Society Consensus; Vascular Disease Foundation. (2006). ACC/AHA 2005 Practice Guidelines for the management of patients with peripheral arterial disease (lower extremity, renal, mesenteric, and abdominal aortic): a collaborative report from the American Association for Vascular Surgery/Society for Vascular Surgery, Society for Cardiovascular Angiography and Interventions, Society for Vascular Medicine and Biology, Society of Interventional Radiology, and the ACC/AHA Task Force on Practice Guidelines (Writing Committee to Develop Guidelines for the Management of Patients With Peripheral Arterial Disease): endorsed by the American Association of Cardiovascular and Pulmonary Rehabilitation; National Heart, Lung, and Blood Institute; Society for Vascular Nursing; TransAtlantic Inter-Society Consensus; and Vascular Disease Foundation. *Circulation*, Vol.113, No.11, (March 2006), pp. e463-654, ISSN 0009-7322

Horrocks, M.; Horrocks, E.H.; Murphy, P.; Lane, I.F.; Ruttley, M.S.; Fligelstone, L.J. & Watson, H.R. (1997). The effects of platelet inhibitors on platelet uptake and restenosis after femoral angioplasty. *Int Angiol*, Vol.16, No.2, (June 1997), pp. 101-106, ISSN 0392-9590

Iida, O.; Nanto, S.; Uematsu, M.; Morozumi, T.; Kitakaze, M. & Nagata, S. (2008). Cilostazol reduces restenosis after endovascular therapy in patients with femoropopliteal lesions. *J Vasc Surg*, Vol.48, No.1, (July 2008), pp. 144-149, ISSN 0741-5214

Jørgensen, B.; Meisner, S.; Holstein, P. & Tønnesen, K.H. (1990). Early rethrombosis in femoropopliteal occlusions treated with percutaneous transluminal angioplasty. *Eur J Vasc Surg*, Vol.4, No.2, (April 1990), pp. 149-152, ISSN 0950-821X

Keller, T.T.; Squizzato, A. & Middeldorp, S. (2007). Clopidogrel plus aspirin versus aspirin alone for preventing cardiovascular disease. *Cochrane Database Syst Rev*, Vol.18, No.3:CD005158, ISSN 0033-8419

Koppensteiner, R.; Spring, S.; Amann-Vesti, B.R.; Meier, T.; Pfammatter, T.; Rousson, V.; Banyai, M. & van der Loo, B. (2006). Low-molecular-weight heparin for prevention of restenosis after femoropopliteal percutaneous transluminal angioplasty: a randomized controlled trial. *J Vasc Surg*, Vol.44, No.6, (December 2006), pp. 1247-1253, ISSN 0741-5214

Mahler, F.; Baumgartner, I. & Do, D.D. (1999). Stenting of the peripheral renal and supraortic arteries and the aorta. *Schweizerische Medizinische Wochenschrift*, Vol.129, No.10, (March 1999), pp. 399-409, ISSN 0036-7672

Mas, J.L.; Chatellier, G.; Beyssen, B.; Branchereau, A.; Moulin, T.; Becquemin, J.P.; Larrue, V.; Lièvre, M.; Leys, D.; Bonneville, J.F.; Watelet, J.; Pruvo, J.P.; Albucher, J.F.; Viguier, A.; Piquet, P.; Garnier, P.; Viader, F.; Touzé, E.; Giroud, M.; Hosseini, H.; Pillet, J.C.; Favrole, P.; Neau, J.P. & Ducrocq, X. for the EVA-3S Investigators. (2006). Endarterectomy versus stenting in patients with symptomatic severe carotid stenosis. *N Engl J Med*, Vol.355, No.16, (October 2006), pp.1660–1671, ISSN 0028-4793

McBride, W.; Lange R.A. & Hillis, L.D. (1988). Restenosis after successful coronary angioplasty. Pathophysiology and prevention. *N Engl J Med*, Vol.318, No.26, (June 1988), pp. 1734-1737, ISSN 0028-4793

Minar, E.; Ahmadi, A.; Koppensteiner, R.; Maca, T.; Stümpflen, A.; Ugurluoglu, A. & Ehringer, H. (1995). Comparison of effects of high-dose and low-dose aspirin on restenosis after femoropopliteal percutaneous transluminal angioplasty. *Circulation*, Vol. 91, No.8, (April 1995), pp. 2167–2173, ISSN 0009-7322

Minar, E.; Pokrajac, B.; Maca, T.; Ahmadi, R.; Fellner, C.; Mittlböck, M.; Seitz, W.; Wolfram, R. & Pötter, R. (2000). Endovascular brachytherapy for prophylaxis of restenosis after femoropopliteal angioplasty: results of a prospective randomized study. *Circulation*, Vol.102, No.22, (November 2000), pp. 2694–2699, ISSN 0009-7322

Norgren, L.; Hiatt, W.R.; Dormandy, J.A.; Nehler, M.R.; Harris, K.A. & Fowkes, F.G.R. on behalf of the TASC II Working Group (2007). Inter-Society Consensus for the Management of Peripheral Arterial Disease (TASC II). *Eur J Vasc Endovasc Surg*, Vol.33, Suppl. 1, (2007), pp. S1-S75, ISSN 1078-5884

Palmaz, J.C.; Sibbitt, R.R.; Reuter, S.R.; Tio, F.O. & Rice, W.J. (1985). Expandable intraluminal graft: a preliminary study. Work in progress. *Radiology*, Vol.156, No.1, (July 1985), pp. 73-77, ISSN 0033-8419

Parmar, J.H.; Aslam, M. & Standfield, N.J. (2010). Significant prostacyclin/thromboxane level imbalance after lower limb arterial angioplasty: a possible platelet function alteration. *J Vasc Interv Radiol*, Vol.21, No.9, (September 2010), pp. 1354-1358, ISSN 1051-0443

Patrono, C.; Bachmann, F.; Baigent, C.; Bode, C.; De Caterina, R.; Charbonnier, B.; Fitzgerald, D.; Hirsh, J.; Husted, S.; Kvasnicka, J.; Montalescot, G.; García Rodríguez, L.A.; Verheugt, F.; Vermylen, J.; Wallentin, L.; Priori, S.G.; Alonso Garcia, M.A.; Blanc, J.J.; Budaj, A.; Cowie, M.; Dean, V.; Deckers, J.; Fernández Burgos, E.; Lekakis, J.; Lindahl, B.; Mazzotta, G.; Morais, J.; Oto, A.; Smiseth, O.A.; Morais, J.; Deckers, J.; Ferreira, R.; Mazzotta, G.; Steg, P.G.; Teixeira, F. & Wilcox, R. European Society of

Cardiology. (2004). Expert Consensus Document on the Use of Antiplatelet Agents. The Task Force on the Use of Antiplatelet Agents in Patients with Atherosclerotic Cardiovascular Disease of the European Society of Cardiology. *Eur Heart J*, Vol.25, No.2, (January 2004), pp. 166-181, ISSN 0195-668X

Peterson, M.B.; Machaj, V.; Block, P.C.; Palacios, I.; Philbin, D. & Watkins, W.D. (1986). Thromboxane release during percutaneous transluminal coronary angioplasty. *Am Heart J*, Vol.111, No.1, (January 1986), pp. 1-6, ISSN 0002-8703

Pilger, E.; Lammer, J.; Bertuch, H.; Stark, J.; Decrinis, M.; Pfeiffer, K.P. & Krejs, G.J. (1991). Nd:YAG laser with sapphire tip combined with balloon angioplasty in peripheral arterial occlusions. Long-term results. *Circulation*, Vol.83, No.1, (January 1991), pp. 141-147, ISSN 0009-7322

Plosker, G.L. & Lyseng-Williamson, K.A. (2007). Clopidogrel: a review of its use in the prevention of thrombosis. *Drugs*, Vol.67, No.4, (2007), pp. 613-646, ISSN 0012-6667

Ranke, C.; Creutzig, A.; Luska, G.; Wagner, H.H.; Galanski, M.; Bode-Böger, S.; Frölich, J.; Avenarius, H.J.; Hecker, H. & Alexander, K. (1994). Controlled trial of high-versus low-dose aspirin treatment after percutaneous transluminal angioplasty in patients with peripheral vascular disease. *Clinical Investig*, Vol.72, No.9, (September 1994), pp. 673–680, ISSN 0941-0198

Rossi, P.; Kuukasjärvi, P.; Salenius, J.P.; Tarkka, M.; Kerttula, T.; Alanko, J.; Mucha, I. & Riutta, A. (1997). Percutaneous transluminal angioplasty increases thromboxane A2 production in claudicants. *Prostaglandins Leukot Essent Fatty Acids*, Vol.56, No.5, (May 1997), pp. 369-372, ISSN 0952-3278

Schillinger, M.; Exner, M.; Mlekusch, W.; Rumpold, H.; Ahmadi, R.; Sabeti. S.; Haumer, M.; Wagner, O. & Minar, E. (2002). Vascular inflammation and percutaneous transluminal angioplasty of the femoropopliteal artery: association with restenosis. *Radiology*, Vol.225. No.1, (October 2002), pp. 21-26, ISSN 0033-8419

Schillinger, M.; Sabeti, S.; Loewe, C.; Dick, P.; Amighi, J.; Mlekusch, W.; Schlager, O.; Cejna, M.; Lammer, J. & Minar, E. (2006). Balloon angioplasty versus implantation of nitinol stents in the superficial femoral artery. *N Eng J Med*, Vol.354, No.18, (May 2006), pp. 1879-1888, ISSN 0028-4793

Schwartz, R.S. (1998). Pathophysiology of restenosis: interaction of thrombosis, hyperplasia, and/or remodeling. *Am J Cardiol*, Vol.81, No.7 Suppl 1, (April 1998), pp. 14E–17E, ISSN 0002-9149

Schweizer, J.; Müller, A.; Forkmann, L.; Hellner, G. & Kirch, W. (2001). Potential use of a low-molecular-weight heparin to prevent restenosis in patients with extensive wall damage following peripheral angioplasty. *Angiology*, Vol.52, No.10, (October 2001), pp. 659–669, ISSN 0003-3197

Sobel, M. & Verhaeghe, R. (2008). Antithrombotic therapy for peripheral artery occlusive disease. American College of Chest Physicians Evidence-Based Clinical Practice Guidelines (8th Edition). *Chest*, Vol.133, No.6 Suppl, (June 2008), pp. 815S-843S, ISSN 0012-3692

SPACE Collaborative Group; Ringleb, P.A.; Allenberg, J.; Brückmann, H.; Eckstein, H.H.; Fraedrich, G.; Hartmann, M.; Hennerici, M.; Jansen, O.; Klein, G.; Kunze, A.; Marx, P.; Niederkorn, K.; Schmiedt, W.; Solymosi, L.; Stingele, R.; Zeumer, H. & Hacke, W. (2006). 30 day results from the SPACE trial of stent-protected angioplasty versus carotid endarterectomy in symptomatic patients: a randomised non-inferiority trial. *Lancet*, Vol.368, No.9543, (October 2006), pp. 1239–1247, ISSN 0140-6736

Strecker, E.P.; Berg, G.; Schneider, B.; Freudenberg, N.; Weber, H. & Wolf, R.D. (1988). A new vascular balloon-expandable prosthesis: experimental studies and first clinical results. *Journal of Interventional Radiology*, Vol.3, No.2, (1988), pp. 59-62, ISSN 1008-794X

Study Group on pharmacological treatment after PTA. (1994). Platelet inhibition with ASA/dipyridamole after percutaneous balloon angioplasty in patients with symptomatic lower limb arterial disease: a prospective double-blind trial. *Eur J Vasc Surg*, Vol.8, No.1, (January 1994), pp. 83-88, ISSN 0950-821X

Taniyama, Y. & Griendling, K.K. (2003). Reactive oxygen species in the vasculature: molecular and cellular mechanisms. *Hypertension*, Vol.42, No.6, (December 2003), pp. 1075-1081, ISSN 0194-911X

Tepe, G.; Zeller, T.; Albrecht, T.; Heller, S.; Schwarzwalder, U.; Beregi, J.; Claussen, C.D.; Oldenburg, A.; Scheller, B. & Speck, U. (2008). Local delivery of paclitaxel to inhibit restenosis during angioplasty of the leg. *N Engl J Med*, Vol.358, No.7, (February 2008), pp. 689-699, ISSN 0028-4793

Timaran, C.H.; Stevens S.L.; Freeman, M.B. & Goldman, M.H. (2001). External iliac and common iliac artery angioplasty and stenting in men and women. *J Vasc Surg*, Vol.34, No.3, (September 2001), pp. 440-446, ISSN 0741-5214

Tsakiris, D.A.; Tschöpl, M.; Jäger, K.; Haefeli, W.E.; Wolf, F. & Marbet, G.A. (1999). Circulating cell adhesion molecules and endothelial markers before and after transluminal angioplasty in peripheral arterial occlusive disease. *Atherosclerosis*, Vol.142, No.1, (January 1999), pp. 193–200, ISSN 0021-9150

Tschöpl, M.; Tsakiris, D.A.; Marbet, G.A.; Labs, K.H. & Jäger, K. (1997). Role of hemostatic risk factors for restenosis in peripheral arterial occlusive disease after transluminal angioplasty. *Arterioscler Thromb Vasc Biol*, Vol.17, No.11, (November 1997), pp. 3208-3214, ISSN 1079-5642

Verheugt, W.F.; Montalescot, G.; Sabatine, M.S.; Soulat, L.; Lambert, Y.; Lapostolle, F.; Adgey, J. & Cannon, C.P. (2007). Prehospital fibrinolysis with dual antiplatelet therapy in ST-elevation acute myocardial infarction: a substudy of the randomized double blind CLARITY-TIMI 28 trial. *J Thromb Thrombolysis*, Vol.23, No.3, (June 2007), pp. 173-179, ISSN 0929-5305

Visonà, A.; Tonello, D.; Zalunardo, B.; Irsara, S.; Liessi, G.; Marigo, L. & Zotta, L. (2009). Antithrombotic treatment before and after peripheral artery percutaneous angioplasty. *Blood Transfus*, Vol.7, No.1, (January 2009), pp.18-23, ISSN 1723-2007

Watson, H.R. & Bergqvist, D. (2000). Antithrombotic agents afeter peripheral transluminal angioplasty: a review of the studies, methods and evidence for their use. *Eur J Vasc Endovasc Surg*, Vol.19, No.5, (May 2000), pp. 445-450, ISSN 1078-5884

Weichert, W.; Meents, H.; Abt, K.; Lieb, H.; Hach, W.; Krzywanek, H.J. & Breddin, H.K. (1994). Acetylsalicylic acid reocclusion prophylaxis after angioplasty (ARPA study). A randomized double-blind trial of two different dosages of ASA in patients with peripheral occlusive arterial disease. *Vasa*, Vol.23, No.1, (1994), pp. 57–65, ISSN 0301-1526

Wentzel, J.J.; Gijsen, F.J.; Stergiopulos, N.; Serruys, P.W.; Slager, C.J. & Krams, R. (2003). Shear stress, vascular remodeling and neointimal formation. *Journal of Biomechanics*, Vol.36, No.5, (May 2003), pp. 681-688, ISSN 0021-9290

Wilson, N.V.; Salisbury, J.R. & Kakkar, V.V. (1991). Effect of low molecular weight heparin on myointimal hyperplasia. *Brit J Surg*, Vol.78, No.11, (November 1991), pp. 1381-1383, ISSN 0007-1323

Wilson, A.M.; Brittenden, J.; Bachoo, P.; Ford, I. & Nixon, G.F. (2009). Randomized controlled trial of aspirin and clopidogrel versus aspirin and placebo on markers of smooth muscle proliferation before and after peripheral angioplasty. *J Vasc Surg*, Vol.59, No.4, (October 2009), pp. 861-869, ISSN 0741-5214

6

Evidence-Based Invasive Treatments for Cerebral Vasospasm Following Aneurysmal Subarachnoid Hemorrhage

Geoffrey Appelboom[1], Adam Jacoby[2], Matthew Piazza[2] and E. Sander Connolly[3]
[1]*Postdoctoral Research Scientist, Department of Neurological Surgery Columbia University, New York, NY*
[2]*Research Fellow, Department of Neurological Surgery Columbia University, New York, NY*
[3]*Bennett M. Stein Professor of Neurological Surgery Columbia University, New York, NY*
USA

1. Introduction

Starting in 1984, the technique of angioplasty was no longer confined to only the treatment of peripheral and coronary arteries. In the original paper investigating the technique of angioplasty in cerebral arteries after cerebral vasospasm from aneurysmal subarachnoid hemorrhage (aSAH) , Zubkov et al. found an overall decrease in headaches and focal neurological deficits after the procedure (Zubkov et al, 1984). Despite advances in both medical and endovascular treatment of cerebral vasospasm since then, vasospasm remains a prominent source of morbidity and mortality for patients in the Neuro-Intensive Care Unit. At an estimated incidence rate of 10-28/100000 people, aSAH is associated with a 20% to 40% risk of development of symptomatic, cerebral vasospasm. Of these patients experiencing symptomatic vasospasm, an estimated 10-15% will die before medical therapy while the other 85-90% will have an overall mortality rate of 32-67% (Weant et al, 2010; Frontera et al, 2009).

In a review of the literature investigating endovascular treatment of cerebral vasospasm, an absence of standardization is present across these studies. Starting from the basics, the literature has not produced a "gold standard" definition of vasospasm. While some groups define vasospasm by a clinical ,neurological deterioration (Andaluz et al, 2002), others use a variety of diagnostic modalities, such as Transcranial Doppler Velocities (Oskouian et al, 2002), digital subtraction angiography (Frontera et al, 2009), and narrowing of vessel diameter via CT angiography (Coenen et al, 1998), to make the same diagnosis. Therefore, assessing the overall efficacy of angioplasty for cerebral vasospasm is difficult when the literature provides different indications for the same treatment.

Once a diagnosis of cerebral vasospasm is confirmed, a lack of standardization continues throughout its treatment. While some groups have associated a good neurological grade upon admission to the hospital and an early, clinical response to initial treatment for vasospasm with improved outcomes, a treatment regimen for vasospasm is far from standardized (Charpentier et al, 1999; Frontera et al, 2010). Although treatment for vasospasm differs from hospital to hospital, most studies examining the management of vasospasm use a combination of hypervolemia, hemodilution, and hypertension (triple-H) therapy as well as the calcium channel blocker nimodipine as their first-line treatments (Frontera et al, 2009). Besides applying these two "core" therapies, recent studies have tried various combinations of endovascular therapies, such as intra-arterial papaverine and verapamil, as well as transluminal balloon angioplasty, first described by Zubkov in 1984 (Frontera et al, 2009; Zubkov et al, 1984). Despite evidence of improved outcomes from papaverine, verapamil, and angioplasty therapies, the absence of a large, prospective, multi-center, randomized, controlled trial, evaluating these treatments has prevented the creation of a gold standard protocol for treatment of vasospasm (Frontera et al, 2009; Zubkov et al, 1984).

2. Definition of vasospasm

Zubkov set the stage for investigating the endovascular treatments of vasospasm after aneurysmal subarachnoid hemorrhage. Epidemiologically, aneurysms are estimated to be present in between 1% and 9% of the population; the incidence of aSAH is around 1 per 10,000 people and increases with age and female sex (Dupont et al, 2010). While the cause of aneurysms and subsequent ruptures are not completely elucidated, risk factors for aSAH include smoking, alcohol use, cocaine use, and hypertension (Dupont et al, 2010).

Cerebral vasospasm after aSAH, macroscopically, is a contraction of smooth muscle in cerebral arteries (Al-Tamimi et al, 2010). This contraction, however, is difficult to measure and define from direct observation. From the articles reviewed, vasospasm definitions can be divided into three categories; groups have defined vasospasm by either clinical indications, Transcranial Doppler Velocity measurements, or by angiographic vessel diameter evidence. While Kaku et al. define vasospasm as a Transcranial Doppler mean flow velocity greater than 100 cm/sec or an increase of more than 30 cm/sec (Kaku et al, 1992) , Firlik et al. report vasospasm by measuring percentage stenosis through angiogram analysis (Firlik et al, 1997). Frontera et al. include a definition for vasospasm, which is defined by the development of new focal neurological symptoms or deficits after other causes have been excluded (Frontera et al, 2011). Below, Table 1 reports the variation in definitions of vasospasm used by different studies in this literature review.

3. Pharmaceutical, non-endovascular treatments of vasospasm

While studies investigating endovascular therapy for cerebral vasospasm are mostly retrospective with a small sample size, a group of prospective, randomized, controlled trials on the efficacy of non-endovascular, pharmaceutical treatment of vasospasm does exist. Recent trials have investigated the efficacy of statins, calcium channel blockers, a nonglucocorticoid aminosteroid, recombinant tissue plasminogen activator, and an endothelin receptor antagonist in vasospasm therapy. Although this review focuses on endovascular treatments for vasospasm, the future of vasospasm therapy also involves non-endovascular treatments.

First Author	Date/Journal	Definition of Vasospasm
Keuskamp	2008, J Neurosurg	Angiographic CT 0, no vasospasm. Mild <20%, Mild Moderate 21-40%, moderate 41-60%, moderate-severe 61-80%. Severe >81% constriction
Firlik	1997, J Neurosurg	Angiographic CT 0, no vasospasm. Mild, <50% stenosis. Moderate 50% stenosis. Severe >50% stenosis.
Kaku	1992, J Neurosurg	Symptomatic (new neurological deficit not attributable to other causes) and TCD velocity >100 cm/sec
Elliott	1998, J Neurosurg	TCD > 120 cm/sec and vessel diameter via CT; >25% narrowing
Coenen	1998, Neurosurgical Focus	25% decrease in the vessel diameter was defined as mild, moderate was 50%, severe was 75%;
Oskouian	2002, Neurosurgical Focus	on TCD measurements alone, VMCA >120 cm/s and HR VMCA/VEC-ICA of more than 3.
Eskridge	1998, Neurosurgery	TCD and Angiography, unclear scales used
Jestaedt	2008, Neurosurgery	TCD > 120 cm/s Retrospective CT angiography 0 , no vasospasm; 1, vessel narrowing less than 70%; 2, vessel narrowing greater than 70%; or 3, subtotal occlusion with high-grade hemodynamic compromise Symptomatic (50% decrease in somatosensory evoked potential amplitutde, increase in somatosensory evoked potential latency or increase of greater than 150 cm/second, or clinical vasospasm by new neurological deficit or loss of two points on GCS), decrease to less than 15 mmHg in tissue oxygenation; also verified via digital subtraction angiography
Beck	2006, J Neurosurg	TCD velocity >120 cm/s in presence of Lindegaard index of>3 and severe vasospasm recorded was >200 cm/s
Zweinenberg-Lee	2008, Stroke	Symptomatic and angiographic >50% narrowing
Frontera	2011, Acta Neurochir Suppl	Symptomatic (delayed neuronal deficits not explained by hydrocephalus, cerebral edema, infection, or other causes)
Katoh	1999, Neurological Focus	TCD velocities; between 150 and 200 cm/s mild vasospasm and >200 moderate and >250 severe
Muizelaar	2001, Acta Neurochir Suppl	Angiographic (mild vasospasm <50% reduction in vessel diameter, moderate = 50% reduction, severe >50% reduction
Kassell	1992, J Neurosurg	Angiographic >50% reduction in diameter
Fujii	1995, Neurosurg Rev	Angiographic; <30% luminal narrowing mild, between 30 and 60% moderate, and over 60% severe
Jun	2010, AJNR	Angiographic; decrease in 50% or more in diameter of vessel segment
Choi	2011, J Korean Neurosurg	Symptomatic (new focal neurological deficit not attributable to seizure, hematoma, brain edema, or hydrocephalus)
Santillan	2011, Neurosurgery	Symptomatic and Angiographic (clinical, not defined greater than 50% constriction of vessel for angiographic)
Murai	2005, Surgical Neurology	Symptomatic defined by onset of delayed neurological deficit with 2 or more decrease on GCS

Table 1.

a. Statin therapy

The statins, or 3-hydroxy-3-methylglutaryl coenzyme A (HMGCoA) reductase inhibitors, have been theorized to have a protective role in the development of cerebral vasospasm. In addition to inhibiting the synthesis of cholesterol, statins are also thought to regulate endothelial and nitric oxide synthase function (Al-Tamimi et al, 2010), and therefore might affect the spasticity of the cerebral vasculature. Two statins, specifically simvastatin and pravastatin, have been investigated in randomized, placebo-controlled, trials. The results on simvastatin treatment of cerebral vasospasm have been mixed. While Vergouwen et al. find that simvastatin treatment provided no improvement on TCD-defined vasospasm (Vergouwen et al, 2009), Chou et al. report that angiographic vasospasm was present in 5/19 patients treated with simvastatin compared with 8/20 patients given a placebo (Chou et al, 2008). No differences, however, are statistically significant. In their meta-analysis, Etminan et al. include only 190 patients and find this number to be too small to make conclusions about the efficacy of statin therapy (Etminan et al, 2011).

b. Calcium antagonist therapy

Nimodipine, a calcium antagonist and part of the current standard of care for treatment of cerebral vasospasm, inhibits calcium entry. However, other pathways exist within the cell that affect calcium utilization and also serve as possible targets for the treatment of vasospasm. In a prospective, randomized, placebo-controlled, double-blind trial, Shibuya et al. investigated the efficacy of AT877, an inhibitor of myosin light-chain kinase, of protein kinases A,G, and C, and of the actions of free intracellular calcium ions (Shibuya et al, 1992). With intravenous therapy of AT877, Shibuya et al. report a statistically significant reduction of angiographic vasospasm by 38% as well as a reduction in symptomatic vasospasm by 30%. Clinically, Shibuya et al. find AT877's effect on outcomes to be similar to nimodipine's; the article reports a significant reduction in poor outcomes associated with vasospasm by 54% and finds no significant adverse side effects (Shibuya et al, 1992). A possible downside of treatment with AT877 is its short half-life. Although Shibuya et al. report that AT877's metabolite still shows spasmolytic qualities, the parent compound has an estimated half-life of under fifteen minutes.

c. Treatment with tirilizad mesylate

In response to the possible connection between free radical-induced lipid peroxidation and vasospasm, the 21 aminosteroid, tirilazad meslyate, was created to inhibit this pathway (Kassell et al, 1996). In a prospective, randomized, double-blind, controlled trial of 1023 patients, Kassell et al. investigated the efficacy of tirilazad mesylate, using symptomatic vasospasm and Glasgow Outcome Scale scores at three months as outcome measures. Although Kassell et al. do not report a statistically significant reduction in symptomatic vasospasm with aSAH after treatment with tirilazad mesylate, they argue for the presence ($p=.048$) of a decrease in vasospasm at higher doses of tirilazad mesylate. The most promising statistics from this article, however, concern the three month outcomes for patients in the treatment group. Kassell et al. report in the highest dosage of tirilazad mesylate, 63% of patients had a good recovery, compared to 53% of the vehicle treated group (Kassell et al, 1996). This difference was statistically significant. Despite minor injection site phlebitis, tirilazad mesylate was not associated with life-threatening or adverse medical events.

d. Endothelin receptor antagonist therapy

Systemic vasoconstriction is controlled by many physiological hormones, including adrenergic agonists, angiotensin II, and antidiuretic hormone. Endothelin, a powerful vasoconstrictor possibly increased after aSAH (Macdonald et al, 2008) and its pathway to vasoconstriction have been investigated for possible targets in the treatment of vasospasm. Specifically, Macdonald et al. looked at the efficacy of the endothelin receptor antagonist, clazosentan, in the prospective, randomized, double-blind, placebo-controlled CONSCIOUS-1 trial. While Macdonald et al. report no significant difference between the treatment and control groups with respect to morbidity and mortality, they find a reduction of moderate or severe vasospasm from 66% in the placebo group to 23% in the highest dosage treatment group (Macdonald et al, 2008). Complications associated with clazosentan administration included anemia, hypotension and pulmonary issues including pneumonia, pleural effusions, pulmonary edema, and acute respiratory distress syndrome. The results of the CONSCIOUS-1 trial point to the disconnect between vasospasm and clinical outcome. While Macdonald et al. report a decrease in vasospasm from digital subtraction angiography after treatment, they find no effect on morbidity and mortality (Macdonald et al, 2008). Like other studies in this review of the literature, this trial calls for further exploration in the connection between vasospasm and clinical consequences.

e. Fibrinolytic therapy

The correlation between subarachnoid clot thickness and degree of vasospasm led to the possibility of fibrinolytic therapy in the treatment of cerebral vasospasm. In a prospective, randomized, blinded, placebo-controlled trial by Findlay, the efficacy of intracisternal, recombinant tissue plasminogen activator for prevention of vasospasm was investigated with angiographic vasospasm serving as the primary endpoint (Findlay, 1995) Although Findlay reports angiographic vasospasm in 74.4% of placebo patients and 64.6% of treatment patients, the difference between the two groups was not statistically significant (P=.31) An interesting, significant finding from the same study comes from the treatment of patients with thick subarachnoid clots. In this group, Findlay finds a 56% relative risk reduction of severe vasospasm in the treatment group, suggesting a very specific indication for treatment with recombinant tissue plasminogen activator. While Findlay also reports a pattern of lower mean velocities on transcranial Doppler, reduced delayed neurological worsening, a lower 14 day mortality rate, and improved 3 month outcome in the treatment group, none of these findings was statistically significant (Findlay, 1995). As with all fibrinolytic treatment, the possibility of treatment associated hemorrhage presents as a risk.

While these studies, investigating the efficacy of pharmaceutical, non-endovascular treatments of vasospasm, are well-designed and have promising results, future larger scale, multi-center trials, with mortality serving as a primary outcome measure, would help determine which therapies should be added to the standard protocol for treatment of cerebral vasospasm.

4. Current institutional protocols for treatment of aSAH and vasospasm

While a standard of care has not been completely established for the treatment of cerebral vasospasm, common themes are ubiquitous throughout a review of the literature. After diagnosis of aSAH, the following treatment can be divided into two sections, common to most recent studies. The first part of therapy involves stabilizing the patient's aSAH while the second focuses on the prevention or management of cerebral vasospasm. Before cerebral vasospasm is even considered, the aSAH is ideally treated surgically by either endovascular coiling or clipping. However, the timing of surgery, similar to the definition of cerebral vasospasm, has not been completely standardized. While Choi et al.'s protocol (Choi et al,

2011) calls for surgery within twenty four hours of the aSAH, Murai et al. include patients whose aneurysms had been clipped or coiled within forty eight hours of aSAH (Murai et al, 2005). After the subarachnoid hemorrhage has been managed surgically, the goal of therapy begins to focus on the treatment of cerebral vasospasm.

Typically after surgery today, patients are then treated with oral nimodipine and a combination of induced hypertension, hemodilution, and volume expansion ("Triple-H") therapy to minimize the effects of cerebral vasospasm (Komotar et al, 2008). Nimodipine, a dihydropyridine calcium channel blocker, which blocks L-type, slow conducting, voltage-dependent, calcium channels, has been shown to reduce cerebral infarction, when compared to untreated patients (Weant et al, 2010) , while triple-H therapy focuses on maintaining high cerebral perfusion pressures to increase cerebral blood flow during vasospasm (Komotar et al, 2008).

These treatments, however, are not applied without controversy. With Triple-H therapy comes the risk of possible organ damage, pulmonary edema, and organ ischemia. On the other hand, the use of nimodipine in the treatment of cerebral vasospasm has raised questions about the connection between cerebral vasospasm and poor outcomes. Mechanistically, the administration of a calcium channel blocker "makes sense"; prevention of an increasing concentration of intracellular calcium should reduce smooth muscle contraction within the cerebral vasculature.

While Pickard et al. do report a significant reduction in cerebral infarction events in those treated with nimodipine after aSAH (Pickard et al, 1989), they do not find a change in Transcranial Doppler Velocities between those treated and the controls. It has been suggested that antithrombotic actions of nimodipine might be responsible for its therapeutic effects (Weant et al, 2010). Nimodpine's clinical benefits without changing Transcranial Doppler Velocities suggests that vasospasm may be correlated with adverse clinical outcomes but may not cause them. Similarly, Frontera et al. report that a Transcranial Doppler Velocity greater than 120 cm/sec, a measurement indicative of vasospasm, is not necessarily a predictor of clinical outcome (Frontera et al, 2009). A recent meta-analysis by Etminan et al., investigating the efficacy of pharmaceutical treatment on delayed cerebral ischemia (DCI), also reported a decrease in radiographic vasospasm without clinical benefit (Etminan et al, 2011). The exact relationship between vasospasm and clinical outcome must still be fully elucidated.

Although nimodipine and Triple-H therapy have been shown to improve clinical outcome, even administration of these therapies are not standardized. While Zweinenberg-Lee et al. report a protocol (Zwienenberg-Lee et al, 2008) of maintaining hematocrit levels between 30-35%, Oskouian et al.'s protocol (Oskouian et al, 2002) calls for a target of 31-35%. Similarly, across these studies on the treatment of vasospasm, a common, unifying goal of hypertensive therapy is not present. Rosenwasser et al. report elevating mean arterial pressure to 130-140 mm Hg (Rosenwasser et al, 1999), while Oskouian et al. present a protocol calling for a perfusion pressure of 70 mm Hg (Oskouian et al, 2002) and Coyne et al. report a maintenance level of 240 mm Hg for systolic blood pressure (Coyne et al, 1994). The methods to achieve high levels of cerebral blood flow and hypertension are also not standardized. While Keuskamp et al. report using neosynephrine, ephedrine, and dopamine in their triple-H therapy (Keuskamp et al, 2008), Murai et al. use dobutamine alone (Murai et al, 2005). Therefore, the current "gold standard," a combination of Triple-H therapy and nimodipine, is not uniformly executed.

5. Experimental endovascular treatments for vasospasm

Besides medical therapy with intravenous or oral nimodipine and Triple-H therapy, cerebral vasospasm after aSAH, has been experimentally treated with methods that are theoretically sound. While nitric oxide donors, phosphodiesterase inhibitors, endothelin antogonists, statins, and magnesium (Weant et al, 2010; Fathi et al, 2001; Shankar et al, 2011) have all been investigated for treating cerebral vasospasm through expected vasodilatory effects, the focus of current endovascular studies has predominantly remained on intra-arterial medical therapy with the calcium channel antagonist ,verapamil ,or the posphodiesterase inhibtor, papaverine, or transluminal balloon angioplasty of the affected vessels.

a. Intra-arterial medical treatment and its efficacy

The methods of administering intra-arterial medical therapy differ slightly from group to group and depend on the specific article from the review of the literature. A representative technique, however, is described by Feng et al . A 5F or 6F guiding catheter is used to infuse the specified drug in the internal carotid or vertebral arteries. With this technique, the physician hopes to deliver medical therapy to the spastic vessels (Feng et al, 2002). Some groups, such as Jun et al., report a slightly different protocol if severe vasospasm is present in the ACA or MCA.; they describe using a microcatheter to reach the spastic portions of the ACA and MCA to deliver medical therapy (Jun et al, 2010).

Although most studies evaluating the efficacy of intra-arterial medical therapy and angioplasty are retrospective with a relatively small sample size, they do show some promise in the treatment of cerebral vasospasm. While Kaku et al. report an improvement in neurological function in 80% of patients treated with intra-arterial papaverine (Kaku et al, 1992), Keuskamp et al. describe a median reduction of 2 units on their vasospasm scale after treatment with intra-arterial verapamil (Keuskamp et al, 2008). However, the data on intra-arterial medical treatment of cerebral vasospasm are not completely straightforward; Coenen et al. report that the benefits from intra-arterial papaverine administration are neither reliable nor sustained. Another problem that arises in comparing studies, evaluating the efficacy of intra-arterial medical treatment, is the dosage of drug administered (Coenen et al, 1998). While Kassell et. al use 100-300 mg of papaverine in their protocol (Kassell et al, 1992) , Firlik et al. report using between 300 and 600 mg of the same drug (Firlik et al, 1997). It is difficult to generalize the efficacy of intra-arterial medical therapy given the variety of dosage protocols across studies in this literature review.

However, intra-arterial treatment of cerebral vasospasm does not come without risk. Investigating the risks of intra-arterial verapamil infusion and papaverine therapy respectively, Feng et al. and Keuskamp et al. find no significant changes in intracranial pressure, heart rate, or hemodynamic parameters after intra-arterial treatment (Feng et al, 2002; Keuskamp et al, 2008). These are not the only parameters, however, by which safety of intra-arterial therapies should be assessed. Intra-arterial administration of papaverine and verapamil have both been associated with case reports of seizures (Zubkov et al, 1984) while papaverine alone has been linked to aphasia, mental status changes, and even respiratory arrest. On the cellular level, papaverine might also adversely affect neuronal mitochondrial respiration (Weant et al, 2010). Although Feng et al. and Keuskamp et al. report that intra-arterial therapy is safe, further research should be conducted before verapamil or papaverine use is widely accepted as treatment for vasospasm.

b. Angioplasty for cerebral vasospasm and its efficacy

Beginning in 1984, the treatment of cerebral vasospasm after aSAH came to include the physical dilation of cerebral arteries using transluminal balloon angioplasty. The original

technique of angioplasty, described by Zubkov et al., involved puncturing the common carotid artery and placing a balloon catheter in the internal carotid artery. In an X-ray room, the balloon catheter was then repetitively inflated and deflated in the proximal part of the affected artery. This procedure then continued distally and after this technique, cerebral blood flow was monitored with a Xe-133 administration (Zubkov et al, 1984).
Since Zubkov's original paper, the actual technique of angioplasty has progressed at a relatively slow rate; today, angioplasty very much resembles the original procedure performed by Zubkov, including the repetitive inflation-deflation cycles. Similar to the description of intra-arterial medical treatment for vasospasm, the current techniques of angioplasty differ slightly from group to group and depend on the specific article from the literature. A representative method of angioplasty for cerebral vasospasm is described by Jun et al (Jun et al, 2010). In this study, Jun et al. report intravenous heparinization prior to angioplasty. Unlike Zubkov et al., they begin treating the distal portions of the spastic artery before the proximal portions. Although angioplasty for cerebral vasospasm has shown promise with respect to clinical outcomes, the technique is not without limitations. Terada et al. and Jun et al. both exclude smaller, distal cerebral arteries as targets of treatment with angioplasty for fear of vessel rupture (Terada et al, 1997; Jun et al, 2010). While each group "sets their own limits" with respect to the smallest vessel they will treat with angioplasty, Jun et al. report treating vasospasm in the supraclinoid ICA, M1 MCA, A1 ACA, intracranial vertebral artery, basilar artery, and P1 PCA (so called "proximal vessels"), while they find treatment of M2 MCA, A2 ACA, P2 PCA (so called "distal vessels") to be too risky (Jun et al, 2010). With every procedure comes the possibility of complications. While the risks of mechanical dilation of spastic cerebral vessels by transluminal angioplasty are lessened by a skilled physician, they are still present. Vessel rupture, thrombosis, and occlusion are possible complications during the angioplasty procedure (Weant et al, 2010).
Since Zubkov's paper, studies have investigated the efficacy of his technique. Overall, the results of cerebral angioplasty have been promising; in a 50 patient pilot study, Eskridge et al. report a 61% sustained neurological improvement after angioplasty (Eskridge et al, 1998). Although most studies in this literature review look positively upon angioplasty for cerebral vasospasm, not all trials have proven to be efficacious. While Fujii et al. and Eskridge et al., respectively, describe an 83% increase in diameters of affected cerebral arteries (Fujii et al, 1995) and a 73% recovery in patients experiencing focal neurological deficits after treatment (Eskridge et al, 1990), Coenen et al. find angioplasty to be an unreliable method of treating cerebral vasospasm. Similar to other conclusions made in this literature review, the results of these retrospective angioplasty trials do not provide a straightforward judgment on its efficacy (Coenen et al, 1998).
Once again, comparing these studies, which assess the efficacy of angioplasty for cerebral vasospasm, is difficult given the absence of standardization of the procedure. One difference, amongst groups, lies in the type and size of balloon used during angioplasty. For example, while Eskridge et al. use a 3 mm. x 12 mm. silicone balloon from Target Therapeutics (Eskridge et al, 1998) , Bejjani et al. report using a 3.5 mm. Cirrus balloon (Bejjani et al, 1998). While these differences might not practically affect the procedure or its results, they should be considered when evaluating the efficacy of this technique.

c. Comparison of angioplasty with intra-arterial medical therapy

Although retrospectively, the efficacy of intra-arterial medical therapy and angioplasty for vasospasm have been compared. Similar to the studies on the efficacy of both of these modes of treatment, the groups comparing these two therapies have produced mixed results. Elliott et al. report a favorable clinical outcome in 67% of patients after angioplasty compared with a 62% favorable outcome after treatment with papaverine (Elliott et al, 1998), while Katoh et al. report a 58% clinical improvement after angioplasty compared with a 25% improvement after papaverine (Katoh et al, 1999). Elliiott et al. also report an increase in Transcranial Doppler velocities on Day 2 after treatment with papaverine, suggesting an absence of sustainable effect from the papaverine (Elliott et al, 1998). Although these studies suggest that angioplasty is a more effective endovascular treatment for cerebral vasospasm, the data are not all one-sided. Coenen et al. report that both angioplasty and papaverine are equivalently ineffective in producing reliable and sustained results (Coenen et al, 1998). Theoretically, an interesting procedure would be combining both angioplasty and intra-arterial medical therapy in the same treatment.

d. Combination therapy with angioplasty and intra-arterial medical treatment

Since it is believed that angioplasty in smaller, more distal vessels, is too risky, it is logical that a combination of intra-arterial medical treatment with angioplasty might be effective in treating both proximal and distal cerebral vasospasm. In a retrospective study by Frontera et al. the group compares combined therapy with chemical vasodilation alone. Frontera et al. find that while 39% of patients undergoing combination therapy developed recurrent angiographic and symptomatic vasospasm, 82% of patients receiving chemical vasodilation, alone, developed vasospasm (Frontera et al, 2011). Future, large-scaled and multicenter trials on the efficacy of combination therapy should help elucidate the most effective combinations of medical endovascular treatment with angioplasty.

Amongst these experimental, endovascular treatments, angioplasty seems beneficial for the larger, more proximal, and more accessible cerebral vessels while treatment with intra-arterial papaverine and verapamil is more appropriate for smaller, more distal, and less accessible arteries where a large risk of rupture is present.

6. Limitations to efficacy comparisons across studies

However, problems with these studies, investigating the efficacy of experimental treatments for cerebral vasospasm, do exist. The small sample sizes and retrospective nature of a vast majority of these studies make it difficult to establish definitive conclusions with respect to efficacy of different endovascular treatments. Also, the criteria to begin endovascular treatment differ from group to group. For example, while Bejjani et al report treating vasospasm with angioplasty only after Triple-H therapy has failed (Bejjani et al, 1998) , Santillan et al. use a decrease in vessel diameter via angiography as one if their indications for treatment (Santillan et al, 2011). Therefore, constructing a meta-analysis, combining the results of these studies, is difficult as different groups make their own decisions about when to treat patients endovascularly. Table 2, below, lists the criteria to treat cerebral vasospasm, from several groups, reviewed in the literature.

7. Recommendations for invasive treatments

Although most experimental studies investigating the efficacy of invasive treatments for cerebral vasospasm after aSAH are retrospective in nature, effective patterns can be extracted from these studies. From the studies in this literature review, it appears that Triple-H therapy combined with administration of nimodipine is the first line of treatment or prevention of cerebral vasospasm. Once the vasospasm is deemed refractory to this

Author/Date	Indication for Endovascular Treatment
Feng, 2002	Verapamil was given "to prevent catheter-induced vasospasm," for treatment of mild vasospasm that did not warrant angioplasty, and for the treatment of moderate to severe vasospasm that could not be safely treated with angioplasty
Firlik, 1997	CBF new region < 20 ml/100 g/minute were treated with angioplasty
Bejjani, 1998	Do angioplasty after failed HHH therapy; digital subtraction angiography performed first.
Kaku 1992	Angioplasty (to deliver papaverine) if onset of new neurological deficit not attributable to other causes, no evidence of infarction on CT, unsuccessful treatment of neurological deficit by conventional medical and pharmacological therapies, mean flow velocity 100 cm/sec or increase in mean flow velocity greater than 30 cm/sec w/in 24 hours in affected vessel by TCD, and vasospasm seen angiographically in location consistent with neurological deficit.
Terada, 1997	Endovascular therapy if new neurological signs appear after SAH, not deriving from hematoma, brain edema, or hydrocephalus, neurological signs are related to vascular territory of vasospasm, vessel diameter is less than 50% of initial diameter angiographically, no low density area is related to vasospasm on CT, clinical signs progress despite medical treatment, and ruptured aneurysm has been treated
Andaluz, 2002	Refractory vasospasm (not clearly defined) to HHH therapy; included if all aneurysm clipped or coiled before Day 3 after SAH, clinical vasospasm defined by the presence of a new neurologic deficit not explained by hydrocephalus, infection, electrolyte imbalance, or other medical complication, clinical vasospasm in patients treated with nimodipine and with symptoms not reversed by maximal HHH treatment, and endovascular therapy instituted w/in 12 hours of onset of symptoms
Eskridge, 1998	hypertensive therapy started if suspicion of vasospasm; angioplasty if new onset of a neurological deficit not attributable to other causes, no evidence of established cerebral infarction on CT scans, deficit persisting despite hypertensive, hypervolemic therapy, and angiographic evidence of vasospasm in a distribution that could explain the deficit
Rosenwasser, 1999	If new deficit, CT scan to eliminate hydrocephalus or bleeding. HHH therapy maximized to elevate MAP to 130-140 mm Hg. If not reversible then go to get angioplasty
Jestaedt, 2008	Clinical symptoms or high grade vessel narrowing (>70%)
Beck, 2006	HHH protocol; symptoms still then get MR; if PW DW mismatch then continue HHH; then DS angiography then TBA
Zwienenberg-Lee, 2008	Randomized to either angioplasty or no angioplasty
Frontera 2011	All patients digital subtraction angiography; vessels which responded to IACV and could not be treated with angioplasty only IACV; accessible vessels with residual vasospasm after IACV then TBA
Eskridge, 1990	Inclusion criteria included new onset of a neurologic deficit after subarachnoid hemorrhage that was not attributable to other causes, such as hydrocephalus, hematoma, mass effect, no evidence of infarction on CT scan, neurologic deficit not reversed by hypervolemic and hypertensive therapy, and angiographically apparent vasospasm in location responsible for deficit
Muizelaar, 2001	All patients had SAH and Fisher Grade III on CT scan w/in first two days of SAH; had to have surgical or neurointerventional treatment of ruptured aneurysm; then TBP could be performed

Fujii, 1995	developed symptomatic vasospasm in spite of intensive medical supportive therapy including hypertension, volume expansion, and administration of brain protective agents, the cases whose showed either consciousness deterioration worse than 30 in Japan Coma Scale and/or distinct neurological deficit, and cases whose angiogram performed as early as possible after emergence of symptoms showed the responsible narrowing in intracranial arteries.
Jun, 2010	Severe proximal CV (luminal narrowing >60%) treated with PTA and distal CV (luminal narrowing >30%) with verapamil
Choi, 2011	CT scan in patients with clinical deterioration; vasospasm defined as increase in TCD flow to 150 cm/second. If greater than 150 cm/second, MRI, DWI and MRA; if infraction or narrowing by MRA, angioplasty was recommended
Santillan, 2011	Indication for TBA neurological deficits were referable to vascular territory of the VSP angiographically, vessel diameter less than 50% of initial diameter angiographically, no evidence of hypodensity on non-contrast head CT scan suggestive of ischemic infarct due to VSP prior to angiogram, and baseline diameter of vessel on initial cerebral angiogram or CT was not less than approximately 2 mm in size.
Murai, 2005	DINDs assumed vasospasm if between 3-14 days after SAH; some had angiograms to determine vasospasm (50% or more narrowing when compared to admission CT); heparinization w/angioplasty if deficit could be related to distribution of vasospasm
Coyne, 1994	Symptomatic vasospasm defined as onset of delayed neurological deficit (2 or more decrease on Glasgow Coma Scale); treated initially with hypervolemia, hypertensive therapy; maintain a capillary wedge pressure of 14 to 18 mm Hg. Maintain a systolic BP of 240 mm HG in clipping or 160 mm HG in unclipped; angioplasty if neurological deficit/CT showed no improvement

Table 2.

treatment, invasive treatments should be employed next. A combination of verapamil or papaverine to treat distal vasospasm with angioplasty to treat proximal vasospasm in larger, more available vessels falls in line with conclusions of many of the studies reviewed. Timing of invasive treatments may also prove to be critical. Rosenwasser's retrospective study finds improved clinical and angiographic outcomes in patients treated with angioplasty within a two hour window (Rosenwasser et al, 1999). Therefore, combined intra-arterial treatment with either papaverine or verapamil and angioplasty within a timely manner appears to be the most effective treatment.

8. Unclear role of vasospasm in clinical outcomes

A review of the literature on invasive treatments for cerebral vasospasm has highlighted a possible disconnect between the presence of cerebral vasospasm and clinical outcome. Frontera's group and Macdonald's group respectively find that Transcranial Doppler Velocities (Frontera et al, 2009) and angiography (Macdonald et al, 2008), consistent with cerebral vasospasm, are not necessarily predictors of a specific clinical outcome. These findings have led to the hypothesis that other mechanisms, after aSAH, may be responsible for poor clinical outcomes. Specifically, early brain injury, before the onset of vasospasm, has been explored. Classically, cerebral vasospasm is thought to occur between four and nine days after the ictus. Early brain injury, defined as injury within 72 hours of the aSAH, may provide insight into poor clinical outcomes after aSAH (Pluta et al, 2009). Within these 72 hours, early brain injury has been associated with an elevation of intracranial pressure, a reduction in cerebral blood flow, blood-brain barrier disruption and neuronal cell death (Pluta et al, 2009). These changes, and not cerebral vasospasm, may be responsible for the subsequent clinical outcome.

Another recently proposed mechanism for the development of poor clinical outcomes has also been suggested. A mixture, similar to that of cerebrospinal fluid after SAH, has been shown to cause spreading cortical depolarization after application to the subarachnoid space (Pluta et al, 2009). This, in turn, has led to eventual ischemia and cortical necrosis. Similarly, 13 out of 18 patients, receiving surgical treatment after aSAH, have been shown to have similar waves of depolarization, consistent with the start of clinical deterioration (Pluta et al, 2009). Therefore, in addition to vasospasm, early brain injury and spreading cortical depolarization should be investigated for their importance in clinical outcomes.

9. Future directions in the treatment of cerebral vasospasm

Theoretically, endovascular therapy for cerebral vasospasm may include treatments other than intra-arterial pharmaceutical administration and cerebral artery angioplasty. Komotar et al. mention the possibility of using intra-aortic balloon counterpulsation to treat vasospasm. In this technique, an aortic balloon is placed distally to the origin of the left subclavian artery endovascularly. During diastole, the balloon inflates, redirecting blood to the coronary, carotid, and vertebral arteries in this part of the cardiac cycle (Komotar et al, 2008). The balloon then deflates during systole. The authors of this study report an average increase in cerebral blood flow by 69.3% (Nussbaum et al, 1998). Since the goal of Triple-H therapy is to improve cerebral blood flow, the intra-aortic balloon might be used in combination therapy with medical treatment for the reduction of cerebral vasospasm and ischemia after aSAH. As this device is implanted in the femoral artery, risks such as hemorrhage and dissection of the femoral artery are present (Komotar et al, 2008). A case report, by Appelboom et al., describes a similar procedure with a Neuroflo, intra-aortic, dual balloon catheter. In this report, two balloons, one above and one below the renal arteries, are inflated to redirect blood flow to the cerebral arteries during refractory vasospasm. An advantage of this technique is the avoidance of complications associated with direct manipulation of cerebral vasculature (Appelboom et al, 2010).

The future of cerebral vasospasm therapy depends on further elucidation of the pathophysiology of this condition. Komotar et al. report initial success with another free radical trapping agent. Just like tirilizad mesylate, disodium 2,4-disulfophenyl-N-tert-butylnitrone inhibits lipid peroxidation and has been associated with improvement in neurological function in primates (Komotar et al, 2008). Other evidence has suggested that the pathogenesis of vasospasm may depend on the immune system. Preventing the interaction between leukocytes and endothelial cells with blocking antibodies has also inhibited vasospasm after aSAH (Baybek et al, 1998). Similarly, patients undergoing therapy with steroids have a lower risk of developing delayed ischemic deficits after aSAH (Chyatte et al, 1987). The interplay between the immune system and development of cerebral vasospasm needs to be further investigated before immune modulating therapy can be directed towards the treatment of vasospasm.

10. Conclusion

A review of the literature on endovascular treatment for cerebral vasospasm has suggested the need for commonly used protocols and definitions to determine the efficacy of these therapies. Although most studies in this review provided protocols that used Triple-H therapy and nimodipine as a first line treatment for cerebral vasospasm, the variation in institutional protocols in these studies made comparisons difficult. Similarly, the absence of a unifying or "gold standard" definition of vasospasm suggests that different indications in each study might call for the same treatment. Given that studies in this analysis use either CT angiography, symptoms, or Transcranial Doppler Velocities to assess for vasospasm, it is difficult to know if each study would treat the same patient for the same degree of vasospasm. It is therefore difficult to compare the results of different studies, investigating the same treatment. Similarly, the actual endovascular therapy, either intra-arterial medical treatment or transluminal angioplasty, was not the same in each study. Both the dosage of intra-arterial drug administered and the type and size of angioplasty balloon differed amongst the studies in this review of the literature.

The retrospective nature and small sample size of an overwhelming majority of the studies in this review call for a newly designed, novel study in the endovascular treatment of vasospasm. Zweinenberg-Lee et al. provide data from a Phase II, Multicenter, Randomized, Clinical Trial assessing the effects of prophylactic angioplasty on infarction rates after cerebral vasospasm. The results of this trial, that prophylactic angioplasty provided an absolute risk reduction of 5.9% for developing an infarction after cerebral vasospasm (Zweienenberg-Lee et al, 2008), may serve as a model for future trials assessing the efficacy of endovascular treatments of vasospasm although not all the data were statistically significant. Future research on endovascular treatment of vasospasm should also follow the study design of trials investigating non-endovascular, pharmaceutical therapy for vasospasm. These studies, included in Etminan's meta-analysis, are prospective, randomized, adequately blinded, and placebo or vehicle controlled (Etminan et al, 2011).

This literature review has highlighted the need for a highly controlled, randomized, multicenter, clinical trial, assessing the efficacy of endovascular treatment. A randomized, controlled, clinical trial placing patients into either an intra-arterial papaverine group, an intra-arterial verapamil group, an intra-arterial papaverine and angioplasty group, an intra-arterial verapamil and angioplasty group, and an angioplasty group alone would provide the groundwork for a standardized protocol for effectively treating cerebral vasospasm endovascularly. Similarly, future studies should investigate vasospasm's role in affecting clinical outcomes and possible novel treatments. The future of vasospasm treatment, however, depends on further elucidation of the pathophysiology of vasospasm after aSAH. The role of the immune system and lipid peroxidation after aSAH should be investigated in the pathogenesis of this condition.

11. References

Al-Tamimi YZ, Orsi NM, Quinn AC, Homer-Vanniasinkam S, Ross SA (2010) A review of delayed ischemic neurologic deficit following aneurysmal subarachnoid hemorrhage: historical overview, current treatment, and pathophysiology. World Neurosurg 73(6): 654-67.

Andaluz N, Tomsick TA, Tew JM, van Loveren HR, Yeh HS, Zuccarello M (2002) Indications for endovascular therapy for refractory vasospasm after aneurysmal subarachnoid hemorrhage: Experience at the University of Cincinnati. Surgical Neurology 58:2 131-138.

Appelboom G, Strozyk D, Hwayng BY, Prowda J, Badjatia N, Helbok R, Meyers PM (2010) Bedside Use of a Dual Aortic Balloon Occlusion for the Treatment of Cerebral Vasospasm. Neurocirt Care 13:385-388.

Bavbek M, Polin R, Kwan AL, Arthur AS, Kassell NF, Lee KS (1998) Monoclonal antibodies against ICAM-1 and CD18 attenuate cerebral vasospasm after experimental subarachnoid hemorrhage in rabbits. Stroke 29(9):1930-5.

Bejjani GK, Bank WO, Olan WJ, Sekhar LN (1998) The efficacy and safety of angioplasty for cerebral vasospasm after subarachnoid hemorrhage. Neurosurgery 42(5): 979-986.

Charpentier C, Audibert G, Guillemin F, Civit T, Ducrocq X, Bracard S, Hepner H, Picard L, Laxenaire MC (1999) Multivariate analysis of predictors of cerebral vasospasm occurrence after aneurysmal subarachnoid hemorrhage. Stroke 30: 7 1402-1408.

Choi BJ, Lee TH, Lee JI, Ko JK, Park HS, and Choi CH (2011) Safety and Efficacy of Transluminal Balloon Angioplasty Using a Compliant Balloon for Severe Cerebral Vasospasm after an Aneurysmal Subarachnoid Hemorrhage. J Korean Neurosurg Soc. 49(3): 157-162.

Chou SH, Smith EE, Badjatia N, Nogueria RG, Sims JR 2nd, Ogilvy CS, Rordor GA, Ayata C (2008) A randomized, double-blind, placebo-controlled pilot study of simvastatin in aneurysmal subarachnoid hemorrhage. Stroke 39(10): 2891-3.

Chyatte D, Fode NC, Nichols DA, Sundt TM Jr (1987) Preliminary report: effects of high dose methylprednisolone on delayed cerebral ischemia in patients at high risk for vasospasm after aneurysmal subarachnoid hemorrhage. Neurosurgery 21(2):157-60.

Coenen VA, Hansen CA, Kassell NF, Polin RS (1998) Endovascular treatment for symptomatic cerebral vasospasm after subarachnoid hemorrhage: transluminal balloon angioplasty compared with intraarterial papaverine. Neurosurg Focus 5 (4): Article 6.

Coyne TJ, Montanera WJ, Macdonald RL, Wallace MC (1994) Percutaneous transluminal angioplasty for cerebral vasospasm after subarachnoid hemorrhage. Can J Surg 37(5): 391-396.

Dupont SA, Wijdicks EF, Lanzino G, Rabinstein AA (2010) Aneurysmal subarachnoid hemorrhage: an overview for the practicing neurologist. Semin Neurol 30(5): 545-54.

Elliott JP, Newell DW, Lam DJ, Eskridge JM, Douville CM, Le Roux PD, Lewis DH, Mayberg MR, Grady MS, Winn, HR (1998) Comparison of balloon angioplasty and papaverine infusion for the treatment of vasospasm following aneurysmal subarachnoid hemorrhage. J Neurosurg 88: 277-284.

Eskridge JM, McAuliffe W, Song JK, Deliganis AV, Newell DW, Lewis DH, Mayberg MR, Winn RH (1998) Balloon Angioplasty for the Treatment of Vasospasm: Results of First 50 Cases. Neurosurgery 42 (3): 510-517.

Eskridge JM, Newell DW, Pendleton GA (1990) Transluminal Angioplasty for Treatment of Vasospasm. Cerebral vasospasm 1(2) : 387-399.

Etminan N, Vergouwen MD, Ilodigwe D, Macdonald RL (2011) Effect of pharmaceutical treatment on vasospasm, delayed cerebral ischemia, and clinical outcome in patients with aneurysmal subarachnoid hemorrhage: a systematic review and meta-analysis. J Cereb Blood Flow Metab 31(6):1443-1451

Fathi AR, Bakthian KD, Pluta RM (2001) The role of nitric oxide donors in treating cerebral vasospasm after subarachnoid hemorrhage. Acta Nuerochir Suppl 110: 93-97.

Feng L, Fitzsimmons BF, Young WL, Berman MF, Lin E, Aagaard BDL, Duong H, Pile-Spellman J (2002) Intraarterially Administered Verapamil as Adjunct Therapy for

Cerebral Vasospasm: Safety and 2-Year Experience. AJNR AM J Neuroradiol 23: 1284-1290.

Findlay JM (1995) A randomized trial of intraoperative, intracisternal tissue plasminogen activator for the prevention of vasospasm. Neurosurgery 37(5): 1026-7

Firlik AD, Kaufmann AM, Jungreis CA, Yonas H (1997) Effect of transluminal angioplasty on cerebral blood flow in the management of symptomatic vasospasm following aneurysmal subarachnoid hemorrhage. J Neuro surg 86: 830-839

Frontera JA, Fernandez A, Schmidt JM, Claassen J, Wartenberg KE, Badjatia N, Connolly ES, and Mayer SA (2009) Defining Vasospasm After Subarachnoid Hemorrhage: What Is the Most Clinically Relevant Definition?

Stroke 40: 1963-1968; published online before print as doi:10.1161/STROKEAHA.108.54470

Frontera JA, Gowda A, Grilo C, Gordon E, Johnson D, Winn RH, Bederson JB, Patel A (2011) Recurrent vasospasm after endovascular treatment in subarachnoid hemorrhage. Acta Neurochir Suppl 110 (Pt 2): 117-122.

Fujii Y, Takahashi A, Yoshimoto T (1995) Effect of balloon angioplasty on high grade symptomatic vasospasm after subarachnoid hemorrhage. Neurosurg Rev (18): 7-13.

Jun P, Ko NU, English JD, Dowd CF, Halbach VV, Higashida RT, Lawton MT, Hetts SW (2010) Endovascular Treatment of Medically Refractory Cerebral Vasospasm Following Aneurysmal Subarachnoid Hemorrhage. AJNR AM J Neuroradiol 31:1911-16.

Kaku Y, Yonekawa Y, Tsukahara T, and Kazekawa K (1992) Superselective intra-arterial infusion of papaverine for the treatment of cerebral vasospasm after subarachnoid hemorrhage. J Neurosurg 77(6): 842-847.

Katoh H, Shima K, Shimizu A, Takiguchi H, Miyazawa T, Umezawa H, Nawashiro H, Ishihara S, Kaji T, Makita K, Tsuchiya K (1999) Clinical evaluation of the effect of percutaneous transluminal angioplasty and intra-arterial papaverine infusion for the treatment of vasospasm following aneurysmal subarachnoid hemorrhage. Neurol Res 21(2): 195-203.

Kassell NF, Haley EC Jr., Apperson-Hansen C, Alves WM (1996) Randomized, double-blind, vehicle-controlled trial of tirilazad mesylate in patients with aneurysmal subarachnoid hemorrhage: a cooperative study in Europe, Australia, and New Zealand. J Neurosurg 84(2):221-8.

Kassell NF, Helm G, Simmons N, Phillips CD, Cail WS (1992) Treatment of cerebral vasospasm with intra-arterial papaverine. J Neurosurg 77(6): 848-852.

Keuskamp J, Murali R, Chao KH (2008) High-dose intraarterial verapamil in the treatment of cerebral vasospasm after aneurysmal subarachnoid hemorrhage. J Neurosurg 108(3):458-463.

Komotar, R, Zacharia, B, Mocco J, Connolly S (2008) Controversies in the endovascular management of cerebral vasospasm after intracranial aneurysm rupture and future direction for therapeutic approaches. Neurosurgery 62(4): 897-905.

Macdonald RL, Kassell NF, Mayer S, Ruefenacht D, Schmiedek P, Weidauer S, Frey A, Roux S, Pasqualin A (2008)Clazosentan to overcome neurologic ischemia and infarction occurring after subarachnoid hemorrhage (CONSCIOUS-1): randomized, double-blind, placebo-controlled phase 2 dose-finding trial. Stroke 39(11):3015-21.

Murai Y, Kominami S, Kobayashi S, Mizunari T, Teramoto A (2005) The long-term effects of transluminal balloon angioplasty for vasospasms after subarachnoid hemorrhage: analyses of cerebral blood flow and reactivity. Surg Neurol 64:122-127.

Nussbaum ES, Sebring LA, Ganz WF, Madison MT (1998) Intra-aortic balloon counterpulsation augments cerebral blood flow in the patient with cerebral vasospasm: a xenon-enhanced computed tomography study. Neurosurgery 42(1):206-13.

Oskouian RJ, Martin NA, Lee JH, Glenn TC, Guthrie D, Gonzalez NR, Afari A, Viñuela F (2002) Multimodal Quantitation of the Effects of Endovascular Therapy for Vasospasm on Cerebral Blood Flow, Transcranial Doppler Ultrasonographic Velocities, and Cerebral Artery Diameters. Neurosurgery 51:1 30-43.

Pickard JD, Murray GD, Illingowrth R, Shaw MD, Teasdale GM, Foy PM, Humphrey PR, Lang DA, Nelson R, Richards P (1989) Effect of oral nimodipine on cerebral infarction and coutcome after subarachnoid hemorrhage: British aneurysm nimodipine trial. Br Med J 298: 636-642.

Pluta RM, Hansen-Schawrtz J, Dreier J, Vajkoczy P, Macdonald RL, Nishizawa S, Kasuya H, Wellman G, Keller E, Zauner A, Dorsch N, Clark J, Ono S, Kiris T, Leroux P, Zhang JH (2009) Cerebral vasospasm following subarachnoid hemorrhage: time for a new world of thought. Neurol Res 31(2):151-8.

Rosenwasser RH, Armonda RA, Thomas JE, Benitez RP, Gannon PM, Harrop J (1999) Therapeutic modalities for the management of cerebral vaso- spasm: timing of endovascular options. Neurosurgery 44: 975–979.

Santillan A, Knopman J, Zink W, Patsalides A, Gobin YP (2011) Transluminal balloon angioplasty for symptomatic distal vasospasm refractory to medical therapy in patients with aneurysmal subarachnoid hemorrhage. Neurosurgery [Epub ahead of print].

Shankar JJ, dos Santos MP, Deus-Silva L, Lum C (2011) Angiographic evaluation of the effect of intra-arterial milrinone therapy in patients with vasospasm from aneurysmal subarachnoid hemorrhage. Neuroradiology 53(2): 123-128.

Shibuya M, Suzuki Y, Sugita K, Saito I, Sasaki T, Takakura K, Nagata I, Kikuchi H, Takemae T, Hidaka H (1992) Effect of AT877 on cerebral vasospasm after aneurysmal subarachnoid hemorrhage. Results of a prospective placebo-controlled double-blind trial. J Neurosurg 76(4): 571-7.

Terada T, Kinoshita Y, Yokote H, Tsuura M, Nakai K, Itakura T, Hyotani G, Kuriyama T, Naka Y, Kido T (1997) The Effect of Endovascular Therapy for Cerebral Artery Spasm, its Limitation and Pitfalls. Acta Neurochir (Wien) 139:227-234.

Vergouwen MD, Meijers JC, Geskus RB, Coert BA, Horn J, Stroes ES, van der Poll T, Vermeulen M, Roos YB (2009) Biologic effects of simvastatin in patients with aneurysmal subarachnoid hemorrhage: a double-blind, placebo-controlled randomized trial. J Cereb Blood Flow Metab 29(8): 1444-53.

Weant KA, Ramsey CN, and Cook AM (2010) Role of Intraarterial Therapy for Cerebral Vasospasm Secondary to Aneurysmal Subarachnoid Hemorrhage. Pharmacotherapy 30:4 , 405-417.

Zubkov YN, Nikirov BM, Shustin VA (1984) Balloon catheter technique for dilatation of constricted cerebral arteries after aneurysmal SAH. Acta Neurochir 70(1-2): 65-79

Zwienenberg-Lee M, Hartman J, Rudisill N, Madden LK, Smith K, Eskridge J, Newell D, Verweij B, Bullock MR, Baker A, Coplin W, Mericle R, Dai J, Rocke D, Muizelaar JP (2008) Effect of Prophylactic Transluminal Balloon Angioplasty on Cerebral Vasospasm and Outcome in Patients With Fisher Grade III Subarachnoid Hemorrhage: Results of a Phase II Multicenter, Randomized, Clinical Trial Stroke 39: 1759-1765.

7

Angiography for Peripheral Vascular Intervention

Yoshiaki Yokoi
Cardiology, Kishiwada Tokushuaki Hospital, Osaka
Japan

1. Introduction

The use of endovascular technique for peripheral vascular disease (PVD) has evolved and new devices and techniques were being developed. Even after recent development of noninvasive diagnosis of PVD, angiography is still the gold standard for the evaluation of stenotic and occluded lesions. Without precise angiographic information, endovascular therapy can not be performed. In this chapter, the angiographic technique to visualize major arteries of atherosclerotic disease is described.

2. Angiography suite for peripheral vascular intervention

Excellent imaging is the key for the success of endovascular therapies. Flat-panel X ray image detectors for use in digital fluoroscopy and angiography are essential for peripheral artery intervention. The ability of three-dimensional (3D) visualization techniques and bolus chasing are also required. Various types of imaging sizes are available but we have to compromise considering of function on the machine. Careful planning and professional expertise is a key factor for choosing every endovascular suite.

2.1 Single plane vs. biplane system

We have two types of our peripheral angiography suite. One is single plane arm with 31cm X 31cm flat panel detector (Fig. Suite1A). And the other biplane with the 30cm X 40cm flat panel detector (Fig. Suite1B). Both machines have its merit and demerit. Single plane machine has the versatile function and more suited for intervention. Biplane system could obtain the multiple images and reduce the dosage of dye. But except for cerebral angiography, it takes time to adjust two images in centred position. For the diagnostic purpose, biplane System has the advantage, but interventional work, the single plane system has more versatile function and much safer for the patient's care during procedure.

2.2 Extra monitor

In angiographic table, operators usually stand on the right side, but for left limb intervention or left brachial approach, operator needs to be positioned on the left side of the table. In these circumstances, the extra monitor is useful for left side operator. Without moving central image monitor, main operator can do the procedure with assistant who are seeing central monitor from right side (Fig. Suite2A). This is the convenient way to intervene right femoropopliteal artery or left subclavian artery. In left below the knee procedure via cross over approach, C-arm is rotated to the left side. Cranial side operator may not see the central image. In this situation, extra monitor can be placed in left cranial side (Fig. Suite2B).

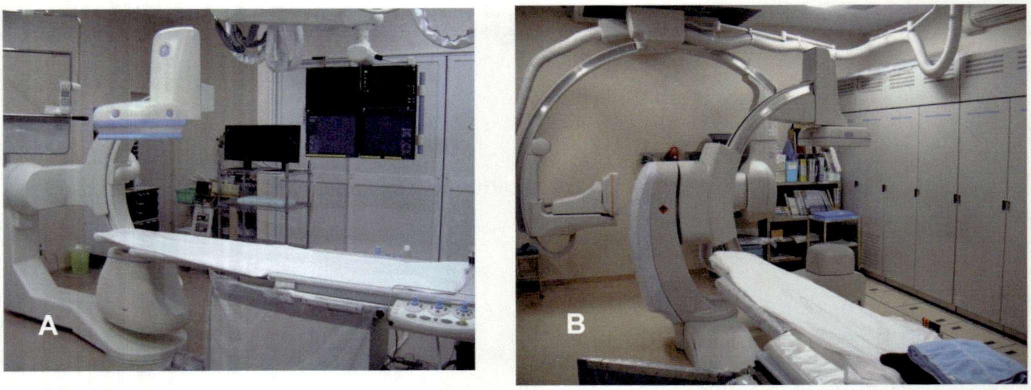

Fig. Angiosuite 1: Peripheral angiography suite
A: Single plane flat panel system.
A single plane system has more versatile function compared to the biplane system. Single system is suited for interventional work
B: Biplane system: Biplane system allows the two images both on fluoro and images. Dye consumption could reduce. However, lateral tube might limit the patient's care. Mostly employed for neuroangiography.

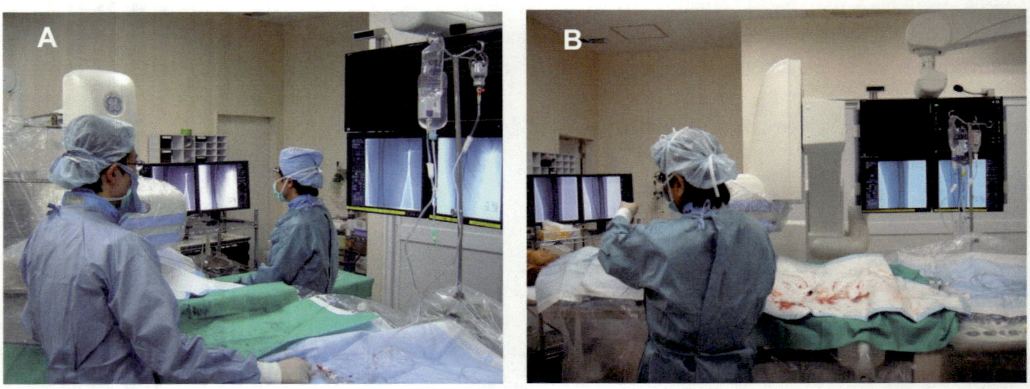

Fig. Angiosuite 2: Extra monitor
A: Operators usually stand on the right side of the table. But for left limb intervention or left brachial approach, operator needs to be positioned on the left side of the table. In these circumstances, the extra monitor is useful for left side standing operator without moving central image monitor
B: In left below the knee procedure via cross over approach, C-arm is rotated to the left side. Cranial side operator may not see the central image. In this situation, extra monitor can be placed in left cranial side. Primary operator could see the image on the cranial side monitor and assistant could see the central monitor.

2.3 Power injectors

For most of small vessel and selective angiography, hand injection is adequate. However, for the optimal opacification of high-flow blood vessels like aorta, the use of power injector is mandatory. Constant and high volume of dye should be injected through electronically calibrated power injector. There are two types of injector. One is old fashioned power injector and the other is the assisted device which could give the small or large amount of dye by the injector attached to catheter table. Any contrast volume is adjusted by manually. Even a small dose of dye can be injected. However, the space of left side of table is occupied by this assisted device. We prefer conventional power injector which is mounted to the celling. This method gives us more space around catheter table.

In the assisted device, the operator is supposed to stand only on the right side of the table and can not be away from the table during injection. To prevent for radiation exposure, conventional use of power injector is more preferable (Fig. Suite4).

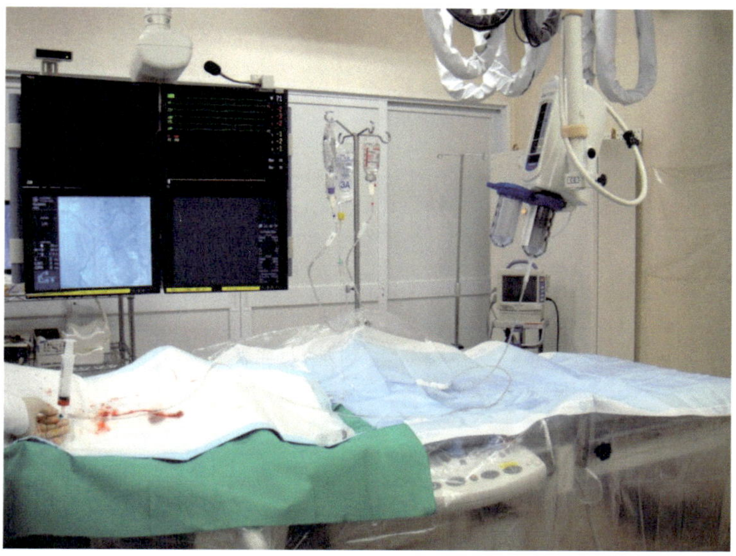

Fig. Angiosuite 3: Celling mounted Power injector
Celling mounted power injector gives more space around catheter table

2.4 Image size and contrast volume

Contrast volume for opacification of the major arteries were listed in Table 1.was listed. These injection volumes are mainly used in our catheter laboratory. But, real contrast volume depends on the patient' condition, catheter size, amount of contrast, speed of injection and et al. Therefore contrast dose should be individurized on each case

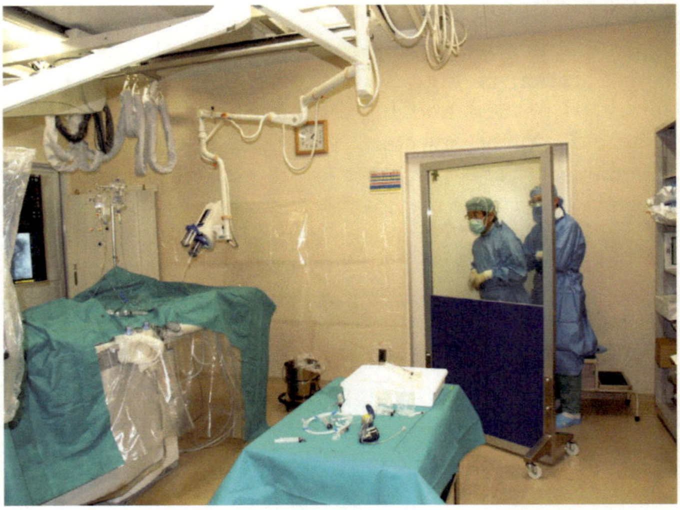

Fig. Angiosuite4: Radiation exposure
Radiation exposure should be minimalized during injection of dye by using power injector

2.5 Table 1 Commonly used imaging size, injection rates and contrast volume for major arteries

Angiogram	Image size	Injection rate	Contrast volume
Aortic Arch	30cm	20cc/s	20-30cc
Carotid (Selective)	20cm	4-6cc/s	7-9cc
Cerebral: AP	20cm	4-6cc/s	7-9cc
Cerebral: Lateral	30cm	4-6cc/s	7-9cc
Abdominal aorta	20-40cm	16-20cc/s	16-25cc
Renal (Selective)	20cm	4-6cc/s (by hand)	4-6cc
Iliac (Selective)	20cm	6-10cc/s	8-10cc
Femoropopliteal-Tibial (Bolus) 30cm	4cc/s	16-20	
SFA	30cm	4-6cc/s	10cc
SFA (Selective)	20–30cm	4-6cc/s	10cc
Below the knee (Bolus)	30cm	3cc/s	7-9cc
Tibial	20cm	3cc/s	5cc
Tibial (Selective)	20cm	1-2cc/s (by hand)	2-3cc

Table 1. Commonly used imaging size, injection rates and contrast volume
AP: antero-posterior, SFA: superficial femoral artery

3. Carotid artery angiography

The atherosclerotic plaque accumulates at the carotid bifurcation. There are a number of factors, including geometry, velocity profile, and shear stress. The carotid bulb forms a focal dilatation. The flow at the bifurcation is considered to be a complex hemodynamics and postulated to lead carotid artery stenosis (Fig. Carotid 1) **(1)**. Carotid disease is one of important cause of ischemic stroke. In symptomatic patients, carotid revascularization is indicated in the presence of a stenosis 50~70% or more **(2)**. There are many arguments about the indication for asymptomatic patients. But asymptomatic stenoses are usually treated only if luminal narrowing exceeds 60%**(2)**. Carotid artery stenting (CAS) is a preferred treatment strategy in high-risk patients requiring Carotid endoatherectomy (CEA). Even though indication of CAS is still controversial, CAS is a less invasive and attractive way for revascularization for carotid artery disease. To indicate carotid artery revascularization, meticulous angiographic approach should be taken to evaluate of carotid artery stenosis.

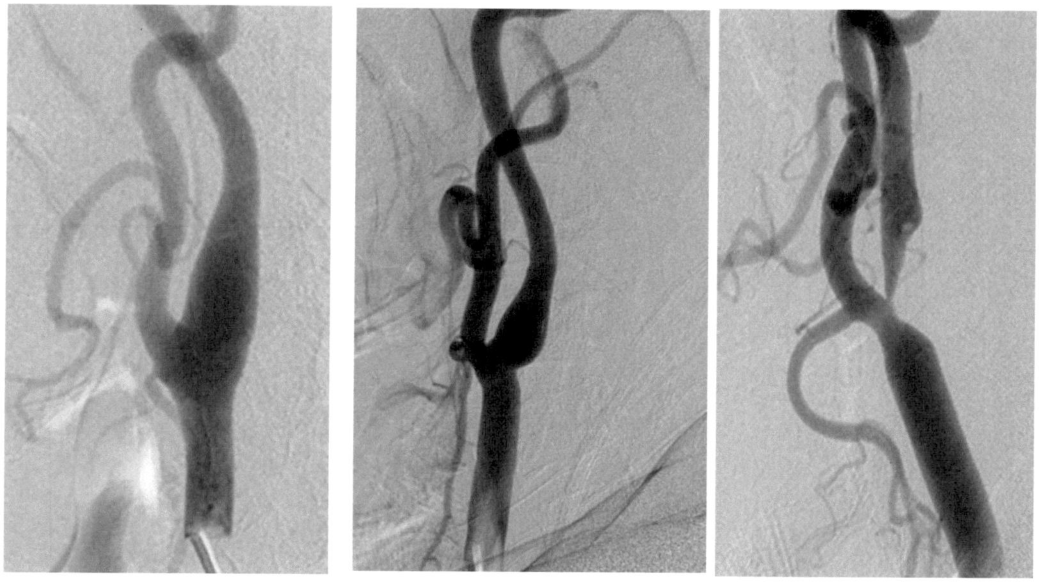

Fig. Carotid 1: Progression of carotid artery disease
A: The carotid bulb forms a focal dilatation
B: Mostly lesion starts at the bifurcation. Mild stenosis is seen
C: In progressive form of atherosclerosis.
Carotid bulb is filled with plaque and the flow at the bifurcation show thc complex hemodynamics. This hemodynamics is postulated to lead carotid artery stenosis

3.1 Aortic arch type

Engagement of catheter to the brachiocephalic or left CCA is required to perform carotid artery angiography. In selecting catheter, the aortic arch anatomy plays an important role for the success of the procedure. In CAS, not only engaging the catheter, guiding sheath have to be placed into common CCA. It does mean the technique of the deep engagement of diagnostic catheter to CCA or external carotid artery (ECA) is the important procedure for carotid artery angiography.
There are classifications that categorize aortic arch anatomy **(3)** (Fig. Carotid 2).
The aortic arch angiography in left anterior oblique view shows three type of aortic arch (Fig. Carotid 3). The vertical distance from the origin of the innominate artery to the top of the arch determines the arch type. In type 3, engagement of catheter, particularly to left common carotid artery is difficult and may account for the failure of carotid artery stenting.

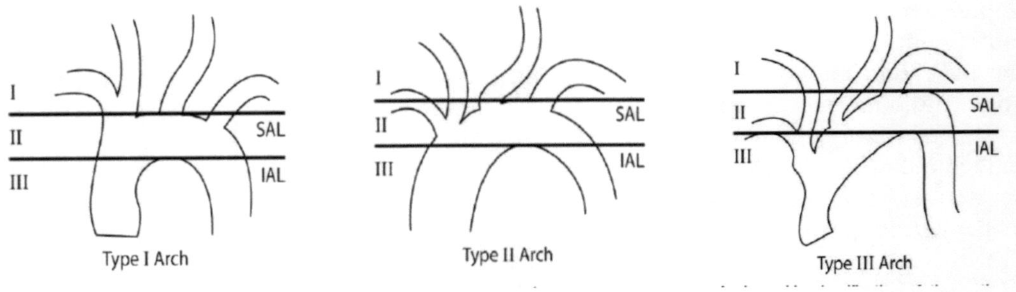

Fig. Carotid 2: Schematic classification of aortic arch (3).
Above figures are quoted from reference 3
A: Type 1 arch: The origins of the great vessels to be catheterized are at the level of the superior arch line
B: Type 2 arch: The origins of the great vessels to be catheterized are between the superior and the inferior arch line
C: Type 3 arch: The origins of the great vessels to be catheterized below the level of the inferior arch line.

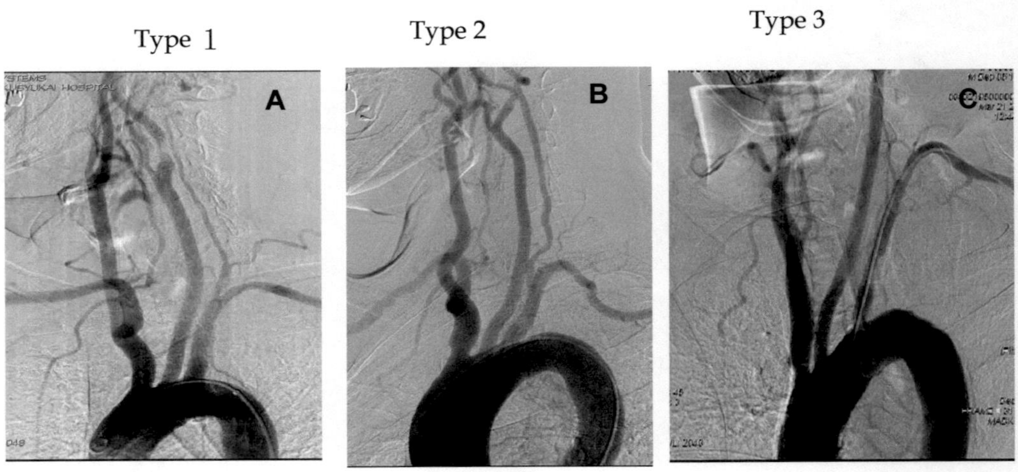

Fig. Carotid 3: Angiographic classification of aortic arch
In Type 1(A) and Type 2(B), catheter can be easily selected. In Type 3(C), steep curve between the top of aortic arch and the origin of arch vessel is shown. This type 3 arch is difficult to negotiate to access to common carotid artery

The anomalies of bovine arch can frequently occur and may lead to prolonged fluoroscopy time to select left common carotid artery (Fig. Carotid 4). Fig. Carotid 4 A and B are the typical bovine arch. Access to left common carotid artery is easy in Fig. Carotid 4A, but In Fig. Carotid 4B, selection to left common may be difficult due to the sharp bend from top of aortic arch Most of the type 3 aortic arch is shaggy and cannulation of selective catheter carries the risks of embolization (Fig. Carotid 5). Even in type 1 aortic arch, horizontally angulated left common carotid artery makes it difficult to engage the catheter from transfemoral approach (Fig. Carotid 6). In recent multi-detector CT angiography, the similar information of aortic arch can be obtained (Fig. Carotid 7).

Since an aortic arch angiogram or CT angiography can accurately reveal aortic arch type, complex anatomic variations and angulated takeoff. The assessment of aortic arch type is important for the success of CAS.

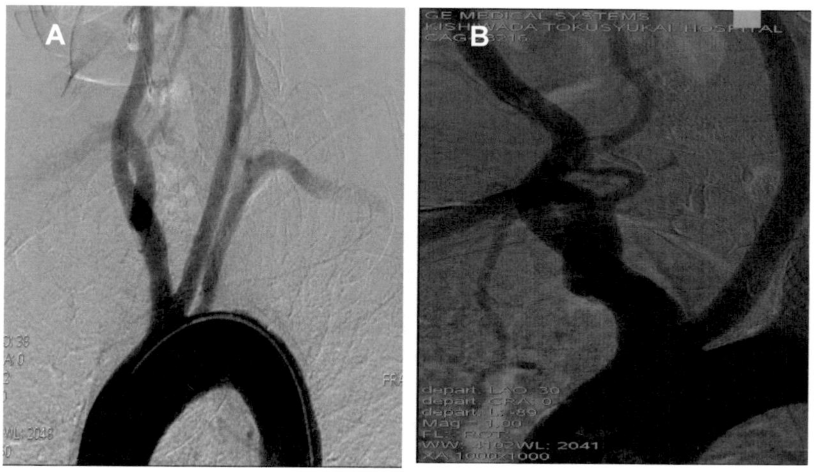

Fig. Carotid 4: Bovine arch
A and B are the typical bovine arch. Access to left common carotid artery is easy in A, but In B, selection to left common may be a difficult due to the sharp bend from top of aortic arch

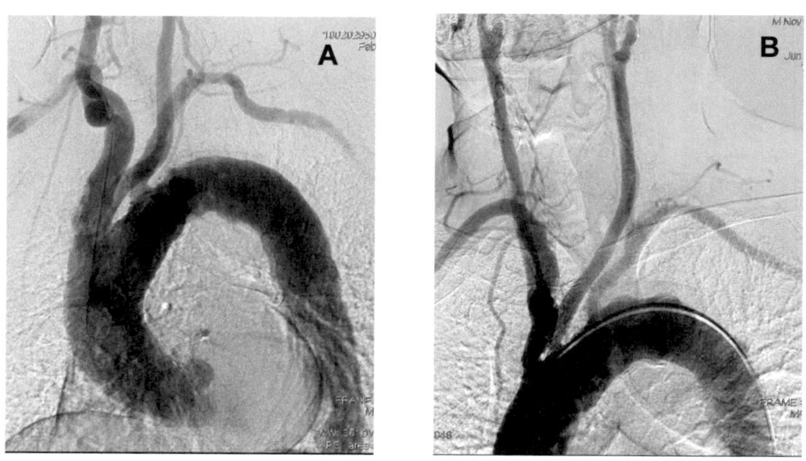

Fig. Carotid 5: Type 3 arch
A and B are typical type 3 arch. Cannulation of catheter to common carotid artery is difficult. Manipulation in these shaggy aortic arch carries the risks of embolization and a predictor of periprocedural complications.

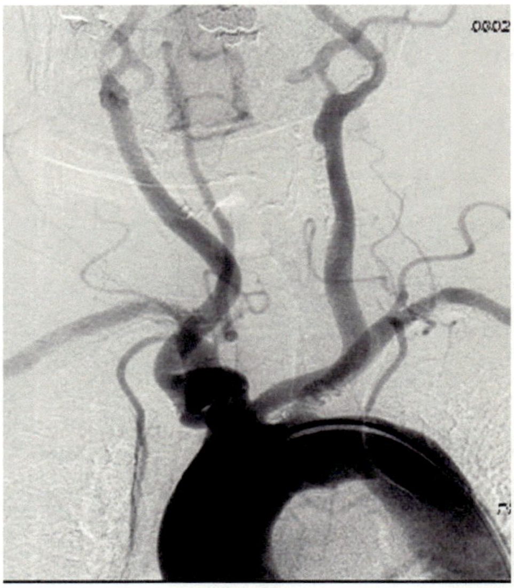

Fig. Carotid 6: Difficult aorta of type 1
Even in type 1 aortic arch, horizontaly angulated left common carotid artery makes it difficult to engage the catheter from transfemoral approach

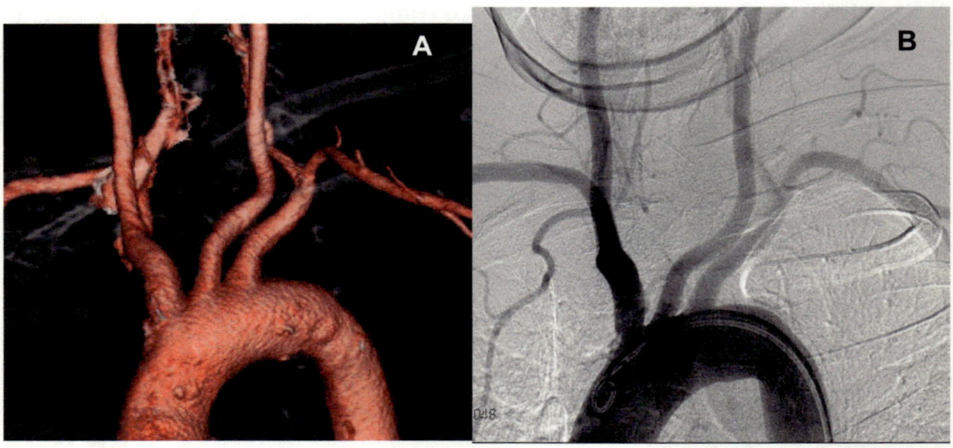

Fig. Carotid 7: Aortic arch assessment by 3D CT angiography and aortic arch angiography
Aortic arch angiogram on the same patient. Similar aortic arch assessment can be obtained on either CT angiography (A) or angiogram(B)

3.2 Selective carotid angiography

3.2.1 CTA vs. DSA

To evaluate carotid stenosis, selective carotid angiography remains the golden standard. But multidetector CT angiography is rapidly becoming the preferred examination for the initial evaluation of carotid artery stenosis **(4)**. CT angiography correlates to DSA. CTA (Fig. Carotid 8A) and DSA (Fig. Carotid 8B) images of left carotid stenosis were compared.

In both images, tight stenosis were seen but CTA overestimates the stenosis. In calcified lesion, CTA does not reveal the real lumen. In Fig.8C,D, CTA image does not clarify the stenosis due to calcification.

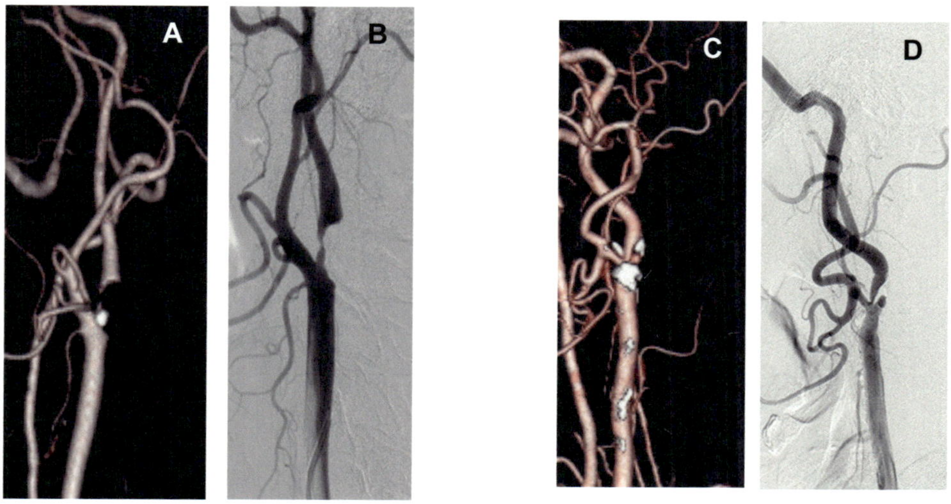

Fig. Carotid 8: Comparison of carotid artery stenosis between CT angiography and angiography
Left internal carotid artery (ICA) stenosis by CT angiography (A) was confirmed by digital subtraction angiography (B). CT angiography overestimates the stenosis.
In calcified lesion, CT angiography failed to show the ICA stenosis (C) and DSA revealed the ulcerated ICA stenosis (D).

3.2.2 Quantitative stenosis measurement

The percentage of stenosis is expressed using the NASCET criteria **(5)**. The NASCET criteria of 70% stenosis is the indication for CEA in symptomatic carotid stenosis. In NASCET, the stenosis calculated as the ratio of the diameter at the narrowest point to the diameter point at which beyond the area of post stentic dilatation. Before intervening carotid artery stenosis, quantitative angiographic assessment is required to measure the stenosis. So called NASCET measurement causes some confusion about the reference point of distal internal carotid artery. To avoid this confusion, minimal lumen Diameter (MLD) should be measured in mm (Carotid 9). In this case, % stenosis based on NASCET was calculated at 87% with MLD 0.7mm.

3.2.3 Angiographic view for carotid artery stenosis

Basic angiographic view for carotid bifurcation can be obtained by anterior-posterior and lateral view. In most of the cases, lateral view shows the stenosis (Fig. Carotid 10). To indicate CAS or CEA, angiographic significant stenosis has to be found in multiple views. In these circumstances, 3D angiography is employed. In Fig Carotid 11, moderate stenosis was seen on either anterior or lateral view. In 3D angiography, right anterior oblique view at 60°could reveal the tight stenosis.

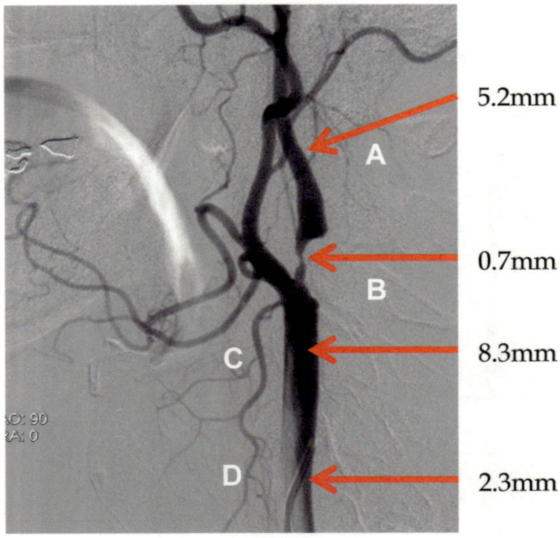

Fig. Carotid 9: Quantitative stenosis measurement
A: Distal internal carotid artery (ICA)
B: minimal lesion diameter (MLD)
C: Common carotid artery (CCA)
D: Reference catheter outer diameter
MLD should be express in mm. Distal ICA, MLD and CCA with reference catheter outerdiametr are needed to caluculate stenosis.

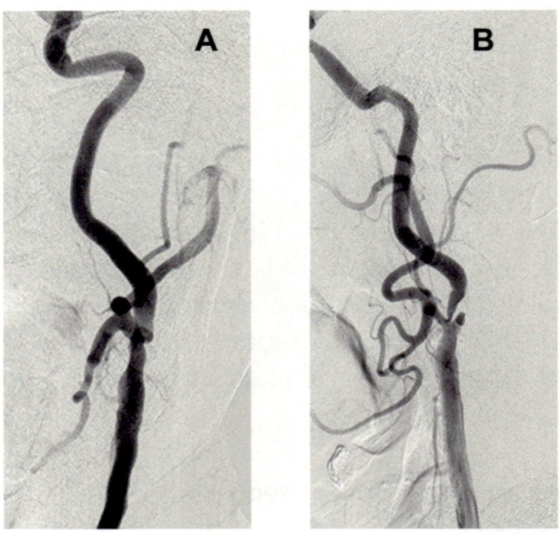

Fig. Carotid 10: Antero-posterior amd lateral view of left carotid artery bifurcation
A: Antero-posterior view
B: Lateral view
Basic angiographic view for carotid bifurcation can be obtained by anterior-posterior (A) and lateral view(B). In most of the cases, lateral view shows the bifurcation stenosis

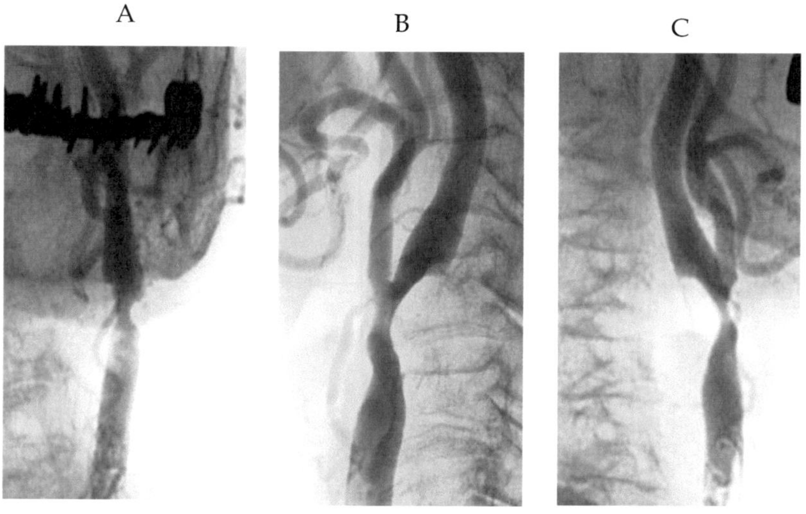

Fig. Carotid 11: 3D angiography for carotid artery stenosis assessment
A: Anterior view
B: Lateral view
C: Right anterior oblique 60° view
Moderate stenosis were seen on either anterior or lateral view. In 3D angiography, right anterior oblique view at 60° could see the tight stenosis.

3.2.4 Level of carotid artery bifurcation and lesion

Carotid artery bifurcates at the level of around C4. To indicate CAS, either anatomical or clinical high risks for CEA have to be clarified. One of the common indications is high position of bifurcation. The level of bifurcation or lesion level must be clearly demonstrated by lateral view. In Fig. Carotid 12A, bifurcation level is normal at the level of C4 In Fig. Carotid 12B, bifurcation is at the C3, but lesion extends to C2. In Fig. Carotid 12C shows the unusually low bifurcation.

3.2.5 Plaque morphology

Carotid artery plaque is evaluated by ultrasound or MRI, but angiogram also could show the large plaque burden (Fig. Carotid 13). Ulcer is commonly seen and the main source of cerebral emboli (Fig. Carotid 13A). Severe long stenosis is seen in Fig. Carotid 13B. This suggests the large plaque burden and CEA is recommended. Severe tight stenosis shows the string sings (Fig. Carotid 13C). This is the near occlusion and shows the sluggish antegrade flow. Real vessel size of distal ICA cannot be determined. In these cases, CEA is better indicated than CAS for thinking of complex plaque morphology.

3.2.6 Tortuosity of ICA

Protection device is placed at distal ICA or petrous portion. Atherosclerotic ICA sometimes shows the tortuosity. To place the protection device by the filter, the landing zone that was relative straight and 3~4 cm away from lesion site must be found. If there is no lamding

A B C

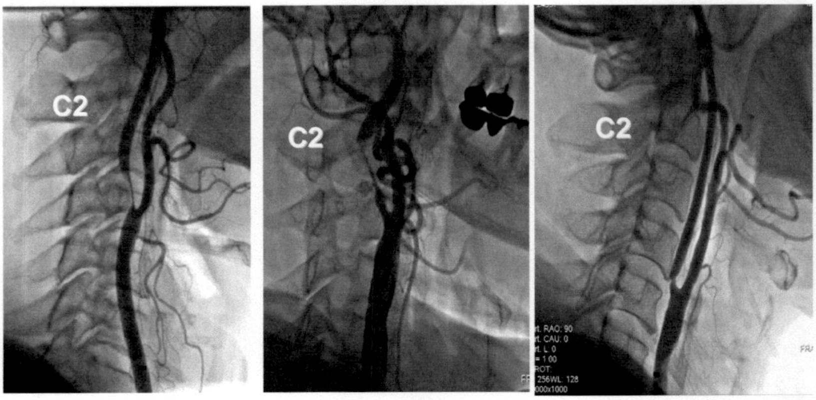

Fig. Carotid 12: Level of bifurcation and lesion
A: Bifurcation level is normal at the level of C4
B: Bifurcation is at the level of C3, but lesion extends to C2.
C: Low bifurcation.

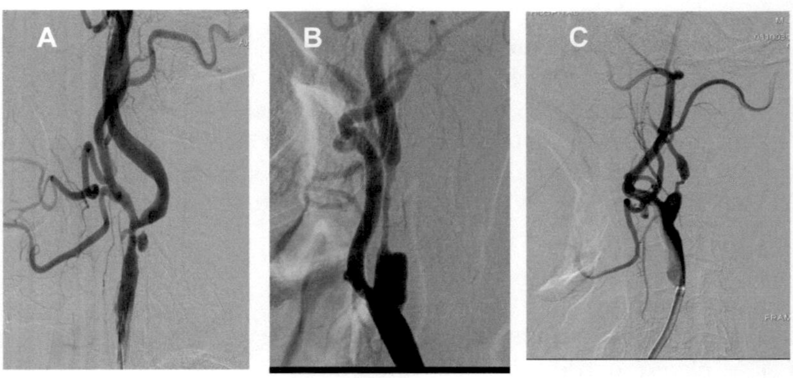

Fig. Carotid 13: Plaque morphology
A: Typical ulcer.
B: Severe long stenosis is seen and this suggests the large plaque burden
C: String sing is the preocclusion and shows the sluggish antegrade flow.

zone for filter, we have to consider proximal protection or balloon occlusion. In Fig. Carotid 14A, there is a landing zone but thinking of stent distal and filter position could be a very close and have the risks of filter trouble. In Fig. Carotid 14B, lesion show the directed to horizontally and upward bending of distal ICA. In this case, conformable stent is desirable and there is a risk of filter retrieval. In Fig. Carotid 14C, ICA shows the extreme tortuosity and CAS shoul be abandoned.

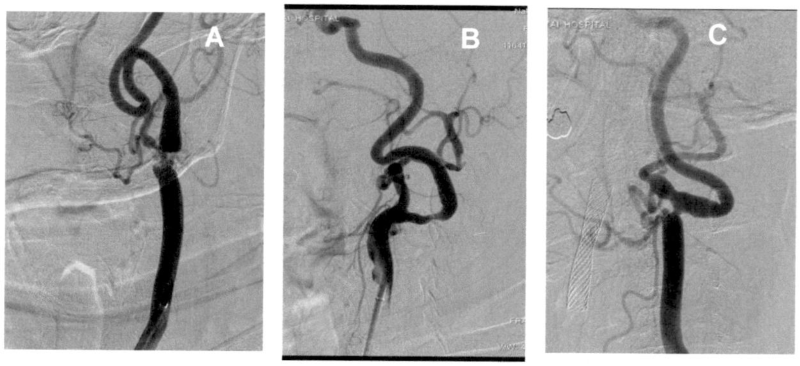

Fig. 14: Tortuosity of internal carotid artery (ICA)
A: S curve of ICA.
B: 90 degree rightward shift of proximal ICA.
C: Marked tortuosity of ICA
These cases suggest carotid artery stenting are not a good indication for anatomical reasons.

3.3 Summary

Internal carotid artery stenosis is an important cause of ipsilateral stroke. CAS is becoming a valid alternative to CEA. Therefore angiography should be taken for thinking of CAS can be possible or not. Precise angiographic stenosis assessment, lesion location and lesion morphology are suitable for CAS. And also, place for filter landing zone have to be taken account.

4. Subclavian artery angiography

Occlusive disease of the supra-aortic trunks still remains an angiographic challenge. Among the proximal supra-aortic trunk disease, atherosclerosis is the most common cause of large artery occlusive disorder in the upper extremity.
In this chapter, angiographic approach for left subclavian artery disease will be discussed.

4.1 Aortic arch angiography for branch disease

Branch disease is defined of innominate, left common carotid, left subclavian artery (SCA) disease. In angiographic assessment of aortic branch disease, left anterior oblique (LAO) projection of aortography is the basic view. However, bony structure of thorathic cage and calcification of aorta made it difficult to obtain the clear image of arch. Severe proximal stenosis of three aortic arch vessels caused by atherosclerosis was shown in In Fig. SCA 1B, proximal left common carotid artery is stenosed. Stenosis or occlusion of innominate and ostium of left common carotid artery are not suited for revascularization by endovascular technique (6). In three aortic arch branch, left SCA stenosis most commonly seen and can be intervened by endovascular approach (Fig. SCA 1C). Atherosclerotic right SCA stenosis is mostly located at the ostium at the bifurcation of right common carotid artery. Aortography by LAO view showed right subclavian artery stenosis at the ostium (Fig. SCA 2A). Selective innominate artery angiography by right anterior oblique (RAO) view reveals that stenosis is located at the bifurcation of right common carotid artery (Fig. SCA 2B). Angioplasty to the right SCA ostium might affect right common carotid artery ostium. Extra caution is needed for right SCA ostium intervention, such as distal protection for right carotid artery territory. Among the three aortic arch branch vessels, atherosclerotic left SCA is commonly found in proximal to vertebral artery and left SCA is most favourable fort endovascular therapy. In this chapter, left SCA angiogram for interventional approach is discribed.

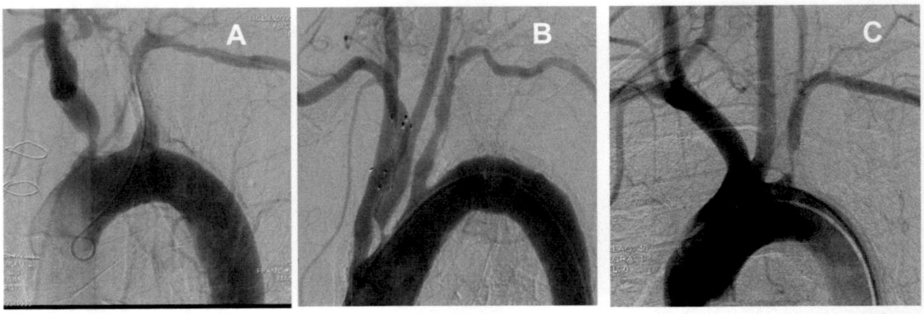

Fig. SCA 1: Aortic arch angiogram of aortic branch disease
A: Innominate, left common, left subclavian artery are diseased.
B: A tight ostial stenosis of left common carotid artery in type 3 arch
C: Typical left subclavian artery stenosis. Bovine arch is noted.

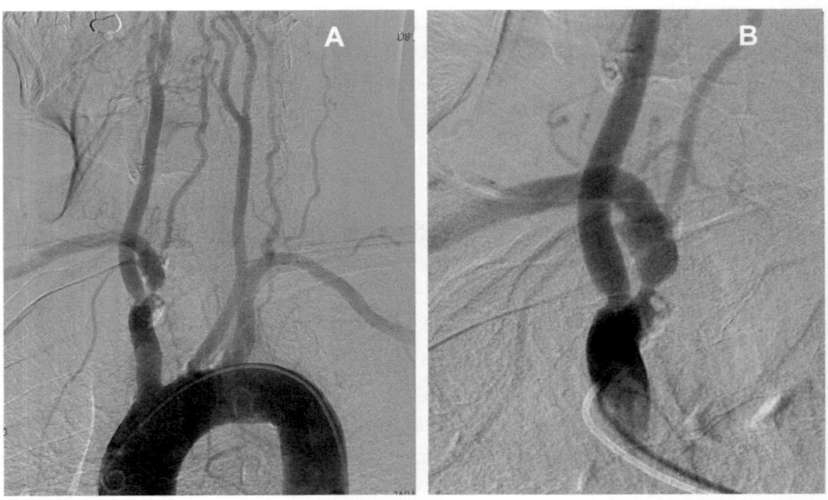

Fig. SCA 2: Ostial location of right subclavian artery stenosis
A: Aortography by left anterior oblique view showed right subclavian artery stenosis at the ostium
B: Selective innominate artery angiography by right anterior oblique view reveals that stenosis is located at the bifurcation of right common carotid artery.

4.2 Aortic arch angiogram for left subclavian artery stenosis

In subclavian artery angiography, nonsubtracted image gives the anatomical information but does not show the detail of subclavian artery stenosis (Fig. SCA 3A). Digital subtraction angiography (DSA) clearly delineates subclavian artery from the background (Fig.SCA3B).

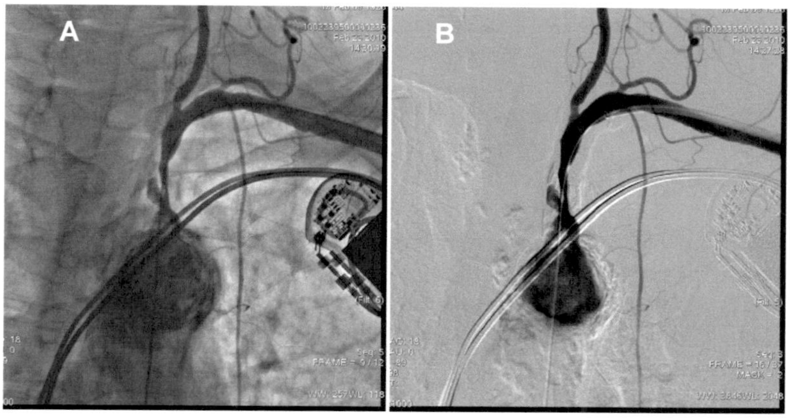

Fig. SCA 3: Non-substracted and subtracted angiogram of left subclavian stenosis
A: Non subtracted angiography gives the anatomical information
B: Digital subtraction angiography (DSA) clearly delineates subclaviar artery stenosis

As the initial angiographic approach for left SCA stenosis or occlusion, aortic arch angiography should be taken in left anterior oblique (LAO) 30~45°view by DSA (Fig. SCA 4A). Contrast volume and speed are at least 18cc/s, total 20~30cc by using 5Fr Pigtail catheter. In Fig. SCA 4A the image was taken by 30cm in size and delayed image reveals the distal SCA via collateral from right vertebral artery (Fig. SCA 4B). Selective right vertebral angiogram proves the reversed flow of left vertebral artery through basal artery (Fig. SCA4C). Image size of aortic arch angiography is usually taken by 30-40cm image (Fig. SCA 5A). Thinking of interventional approach, 20cm image is more practical to cannulate catheter to left SCA (Fig. SCA 5B). But to confirm the exact location of stenosis, selective left subclavian artery angiogram is required (Fig. SCA 5C). In Fig. SCA 6A, aortogram showed the total occlusion of proximal left SCA, but

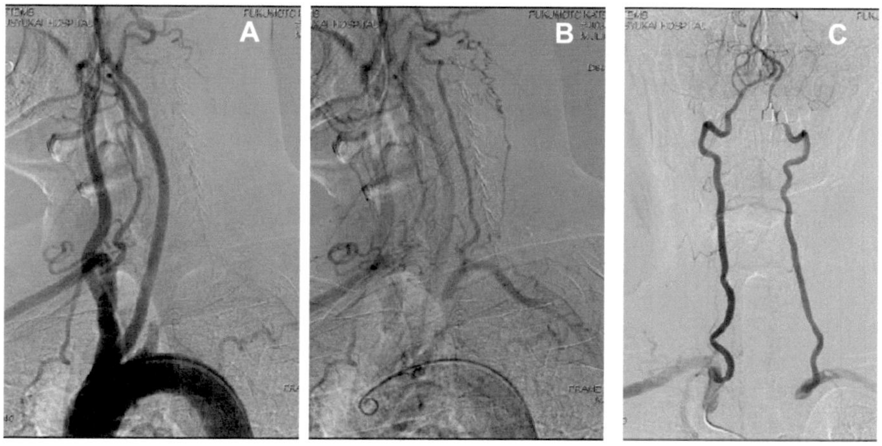

Fig. SCA 4: Angiogram of left subclavian artery occlusion
A: Aortography by LAO 45°by 30cm image size
B: Delayed image reveals the distal SCA via a collateral from right vertebral artery
C: Selective right vertebral angiogram proves the reversed flow of left vertebral artery through basal artery

selective injection revealed the 95% stenosis (Fig. SCA 6). To determine subtotal or occlusion, selective angiography is needed.

30 cm 20 cm selective

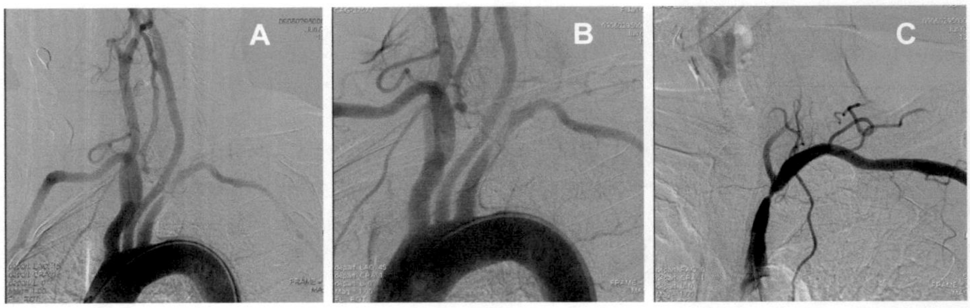

Fig. SCA 5: Angiographic image size of for left subclavian artery disease
A: Aortic arch angiography is usually taken by 30cm image
B: To cannulate catheter selectively to left subclavian artery, 20cm image of angiogram is appropriate
C: Selective left subclavian artery angiogram is needed to confirm the stenosis.

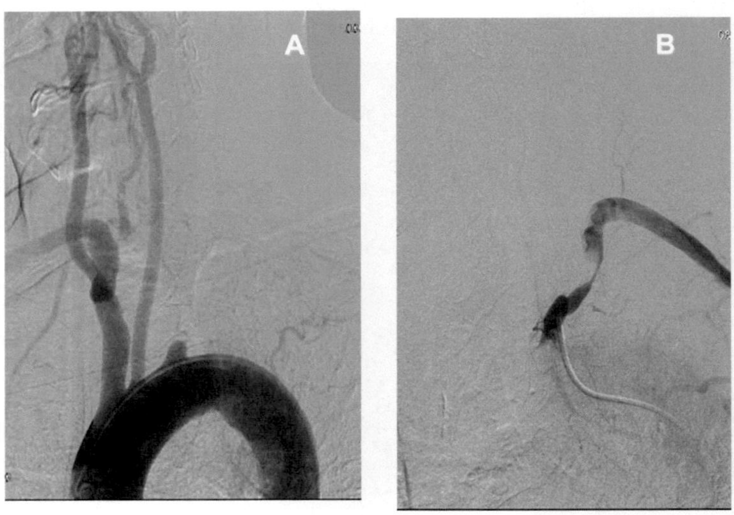

Fig. SCA 6: Aortography and selective angiography
A: Aortagram showed the total occlusion of proximal left subclavian artery
B: Selective left subclabian artery angiogram showed subtotal stenosis.
Selective angiography is necessary to intervene the lesion.

4.3 Angiography for subclavian artery intervention.

Although there is a paucity of long-term data of endovascular therapy, subclavian artery stenting is now the standard approach and offer many advantage over surgery in terms of morbidity and mortality. To succeed in left SCA stenting, a precise location of stenosis or occlusion must be visualized.

Fig. SCA 7 shows the typical left SCA stenosis. Initial aortogam by LAO view reveals left SCA stenosis (Fig. SCA 7A). To intervene left SCA stenosis, stenosis should be exactly located. Selective angiography combined with brachial artery catheter injection of dye clearly demonstrates the tight stenosis of left SCA (Fig. SCA 7B). Based on this angiogram, further stenting became the straightforward procedure (Fig. SCA 7C). The simultaneous injection of dye from distal and proximal SCA is very useful technique for subclavian artery intervention. To confirm SCA occlusion, the similar technique is applied during aortography. Selective SCA angiogram by injecting dye through catheter from brachial artery at the time of aortography showed the exact occlusion site (Fig. SCA 8A). This kind of angiogram leads to the successful intervention. Same angiographic technique was taken after stenting (Fig. SCA 8B).

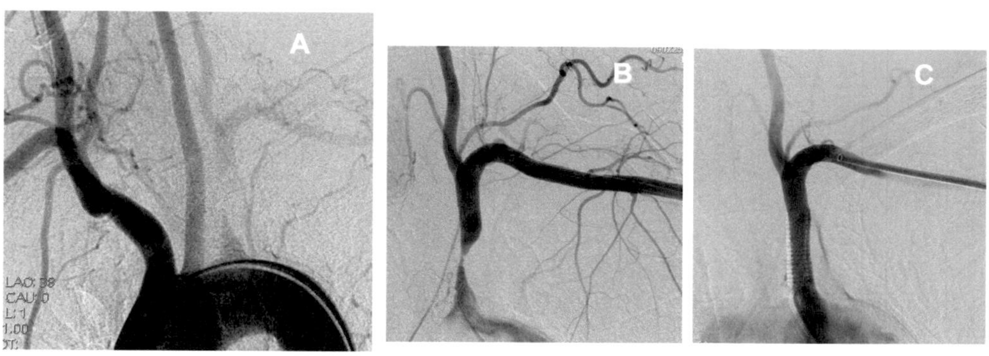

Figure. SCA7: Angiographic technique to assess left subclavian stenosis
A: Initial aortagram by LAO view reveals left SCA stenosis
B: Selective angiography combined with brachial artery catheter injection of dye clearly demonstrates the tight stenosis
C: Selective angiogram of post stenting. Distal and proximal injection of dye clearly demonstrate successful stent implantation

Not all angiogram could show the clear image of subclavian stenosis. In these cases, hemodynamic assessment is the useful to confirm a significant stenosis. In Fig. SCA 9A, simultaneous pressure recording was performed and showed 40mmHg peak systolic gradient and left SCA stenosis was located at the ostium. After stenting, no gradient was detected and successful stent placement was confirmed (Fig. SCA 9B).

4.4 Angiographic assessment for coronary- internal mammary steal

The increased employment of internal mammary artery (IMA) grafts for coronary revascularization, proximal SCA stenosis is becoming well known cause of coronary-

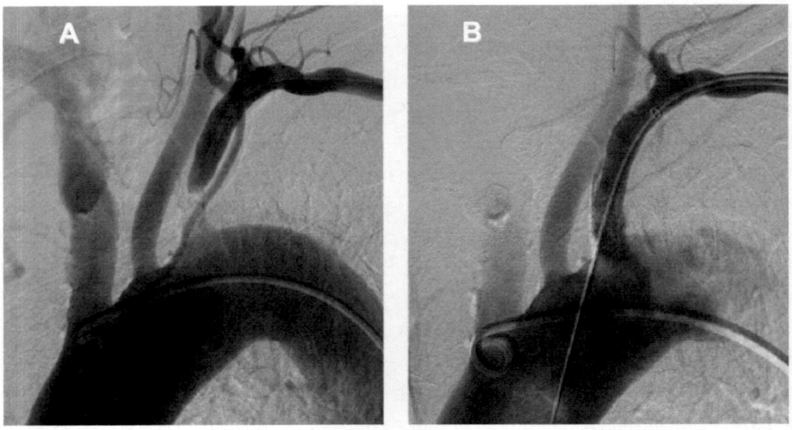

Fig. SCA 8: Angiographic technique for left subclavian occlusion
A: Aortography with simultaneous injection of dye through the catheter from brachial artery. This angiogram gives the precise morphologic information of occlusion.
B: Aortography of post stenting.
Same angiographic technique was taken and shows the successful stent placement.

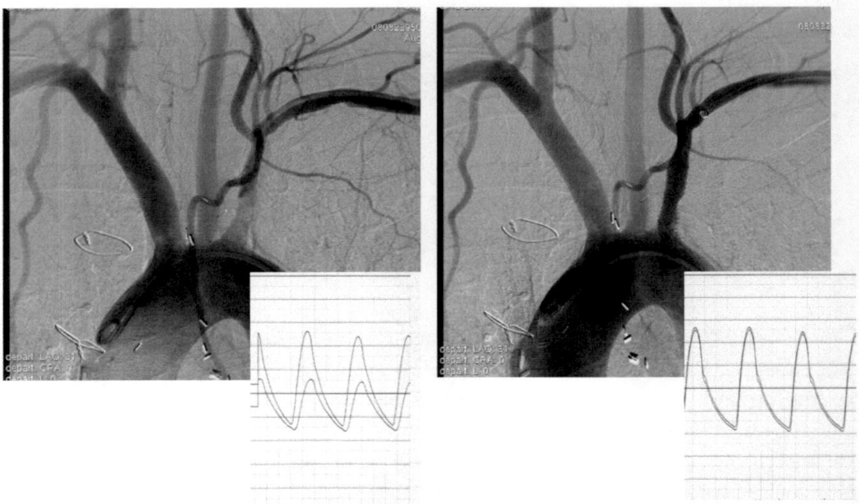

Fig. SCA 9: Simultaneous pressure tracing for subclavian artery stenosis
A: Aortography with selective distal SCA angiogram. Angiogram does not clearly reveal SCA stenosis. Simultaneous pressure tracing confirmed the siginificant stenosis.
B: Aortography of post stenting. Distal and proximal pressure were equalized and successful stenting was proven by hemodynamic study.

subclavial steal. Left SCA stenting is the good indication for coronary to left IMA steal **(7)**. In coronary steal to left IMA, selective left coronary angiogram is needed to prove reversed flow of IMA. The 70-year-old patient with suspected coronary steal was shown in Fig. SCA 10A. The left coronary angiogram showed the typical coronary steal which left IMA shows reversed flow and draining into left SCA is seen. This image was taken by coronary mode, but point is to prove coronary to left SCA steal phenomenon and DSA image can be used with 30cm image (Fig. SCA10B).

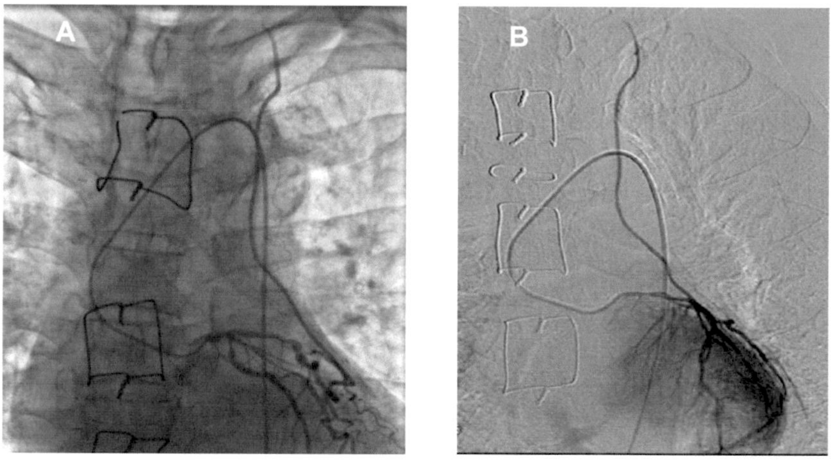

Fig. SCA10: Left coronary angiography for coronary-subclavian steal
A: Suspected coronary steal patient. Left coronary angiogram showed revealed reversed flow of left IMA. This angiogram was taken by coronary mode.
B: Similar left coronary angiogram was taken by digital subtraction angiography. IMA is more well visulalized. Either method can be used to prove IMA to left SCA. 30cm of image is preferable.

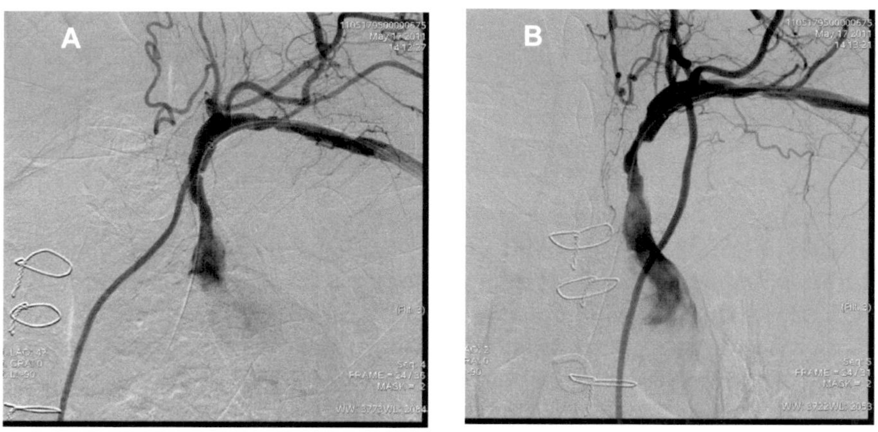

Fig. SCA 11: Relation between proximal left subclavian artery stenosis and origin of left internal mammary artery (IMA)
A: Left subclavian artery angiogram by left anterior oblique (LAO) view. Origin of left IMA is not identified by LAO view.
B. Left subclavian artery angiogram by antero-posterior view.
Relation between left IMA and proximal SCA stenosis is well seen.

Most of the initial left SCA angiogram is taken by LAO view. However, in this view, in some cases, left IMA origin is not well seen (Fig. SCA 11A). Relation between left SCA stenosis and IMA is very important for stent placement. The left SCA selective angiogram was taken by anterior-posterior (AP) view (Fig. SCA 11B). In AP view, origin of left IMA is visualized and relation between left SCA stenosis and IMA is well understood. This could lead to successful stent placement.

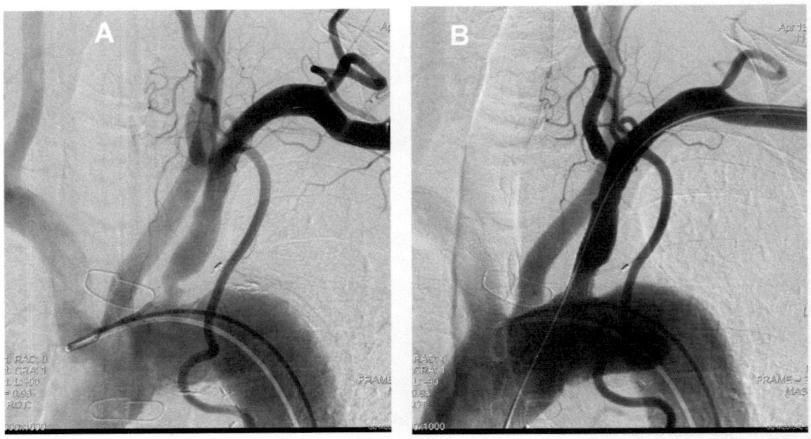

Fig. SCA12: Pre and post left subclavian artery stenting in coronary-subclavian steal
A: Aortic arch angiogram.
A 65 year-old female post coronary bypass patient, lesion was located at left SCA ostium.
B: Aortic arch angiogram post stenting. This angiogram showed the successful stenting.

In left SCA ostium disease, precise lesion location is mandatory. In Fig. SCA 12, a 65 year-old female post coronary bypass patient, lesion was located at left SCA ostium. This was confirmed aortography combined with brachial side simultaneous injection of dye (Fig. SCA 12A). Based on the angiogram, stent was precisely implanted and same angiographic technique was repeated to confirm successful procedure.

4.5 Summary

Primary stenting for a symptomatic SCA stenosis can be performed with relatively safe procedure risks. However, to succeed SCA stenting, the stenosis or occlusion must be clearly visualized by angiography. Aortic arch angiography with selective angiography by using distal injection of dye gives the precise lesion location and could lead to successful intervention. When patient presents after coronary bypass with coronary-subclavian steal, SCA stenting is the good option. But, origination of IMA must be precisely identified. Thereis no clinical randomized study about SCA stenting. To intervene to subclvian artery, a meticulous angiographic assessment is required.

5. Renal artery angiography

Atherosclerotic renal artery stenosis (ARAS) is an increasingly recognized cause of severe hypertension and declining kidney function **(8)**. Typically involving the renal artery ostium or proximal segment of the renal artery. Patients with ARAS have been demonstrated to have an increased risk of adverse cardiovascular events **(9)**. However, the efficacy of renal artery stenting for ARAS is a bit of controversial since ASTRAL trial was published **(10)**. Discordance exists between the procedural success rate and the equivocal clinical response rate after renal stent placement, which is likely to be a result of poor patients selection and inadequate angiographic assessment of lesion severity. Angiographic technique for ARAS will be discussed in this chapter.

5.1 Aortography for renal artery stenosis

Aortography and selective renal artery angiography considered to be the gold standard for assessing renal artery anatomy and renal artery stenosis. 3D CT angiography consists of a continuously overlapping transaxial images and is now replacing aortography for the diagnostic purpose. The drawback of aortography, only one shot image can be obtained and the image may not be in a single plane to see the both renal artery ostium. We usually take left anterior oblique view 15~30° for initial aortography (Fig. Renal 1). In Fig. Renal 1, bilateral renal artery stenosis is well visualized in one flame.

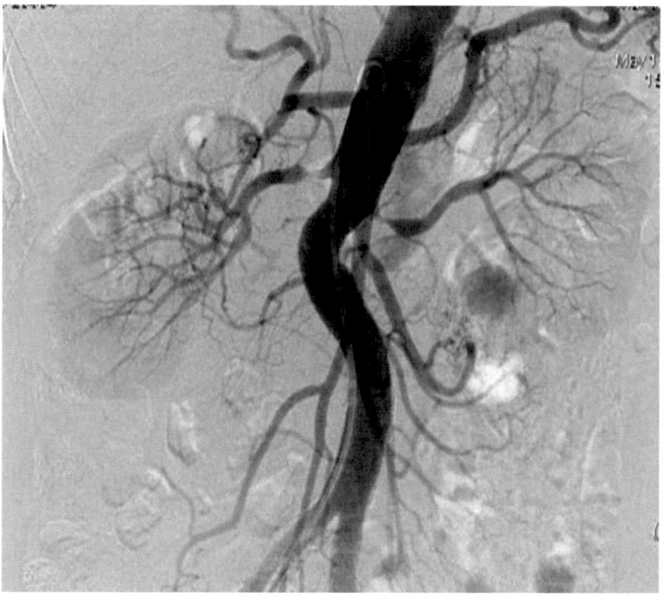

Fig. Renal 1: Aortography for the assessment of renal artery stenosis
Aortography was taken by left anterior oblique view 30°. Typical bilateral atherosclerotic renal artery stenosis is shown in one flame.

- **Multiple renal arteries:** Computed tomography angiography (CTA) with multiple detector-row CT (MDCT) has evolved into an established technique for imaging of renal and mesenteric vessels. Particularly, in multiple renal arteries, MDCT is superior to DSA to detect all renal arteries. To make a correct diagnosis of multiple renal arteries, MDCT and DSA could be used complimentary. In Fig. Renal 2, a case of multiple renal arteries are shown in both MDCT and DSA. In DSA, many other arteries were shown and we might miss to identify all 4 renal arteries. With the information of MDCT image, all renal arteries were confirmed.

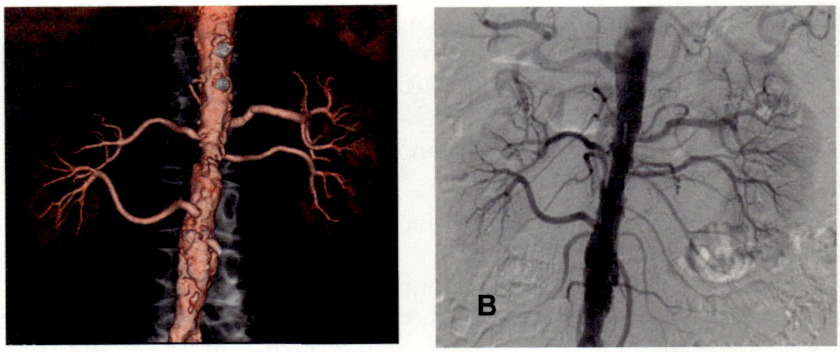

Fig. Renal 2: CT angiography and angiography for multiple renal arteries
A: CT angiography showed two renal arteries on both kidney.
B: The same view was taken by angiography. 4 renal arteries were seen but many other arteries are included and might miss multiple renal arteries.

- **Right renal artery ostium and super mesenteric artery:** Often times, right renal artery overraps to superior mesenteric artery (SMA) by antero-posterior view and proximal right renal is not visualized (Fig. Renal 3A). Selective right renal artery angiography confirmed the tight stenosis in right renal artery ostium (Fig. Renal 3B). There are reports about the detection of renal artery stenosis by aortography at the time of coronary angiography. But in reality, the simple aortogram might not identify the stenosis of right renal artery proximal stenosis.

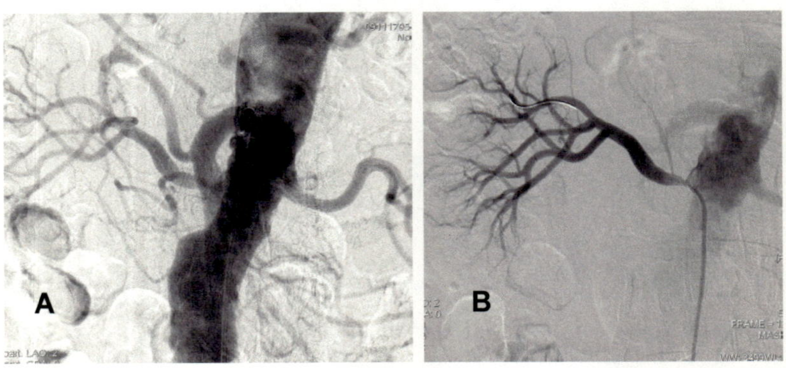

Fig. Renal 3: Relation between right renal artery ostium and super mesenteric artery
A: In aortography of left anterior oblique view, right renal artery overraps to superior mesenteric artery and proximal right renal artery is not shown
B: Selective right renal artery angiography confirmed tight stenosis in proximal right renal artery ostium

- **Access for selective renal artery catheter placement:** Aortography gives the important information about the access to selective renal artery angiography. The straight aorta with minimal atherosclerotic change is seen in Fig. Renal 4A. This suggests easy access for left renal catheter engagement. In Fig. Renal 4B, there is a marked tortuosity of aorta and tranfemoral approach may face difficulty to reach both renal artery ostium. In this case, transbrachial or transradial approach should be considered.

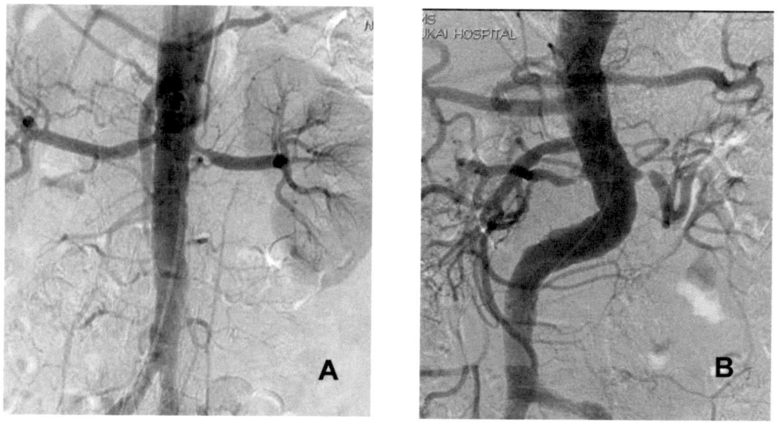

Fig. Renal 4: Access for selective renal artery catheter placement
A: The straight aorta with minimal atherosclerotic change is seen. This suggests easy access for left renal catheter engagement.
B: There is a marked tortuosity of aorta. Selective angiography by tranfemoral approach might be difficult procedure to reach both renal artery. In this case, transbrachial or transradial approach is recommended.

5.2 Selective renal artery angiography

Selective renal artery angiography is the definitive gold standard for the diagnosis of the significant renal artery stenosis. In aortography, clear relation between aorta and renal artery ostium is shown (Fig. Renal 5A). However, in aortography, information of intrarenal arteries is not obtained. Only selective renal artery angiography could show the picture of intrarenal artery as well as proximal stenosis (Fig. Renal 5B).

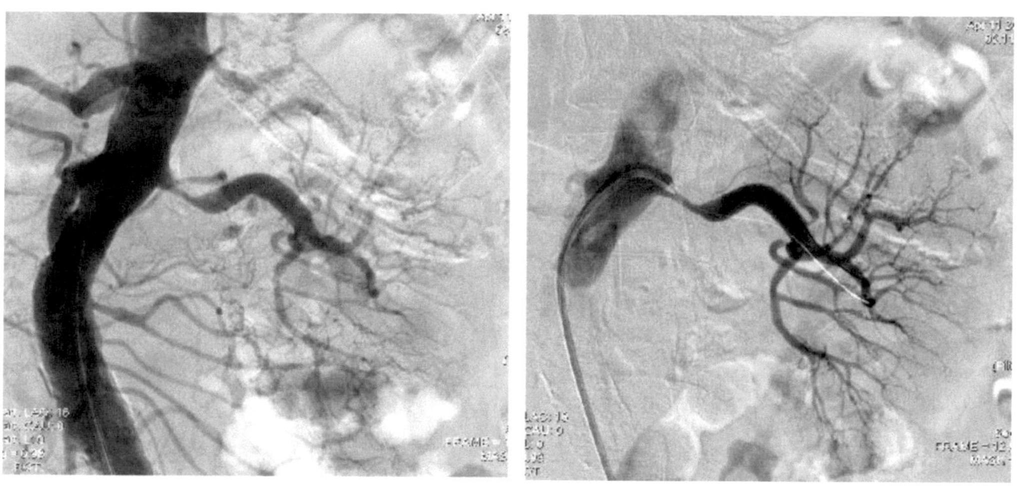

Fig. Renal 5: Aortography and selective renal artery angiography
A: Aortography shows the clear relation between aorta and renal artery ostium stenosis.
B: Selective renal artery angiography could show precise renal artery stenosis and anatomy of intrarenal arteries.

5.2.1 Digital subtracted image

By using digital subtraction angiography (DSA), the excellent renal artery angiography is Taken (Fig. Renal 6A). But in reality, it is very difficult to take excellent DSA image. Recent advances of digital image, distinction between subtracted and non subtracted image are relatively small (Fig. Renal 6B). Non DSA image is more important for renal artery intervention. In the near future, good quality digital image might replace DSA at least in renal artery.

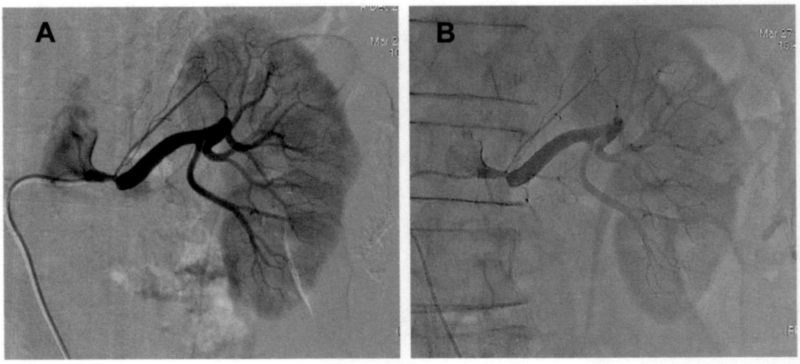

Fig. Renal 6: Digital subtracted and non subtracted selective renal artery angiography
A: Digital subtracted renal artery angiography.
B: Non subtracted image
Digital subtraction angiography (DSA) gives excellent image of renal artery vasculature(A). Recent advances of digital angiography shows that image quality between subtracted and non subtracted image are relatively small(B).

5.2.2 Ideal renal artery angiography

In selective renal artery angiography, catheter tip is in the renal artery ostium, but most of catheter goes into distal to stenosis and relationship between ostium and stenosis is not clarified. Aortagraphy of typical bilateral ARAS is shown in Fig. Renal 7A). In selective right renal artery angiography, catheter tip goes further to stenosis (Fig. Renal 7B) and relationship between ostium and stenosis is not clear. The ideal selective renal artery angiography is shown in Fig. Renal 8. In Fig. 8A, catheter tip attached to stenosis and is not recommended to inject dye. The ideal renal artery angiography is catheter tip located in aorta and could see the proximal stenosis (Fig. Renal 8B). To take the good quality renal artery angiogram, lesion is crossed by soft coil 0.014inc. wire. After confirming normal aortic pressure pattern, dye should be injected. If the catheter is too close to stenosis, slight drawback of catheter is needed to take the good quality angiogram. By doing this procedure, correct stenosis assessment can be made.

5.2.3 Lesion location

In ARAS, stenosis is basically localized in proximal renal artery. There are 3 types of lesion locations **(11)**. One is typical ostial stenosis (Fig. Renal 9A). Lesion located in middle of the proximal renal artery is called renal type (Fig. Renal 9B). In most of the cases, mixed type of stenosis is seen (Fig. Renal 9C).

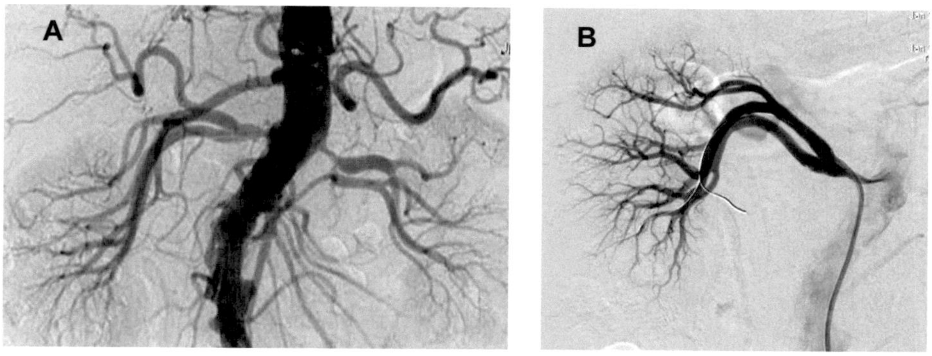

Fig. Renal 7: Catheter tip position of selective renal artery angiography
A: Aortography of typical bilateral ARAS
B: Selective right renal artery angiography.
In selective angiography, catheter tip goes into further stenosis. Relation between ostium stenosis and aortic wall is not elucidated.

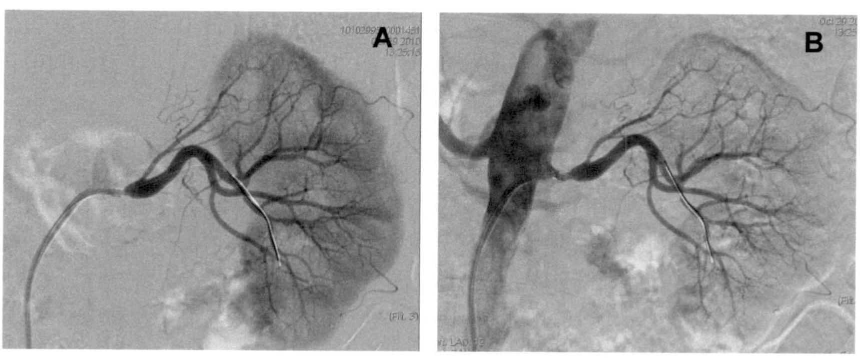

Fig. Renal 8: Ideal selective renal artery angiography
A: Catheter tip attached to stenosis and injection of dye at this place might damage the vessel.
B: The ideal renal artery angiography. Catheter tip is located in aorta and could see the proximal stenosis with distal renal vasculature.

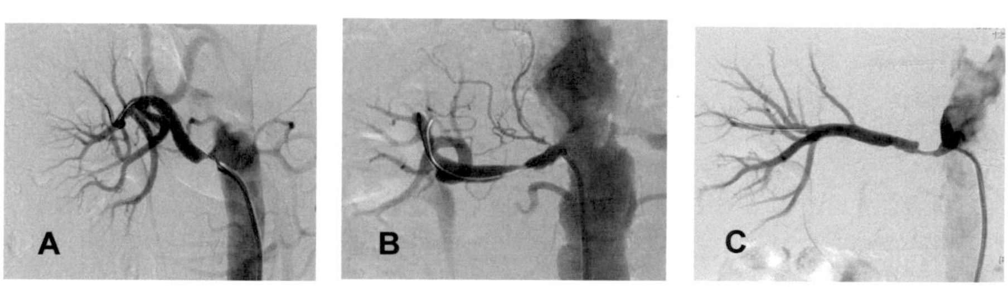

Fig. Renal 9: Lesion location of atherosclerotic renal artery stenosis. Atherosclerotic renal artery stenosis is basically localized in proximal renal artery. There are 3 types of lesion locations. One is typical ostial stenosis (A). Lesion located in middle of the proximal renal artery is called renal type(B). In most of the cases, mixed type of stenosis is seen (C).

5.2.4 Reference vessel

To select the correct stent size, accurate vessel diameter must be measured **(12).** To make a correct assessment of stenosis and vessel size, reference point is chosen. In Fig. Renal 10A, reference vessel is considered to be about 2cm distal to stenosis. However, in Fig. Renal 10B, post-stenostic dilatation is seen and bifurcation follows (Fig. Renal 10B). In this case, reference vessels cannot be determined. The bifurcation located at the ostium, real vessel size is not known (Fig. Renal 10C). This fact is not well understood and this is the main cause of recent confusion of stenosis evaluation.

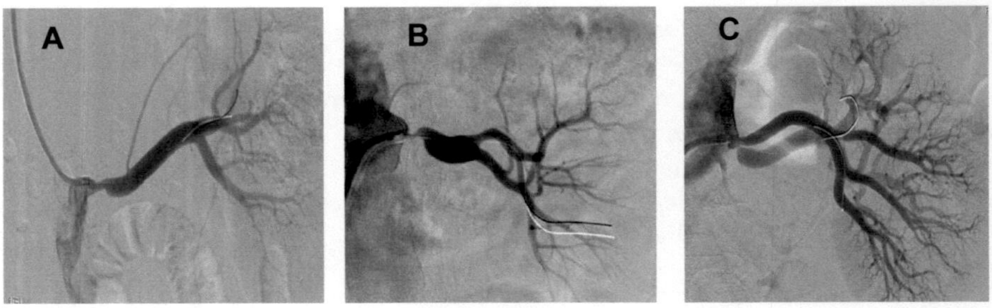

Fig. Renal 10: Reference vessel
To calculate % diameter stenosis or minimal lesion diameter, reference vessel must be determined.
A: Reference vessel can be determined about 2cm distal to stenosis.
B: Typical post-stenostic dilatation is seen and bifurcation follows. In this case, reference vessels can not be determined.
C: The bifurcation located at the ostium and real vessel size is not known.

- **Summary:** Renal artery angiography is the gold standard diagnostic test.

However, to make a correct diagnosis of ARAS, excellent visualization of renal vasculature should be performed. Aortography is now replacing to CT angiography. But in placing catheter to renal artery ostium, we still need aortography for the safe catheter manipulation. Selective angiography identifies the severity of stenosis with intra renal vasculature information. Confusion for the indication of renal artery stenting is mostly coming from poor angiographic image of renal artery stenosis.

6. Iliac artery angiography

Peripheral arterial disease at the level of iliac artery is well known for good indication of angioplasty. Currently, stenting for the treatment of iliac occlusive disease is the most effective modality and endovascular treatment of iliac artery disease should be considered as a first-line therapy for symptomatic PAD. The most commonly quoted classification of iliac lesions has been set forth by the TransAtlantic inter-Society Consensus (TASC II) group with recommended treatment options **(13)**. The type A and B lesions are treated preferentially by endovascular techniques and typed C and D lesions are more suited for surgical treatment. However, recent development of endovascular technique, even type D lesions sometimes is treated by endovascular procedure. To maximize the success of iliac artery stenting, good quality angiogram is needed.

6.1 Aortography for iliac artery disease

artery. The image field at least 30cm is needed. In Fig. Iliac 1, 31X31 cm and 30X40 cm image field are shown (Fig. Iliac 1). In both angiogram show from terminal aorta to common femoral artery. However, in 31cm image field, we are lifting a table to maximize image field (Fig. Iliac 2). Typical long left iliac artery total occlusion is shown in Fig Iliac 2A. This image was taken by lifting table to obtained collateral vessels to common femoral artery (Fig. Iliac 2B). DSA image is considered to be the standard angiography for iliac artery disease, but pelvic vessels often times interfered by bowel movement and gas. In recent advanced digital angiography, similar image to subtracted angiogram can be obtained. In Fig. Iliac 3, subtracted (In Fig. Iliac 3A) and non-subtracted (In Fig. Iliac 3B) are shown. Even nonsubtracted image is acceptable with bony landmark.

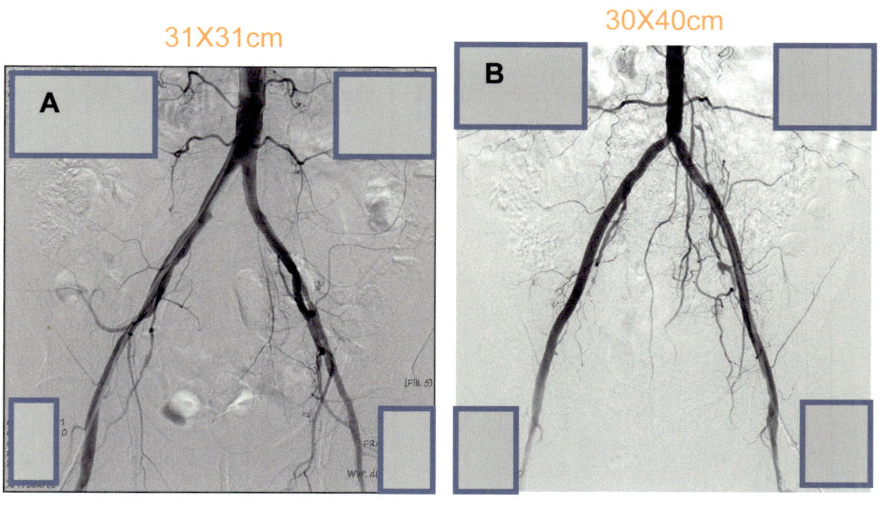

Fig. Iliac 1: Aortography for iliac artery
A: 31X31cm image,
B: 30X40cm image
Both angiogram could show from terminal aorta to common femoral artery.

6.2 Image size

To visualize aorto iliac disease, more than 30 cm image field is required. But in reality, image of 30 cm often times misses the complicated stenostic lesion. In Fig. Iliac 4A, there is a tight stenosis in left external iliac artery. In 20cm image, ulcerated tight stenosis in left common iliac artery clearly visualized (Fig. Iliac 4B). To intervene the iliac artery disease, the information of vessels size and lesion length is needed. 30cm image could confirm the disease of common femoral artery, but to obtain the precise lesion morphology, 20cm image is better than 30cm image.

6.3 Basic 3 views for iliac artery

The anteriorposterior (AP) pelvic angiogram is the basic angiogram. The oblique images should be obtained. If contrast load permits, basically we are taking three view of aortogram

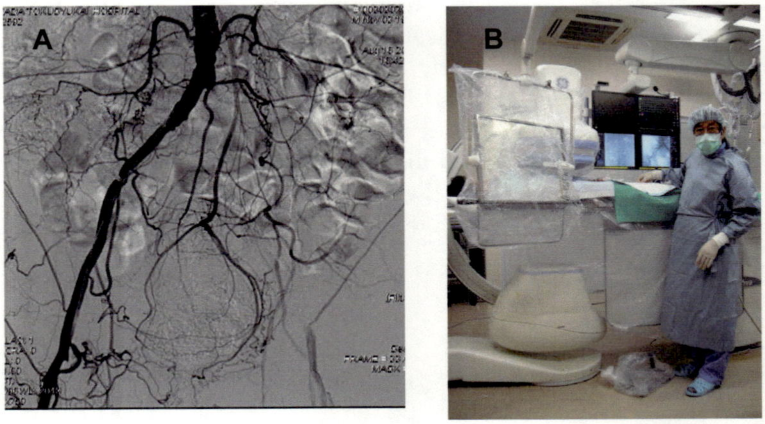

Fig. Iliac 2: Aortography by 31X31cm image field
A: Aortography of 31X31cm image. Left common femoral artery is visulaized through collateral.
B: Catheter table is lifted to maximize image field

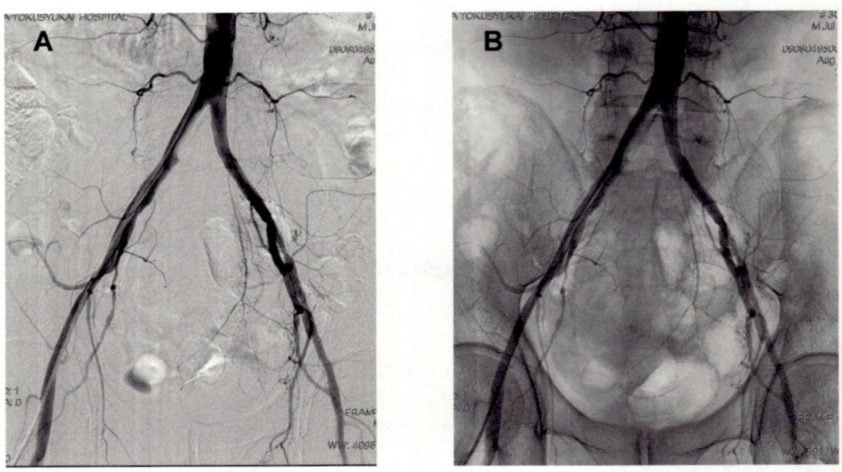

Fig. Iliac 3: Subtracted and non subtracted Aortography
A: Image of digital subtraction angiography
Image of digital subtraction angiography is considered to be the standard for the visualization of iliac artery disease
B: Non subtracted image
Pelvic vessels are interfered by bowel movement and bowel gas. Recent digital angiography could give the similar image to subtracted angiogram.

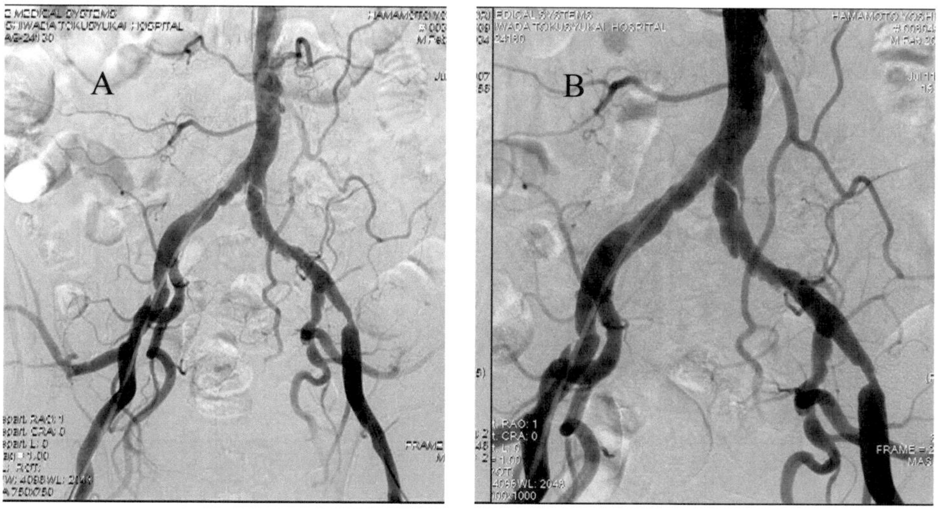

Fig. Iliac 4: Image size of Iliac artery disease
A: 31cm of image
B: 20cm of image
To visualize iliac artery disease, more than 30 cm image field is required. But for the purpose of interventional work, image of 30 cm often times misses the complicated stenotic lesion. There is a tight stenosis in left external iliac artery(A). In 20cm image, ulcerated tight stenosis in left common iliac artery clearly visualized (B).

(Fig. Iliac 5). In a right anterior oblique view, the left iliac artery is best visualized and could separate bifurcation of internal iliac artery (Fig. Iliac 5A). Similarly, right iliac artery is taken by left anterior oblique (Fig. Iliac 5C) with the projection 30°. In complex disease anatomy, this approach is very important before intervention. In Fig. Iliac 6, severely diseased bilateral external iliac artery are shown in three views. In AP view, right external iliac artery over rap and left external iliac artery is not well visualized (Fig. Iliac 6B). The right internal anterior oblique view shows occlusion of left external iliac artery iliac artery (Fig. Iliac 6A). Left anterior view clearly delineate right external and internal iliac artery (Fig. Iliac 6C).

6.4 Working image for intervention

In iliac artery disease, primary iliac stenting is performed in most of the cases. To stent, exact lesion location must be visualized. In Fig. Iliac 7, left external iliac artery focal stenosis is shown (Fig. Iliac 7A). In DSA image, bony landmark is not seen and DSA image converted to non-subtracted image (Fig. Iliac 7B). By seeing femoral head, precise stenting was performed (Fig. Iliac 7C).

6.5 Contrast injection from sheath

Iliac artery stenting is becoming the routine procedure and angiography can be simplified. In ipsilateral retrograde femoral approach, sheath is placed and this sheath can be used

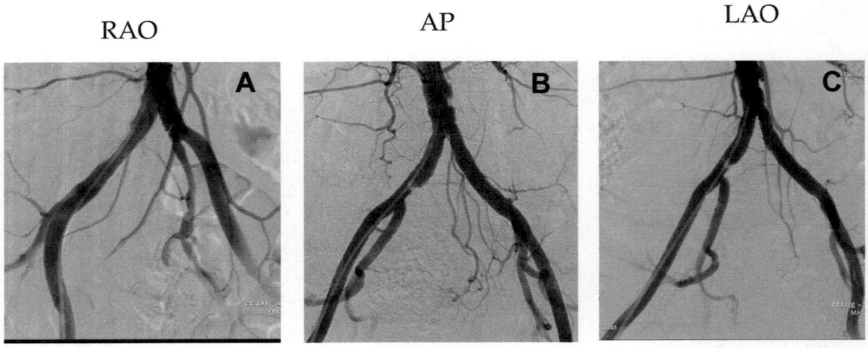

Fig. Iliac 5: Basic 3 views for iliac artery
A: 30° right anterior oblique view
B: Anteriorposterior (AP) view
C: 30° left anterior oblique view
In a right anterior oblique view, the left iliac artery is best visualized and separate bifurcation of internal iliac artery (A). In AP view, both external iliac artery are shortened(B) Similary the right iliac artery is taken by a left anterior oblique with the projection 30°angle(C).

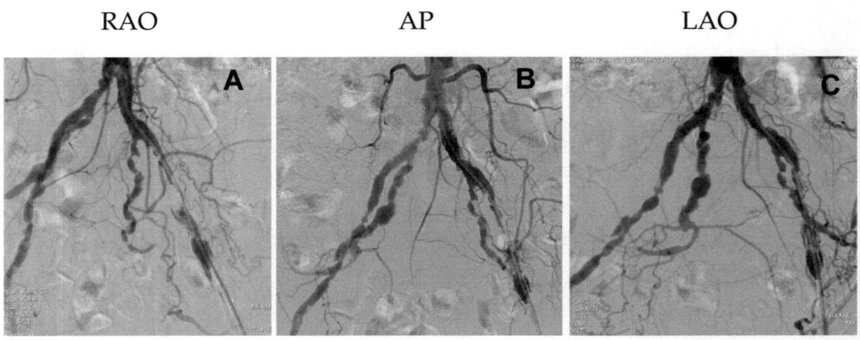

Fig. Iliac 6: Basic 3 views for iliac artery diease
A: 30° right anterior oblique view
B: Anteriorposterior (AP) view
C: 30° left anterior oblique view
The right internal anterior oblique view shows occlusion of left external iliac artery iliac artery (A). In AP view, right external iliac artery over rap with right internal iliac artery and left external iliac artery is not well visualized (B). The left anterior view clearly delineate right external and internal iliac artery and shows diffusely diseased right external iliac artery (C).

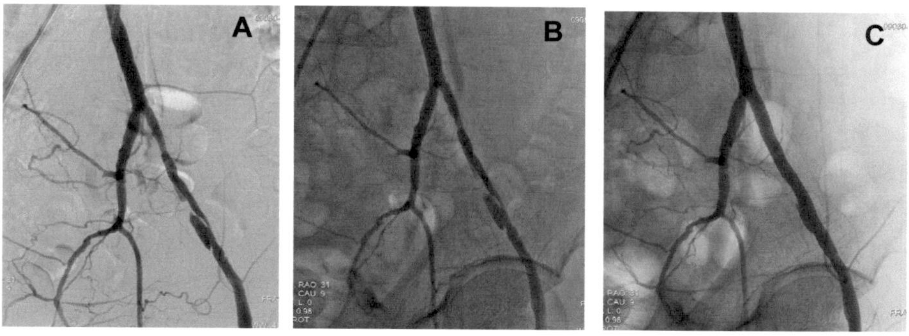

Fig. Iliac 7: Working image for intervention
A: Subtracted image
B: Non subtravted image
C: Post stenting
To stent, exact lesion location has to be visualized. Foca stenosis in left external iliac artery is shown by DSA image (A). Bony landmark is not seen and DSA image converted to non-subtracted image (B). By seeing femoral head, precise stenting was performed (C).

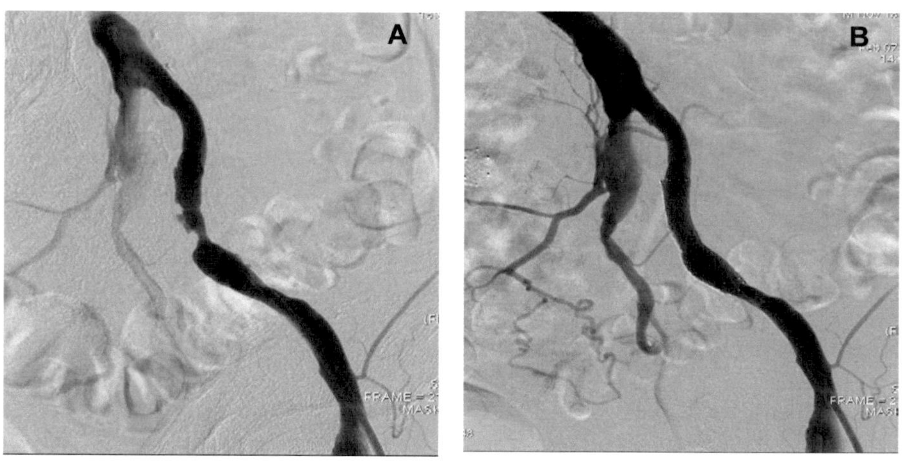

Fig. Iliac 8: Ipsilateral contrast injection from sheath
A: Angiogram by injecting dye through left femoral artery sheath
B: Post stenting angiogram
In ipsilateral retrograde femoral approach, sheath can be used to injection of dye. There is a focal stenosis in left external iliac artery (A). Angiogram was performed through this sheath and ballooning and stenting was performed. (B).

to injection of dye. There is a focal stenosis in left external iliac artery (Fig. Iliac 8A). Angiogram was performed through this sheath and ballooning and stenting was performed. (Fig. Iliac 8B). However, in retrograde approach, hand injection cannot visualize proximal iliac artery. Power injector should be employed and test injection is needed to check the tip of sheath position is in vessel lumen.

6.6 Summary

Iliac artery stenting is recognized as an effective treatment and became the standard therapy for iliac artery disease. CTA and vascular echo can be utilized for diagnostic purpose and diagnostic angiography is less performed. But pelvic vessels are difficult to diagnose by echo. CTA can be misread by calcification. The angiogram is still the golden standard for final decision making of iliac artery stenting.

7. Femoropopliteal artery angiography

Patients with disease limited to superficial femoral artery (SFA) usually present with claudication. However, most of severe claudication shows multi level involvement. In SFA, popliteal and infrapopliteal artery disease could be a cause of critical limb. Interventional approach to SFA is much easier than infrapopliteal artery and precise assessment of femoropopliteal artery disease in very important to deal with severe claudication and critical limb.

7.1 Proximal femoral artery

proximal femoral artery disease. In AP view, profunda femoral override to SFA (Fig. SFA 1A). In ipsilateral oblique view, separation between SFA proximal and profund femoral are well seen (Fig. SFA 1B). This view is particular important for diseased proximal femoral artery. The SFA proximal stenosis is not delineated by anterior posterior (AP) view (Fig. SFA 2A). Left anterior oblique view shows SFA ostial stenosis and found that lesion length of proximal profunda artery is longer than AP view (Fig. SFA2B). This angled view is particular useful to guide the wire into SFA ostial occlusion. In Fig SFA 3 shows the typical SFA long occlusion originating from SFA ostium (Fig. SFA 3A). In AP view, SFA ostium is not identified (Fig. SFA 3B). In left anterior oblique view, SFA ostium occlusion is well visualized (Fig. SFA 3C).

7.2 Bolus chase for limb artery angiography

To see the entire limb artery, a bolus chasing angiography is very useful method. In some angiographic system, this angiography can be done by digital subtraction with small amount contrast. We usually give 4cc/second, total 16~18cc of contrast to visualize from femoral to tibial artery. In Fig SFA 4A is the bolus chase of right limb. Infrapopliteal arteries are not well seen, but this angiogram give the right limb is not severely diseased. In Fig. SFA 4B shows the two focal stenosis with three tibial vessels run-off. The typical SFA occlusion with well developed collateral via profunda femoral artery is well seen (Fig. SFA4C).

7.3 Lesion length

marking is placed in SFA. Tape measurement is fairly consistent with marker wire and this tape can be used to measure lesion length (Fig. SFA 5). By using this tape, lesion length can be measured. Short focal lesion was measured at 1cm (Fig. SFA 6A). The lesion length of short CTO is measured at 6.5cm. In Fig. SFA 6C, 20cm long CTO is shown. In long diffuse lesion, another way to measure lesion length is to employ balloon marker. In Fig. SFA 7A, long SFA lesion is shown. By using 10cm balloon marker (Fig. SFA 7B), lesion was calculated about 20cm and two 6mmX100mm stent were implanted (Fig. SFA 7C).

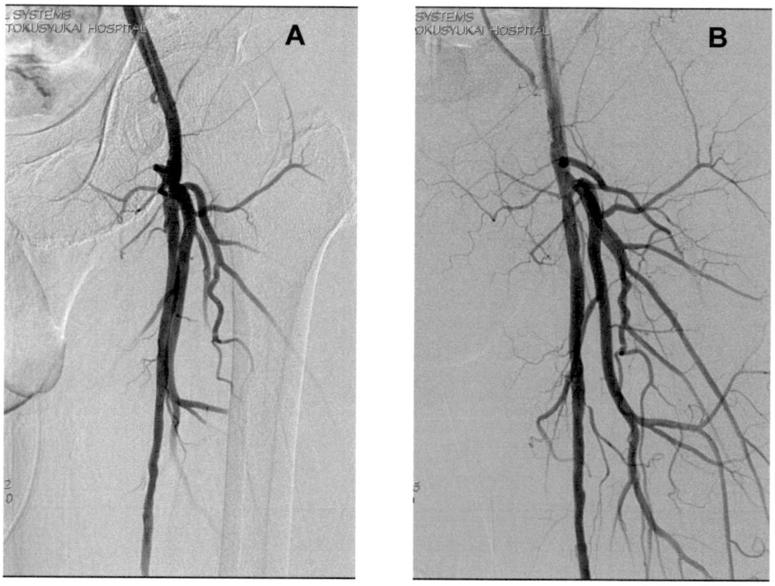

Fig. SFA 1: Anteroposterior view and left anterior
oblique view for proximal left femoral artery
A: AP view shows that profunda femoral override to SFA
B: In left anterior oblique view, separation between SFA proximal and prfund femoal are well seen

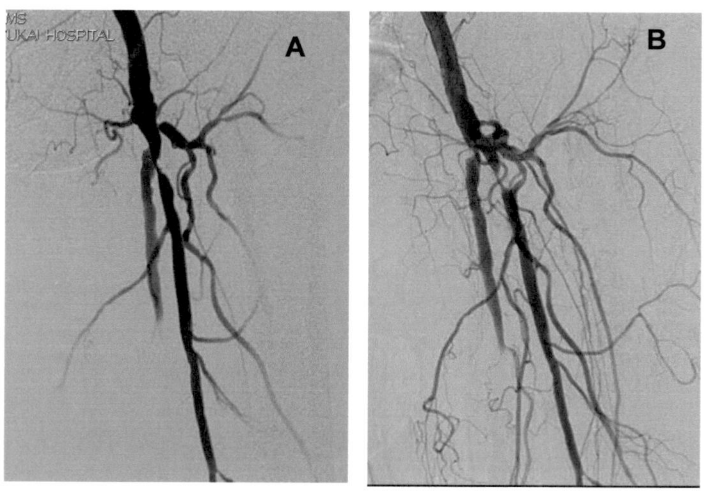

Fig. SFA 2: Anteroposterior view and left anterior
oblique view for proximal left femoral diseased artery
A: The SFA proximal stenosis is not delineated by anterior posterior (AP) view
B: Left anterior oblique view shows SFA ostial stenosis and lesion length of proximal profunda artery is longer than AP view

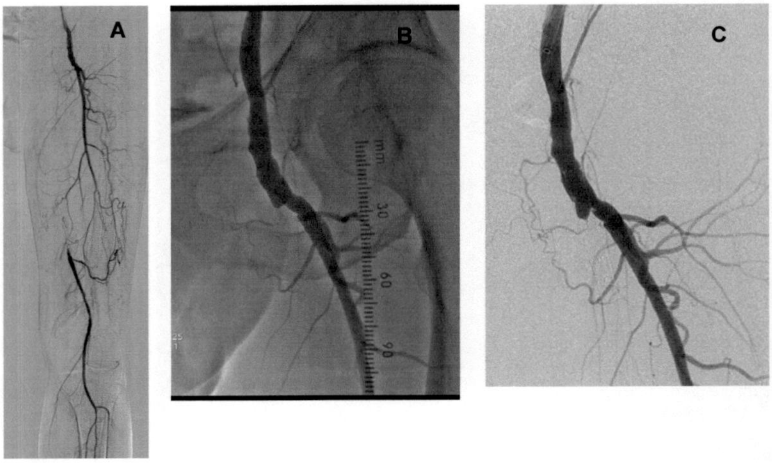

Fig. SFA 3: Anteroposterior view and left anterior oblique view for proximal left femoral artery occlusion
A: Typical SFA long occlusion originating from ostium
B: In AP view, SFA ostium is not clearly seen
C: In left anterior oblique view, the stump of SFA ostium occlusion is well visualized

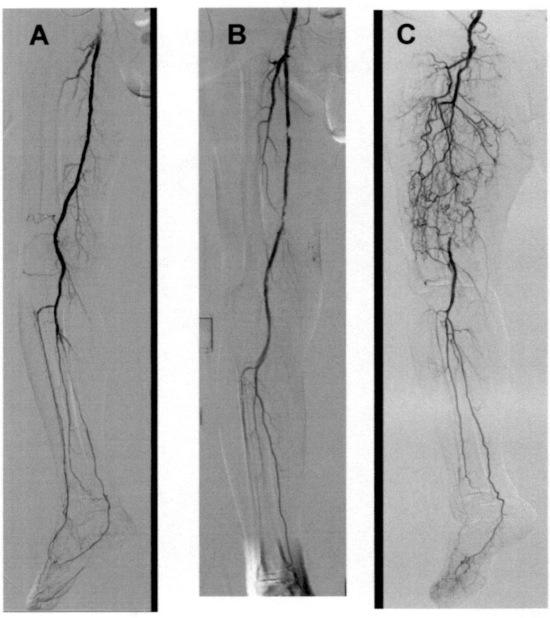

Fig. SFA 4: Bolus chase for limb vessel angiography
To see the entire limb artery, bolus chasing is very useful method. This angiogram can be obtained by digital subtraction with small amount dye.
A: Bolus chase of right limb. Infrapopliteal arteries are not well seen, but this angiogram shows the right lower limb is not severely diseased.
B: Two focal stenosis with three vessels run-off is shown
C: Typical SFA occlusion with well developed collateral via profunda femoral artery is well seen

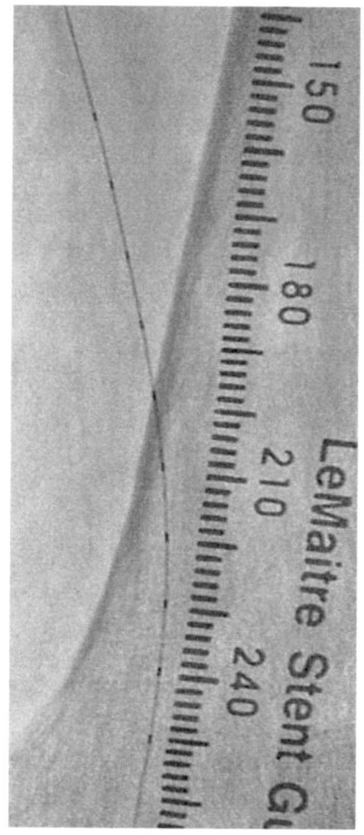

Fig. SFA 5: Marker wire and measure tape
To measure lesion length, maker tape is attached to frontal leg muscle. This tape is validated with marker wire placed in SFA. This tape can be used to measure lesion length.

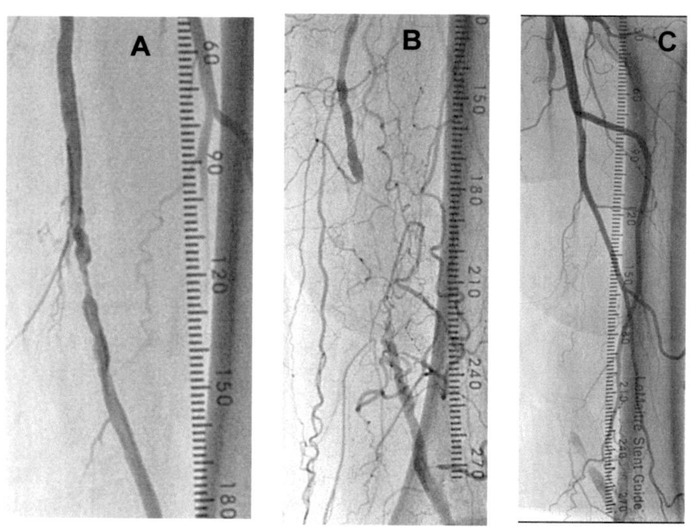

Fig. SFA 6: Lesion length of SFA disease
A: Focal lesion was measured at 1cm
B: Short CTO was measured at 6.5cm.
C: SFA long CTO was measured at 20cm

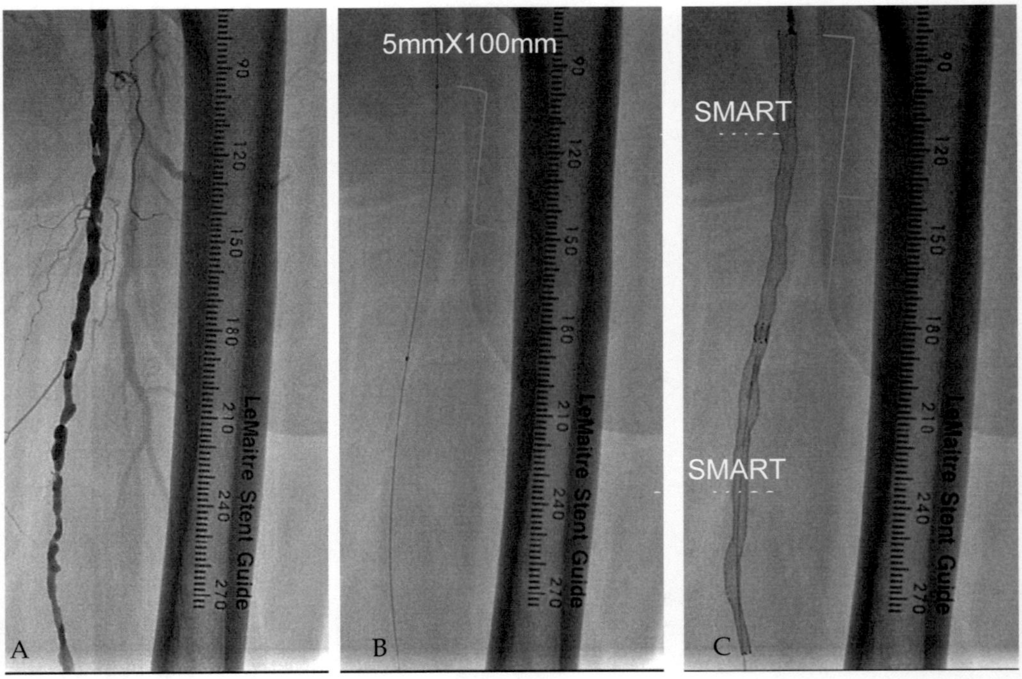

Fig. SFA 7: Lesion length measured by balloon marker
A: SFA long diffuse lesion
B: Measring lesion length by using 10cm balloon marker
C: Lesion was calculated about 20cm and two 6mmX100mm stent were implanted

7.4 TASC II Classification(13)

Before intervening the lesion, lesion length and morphology can be classified according to TASC II guideline (13). It will give the standard indication of interventional treatment or bypass surgery. Fig. SFA 8A shows a single focal lesion less than 10 cm in length and did not involve the origins of SFA. This lesion is classified into type A (Fig. SFA8A). Fig. SFA 8B is a single CTO lesion less than 15cm and considered to be type B (Fig. SFA 8B). Fig. SFA 8C shows multiple stenosis more than 15cm lesion length and a typical example of type C (Fig. SFA 8C). Fig. SFA 8D shows the long CTO and lesion length is more than 20cm (Fig.SFA 8D). This is the typical type D and stenting for this kind of lesion could be a high chance of restenosis.

7.5 Ballooning or stenting

In iliac artery disease, primary stenting is firmly established. In femoropopliteal artery disease, it is still controversial about primary stenting. In short lesion, the initial approach is still balloon angioplasty (Fig. SFA 9A, B). Angiogram of post balloon angioplasty shows suboptimal result (Fig. SFA 9C). But in reality, most of the lesion needs to be stented. Fig. SFA 10A shows the typical 5cm stenostic lesion and balloon angioplasty was performed (Fig. SFA10B). Balloon dilatation resulted in dissection and bail out stenting was performed. Nitionol stenting could seal dissection with no residual stenosis (Fig. SFA 10C).

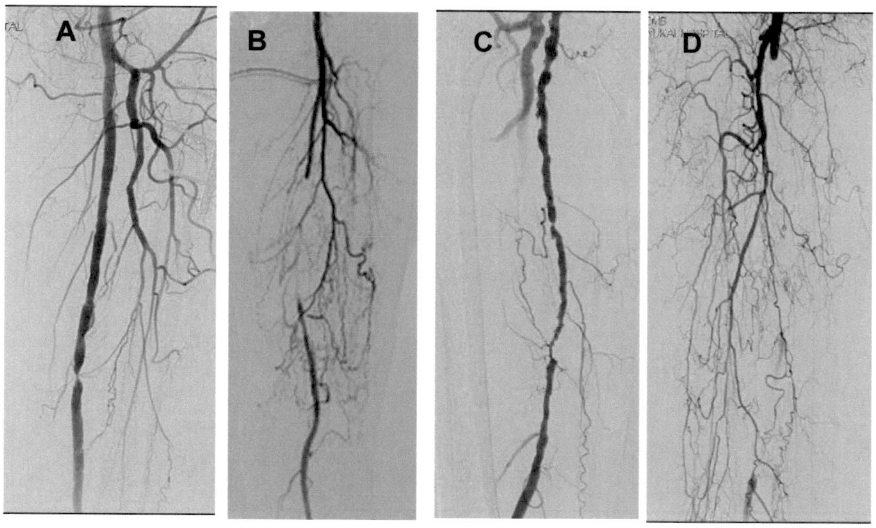

Fig. SFA 8: Lesion classification based on TASC ll guideline (13)
TASC II guideline gives the standard indication of interventional treatment or bypass surgery.
A: TASC A is a single focal lesion less than 10 cm in length
B: TASC B is a single CTO lesion less than 15cm
C: TASC C is multiple stenosis more than 15cm lesion length
D: TASC D is a long CTO and lesion length is more than 20cm

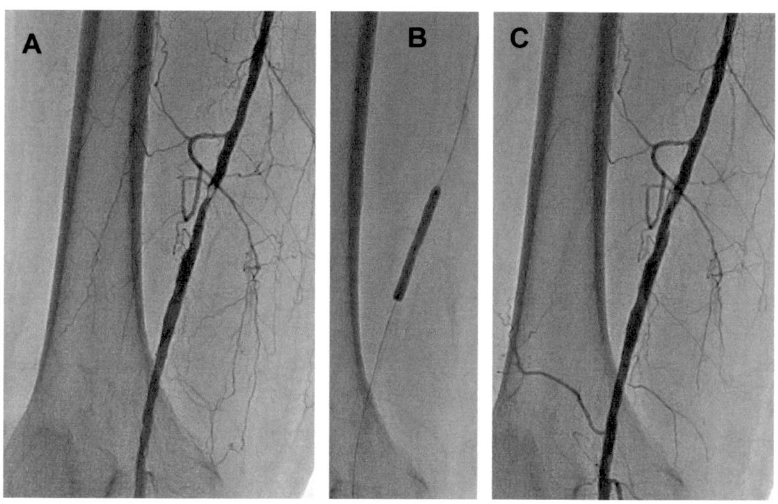

Fig. SFA 9: Balloon angioplasty
In short lesion, initial approach is the balloon angioplasty
A: A sort focal lesion in distal SFA
B: Balloon angioplasty was performed 5X40mm balloon at 8 ATM
C: Post balloon angioplasty showed a residual less than 50% stenosis at ballooning site

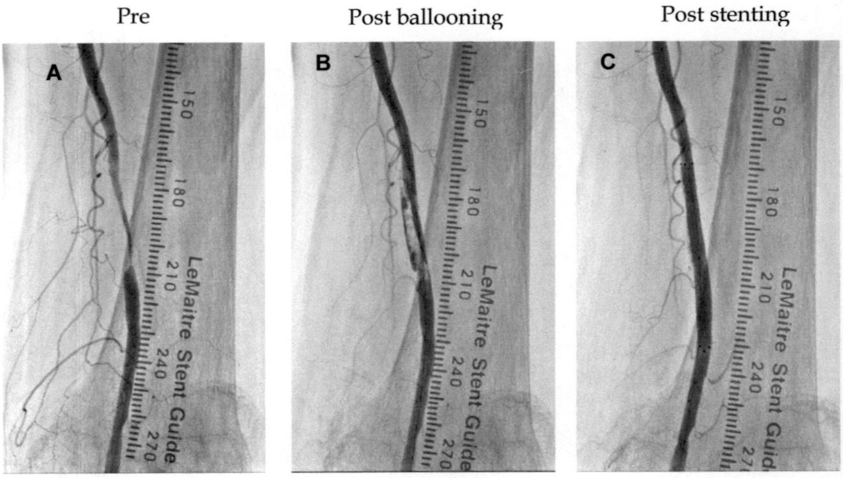

Fig. SFA 10: Bail out stenting post balloon angioplasty
A: 5cm stenostic lesion
B: Balloon angioplasty was performed and resulted in dissection
C: Nitinol stenting for bail out purpose succeeded to seal the dissection

7.6 Stent fracture

Stent fracture in SFA is a growing concern **(14)**. In most of the cases, stent fracture are not related to restenosis. Wall stent was implanted at 8 years ago (Fig. 10A). The stent showed complete traverse liner separation without stent displacement. This is called type 3 stent fracture. But there is a stent fracture related to restenosis. In Fig. SFA 11A, there is a focal restenosis at SMART stent implanted site. In plain view, multiple separation of strut is seen (Fig. SFFA 11B). Magnified view shows, multiple stent strut were separated (Fig. SFA 11C). This stent fracture could be a cause of restenosis.

7.7 Stent restenosis

In recent years, studies have demonstrated the superiority of stents over balloon angioplasty as far as primary patency is concerned **(15)**. In some center, SFA Nitinol stent is empoloyed as primary use. However, stent restenosis is still the big issue for primary stenting. SFA long CTO originating from SFA ostium was shown in Fig. SFA 12A. Successful recanalization was obtained with stenting (Fig. SFA 12B). Angiogram at 6 months showed stent restenosis with new stenosis in profund femoral artery (Fig. SFA 12C). This restenosis is clearly seen in non subtracted angiogram (Fig. SFA12D). This suggest stent affecting to other vessel as the chronic cell proliferation.

7.8 Summary

SFA is the longest vessel and is difficult to visualize entire vessel. In proximal part of SFA should be taken by ipsilateral view. To evaluate lesion severity, lesion length is the important factor for endovascular approach. The precise lesion length measurement must be made. Stent restenosis after endovascular treatment of SFA obstructions is still the big concern.

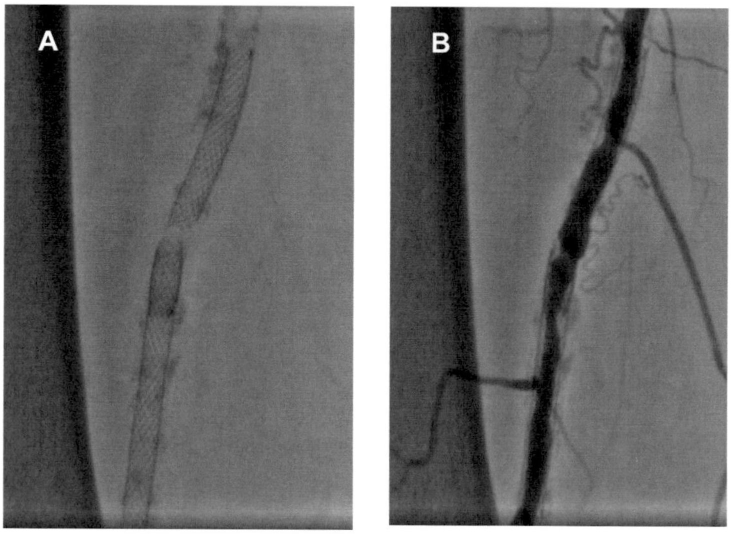

Fig. SFA 11: Stent fracture
A: Wall stent was implanted at 8 years ago. The stent showed complete traverse liner separation without stent displacement. This is called type 3 stent dissection.
B: There is no restenosis at fractured site

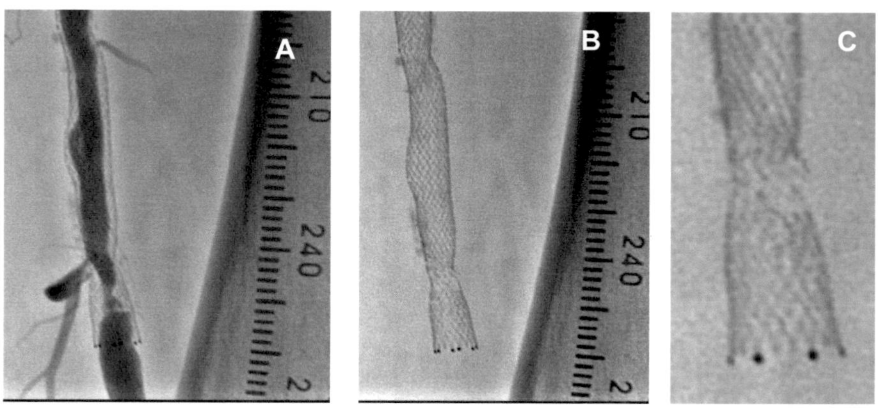

Fig. SFA 12: Stent fracture with restenosis
A: There is a focal restenosis at SMART stent implanted site.
B: In plain view, multiple separation of strut are seen
C: More magnified view shows, multiple stent strut were separated

8. Below the knee angiography

Infrapopliteal atherosclerotic lesions are common in critical limb ischemia and to assess these lesions, a meticulous angiographic technique should be taken. In Below the knee (BTK) angiogram, 4 BTK arterial segments (tibioperoneal trunk, anterior tibial, posterior tibial arteries and peroneal artery) must be separated and identified. And also, continuation

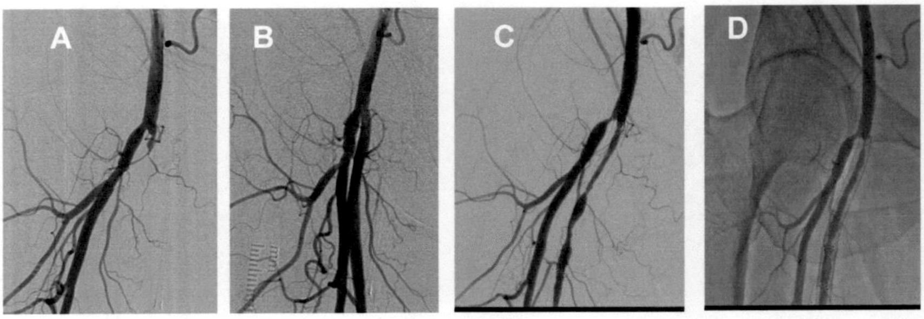

Figure SFA 13: Stent restenosis
A: SFA occlusion originating from ostium
B: Succeful recanalization was obtained with Nitinol stenting
C: At 6 months, angiography showed SFA stent restenosis with a new stenosis in profund femoral artery.
D: This restenosis is clearly seen in non subtracted angiogram

from anterotibial artery to dorsal pedis and posetotibial to planter artery have to be delineated. BTK arteries are most complicated vessels and difficult to identify each three vessels. Meticulous angiographic approach should be taken to visualize three tibila arteries.

8.1 Basic angiography for BTK

Femoropopliteal artery angiogram must be taken to rule out inflow disease (Fig. BTK 1A). After confirming no inflow disease is present, BTK angiography is performed through the catheter located at distal popliteal artery (Fig. BTK 1B). This BTK angiogram is to show three tibial arteries and antero tibial artery is occluded. To locate exact lesion location, we take 4 views. These are two right anterior oblique view (RAO) (Fig. BTK 1C, 1D)and two left anterior oblique view (LAO) taken (Fig. BTK 1E, 1F). In upper RAO, proximal left anterotibial artery is well seen (Fig. BTK 1C). In lower RAO view, distal three tibial arteries are well seen (Fig. BTK 1D). In this case, distal anterotibial artery is occluded. In upper LAO, three tibial arteries are separated (Fig. BTK 1E). In lower LAO view, anterotibial and peroneal artery overrap and could not separate these two vessels (Fig. BTK 1F).

8.2 Anatomical variation of infrapopliteal arteries

Branching variations of the popliteal artery are not uncommon. A practical triad classification of the anatomical variation in the branching pattern is reported **(17)**. Type 1 indicates a normal level of popliteal arterial branching, including the usual pattern (Fig. BTK 2A) and trifurcation (Fig. BTK 2B). Type 2 indicates a high division of popliteal artery branching. In Fig. BTK 2C, anterotibial artery arises at the knee joint. Type 3 indicates hypoplastic or branching with an altered distal supply, including a hypoplastic posterotibial (Fig. BTK 2D) and a hypoplastic antrotibial (Fig. BTK 2E) .There are more other variation, but we have to keep in mind variant tibial arteries are not uncommon.

8.3 Numbers of patent tibial arteries

After completing initial angiogram, we have to evaluate how many tibial arteries are patent. In normal BTK arteries, three vessels are patent (Fig. BTK 3A.) In Fig. BTK 3B, peroneal

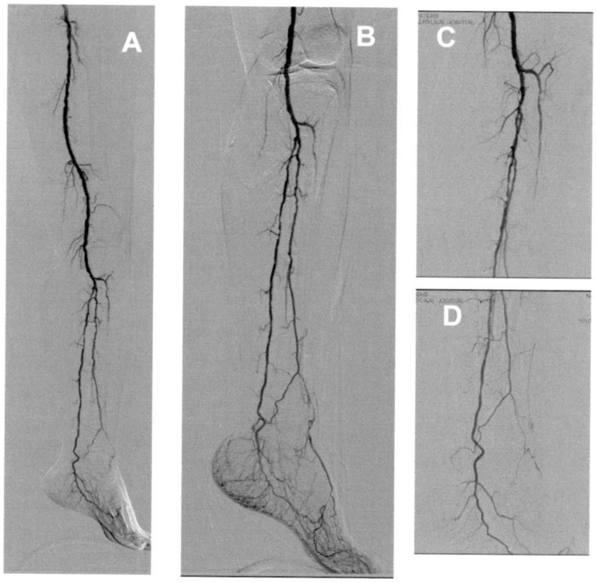

Figure BTK 1: Basic below the knee angiography
A: Ipsilateral left femoropopliteal to infrapoplital artery angiogram. This angiogram could rule out the inflow disease.
B: BTK angiography shows the entire three tibial arteries.
C: Upper right anterio oblique view.
Proximal left anterotibial artery is well seen. But posterotibial and peroneal artery are over rapped.
D: Lower right anterio oblique view. In this view, distal 3 tibial arteies are separated.
E: Upper left anterior oblique view.
Proximal three tibial arteries are well separated.
F: Lower left anterior oblique view.
Distal Posterotibial artery is well seen.

artery is not seen and considered two vessels run off. In Fig. BTK 3C, peroneal and posterotibial artery are patent and means two vessel runoff., In Fig. BTK 3D, only personal artery is patent and shows the one vessel run off.

8.4 Single vessel run off of peroneal artery

In Fig. BTK 4, both cases are single vessel disease with peroneal artery patent. These 2 cases, one peroneal artery is patent, but have active ulcer. It means that peroneal artery is not good enough for supplying foot arteries.(Fig. BTK 4). Peroneal artery terminates at the ankle and gives collateral to planter artery (Fig. BTK 4A). In Fig. BTK 4B, peroneal artery gives the collateral to dorsal pedis. This means to revascularize either anterotibial or posteriotibial artery must be recanalaized for the successful angioplasty.

8.5 BTK angiogram of pre and post balloon angioplasty

Before intervening BTK vessels, target vessel have to be clearly identified. In Fig. BTK 5, patient is a 65 year old man with diabetes and presented with right 4th and 5th toe ulcer. Pre

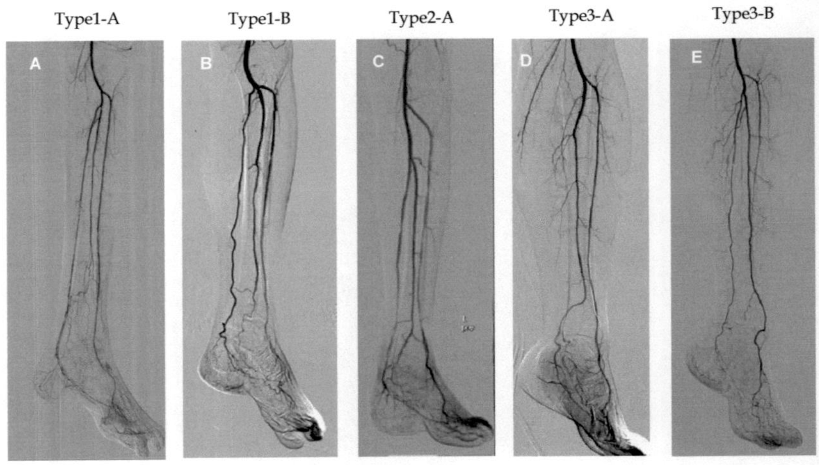

Fig. BTK 2: Anatomical variation of tibial arteries
A: Type 1-A
A normal level of arterial branching and most common pattern. The first brach is antrotibial artery and peroneal trunk separate to peroneal and posterotibial artery.
B: Type 1-B
A normal level of arterial branching. The three tibial arteries show trifurcation.
C: Type 2-A
A high division of popliteal artery branching and antrotibial artery arises at the knee joint.
D: Type3-A
Hypoplastic posterotibial artery and peroneal artery is giving a distal supply.
E: Type 3-B
Hypoplastic anterotibial artery and peroneal artery is giving a distal supply.
D: One vessel, peroneal arterry is patent

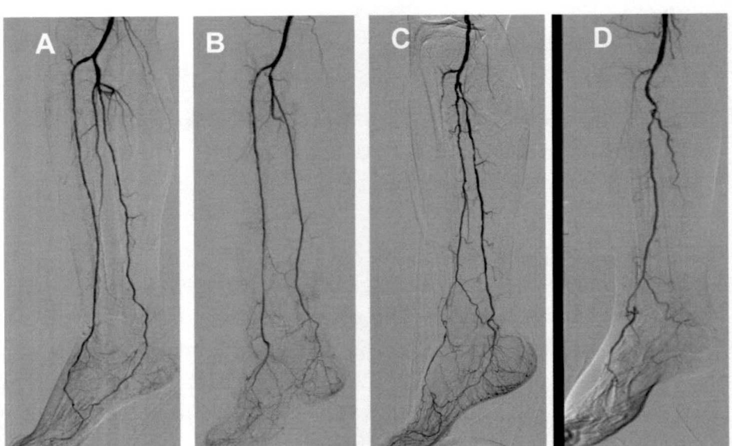

Fig. BTK 3: Number of patent tibial arteries
A: Three vessels are patent
B: Two vessels are with occluded peroneal artery
C: Two vessels are with occluded anterotibial artery

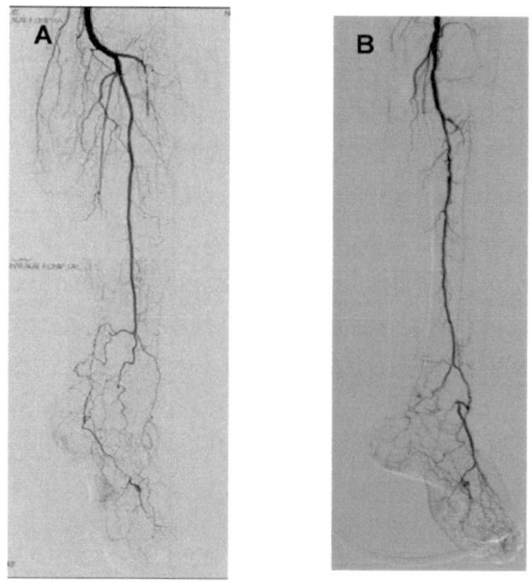

Fig. BTK 4: Single vesses runoff of peroneal artery in patients with critical limb
A: Peroneal artery terminates at the ankle and gives collateral to planter artery
B: Peroneal artery terminates at the ankle and gives collateral to dorsal pedis.
In these two cases, single vessel are patent but ulcer does not heal. Peroneal artery is not giving sufficient flow distal to ankle.

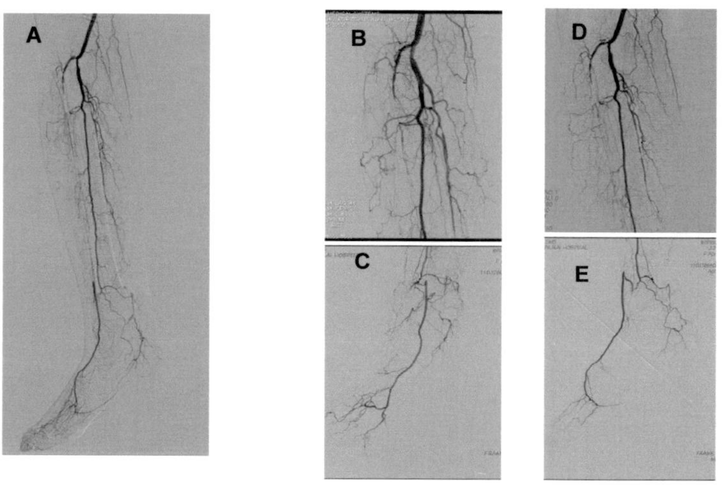

Fig. BTK 5: Pre interventional BTK angiography for critical limb ischemia
A 65 year old man with diabetes and presented with right 4th and 5th toe ulcer.
A: Bolus chase
Right anterotibial and posterotibial arteries were occluded and peroneal artery is patent
B: The upper RAO view
Three tibial arteries and right antrotibial artery was occluded at proximal portion
C: The lower RAO view
Right dorsal pedis was patent; D: The upper LAO view - Only peroneal artery is patent
E: The lower LAO view - Right antrotibial artery was occluded at the ankle and dorsal pedis artery is getting collateral through peroneal artery. Right planter artery is not well seen

intervention angiography showed right anterotibial and posterotibial arteries were occluded (Fig. BTK 5A). Two right anterior oblique view (RAO) (Fig. BTK 5B, C) and two left anterior oblique (LAO) (Fig. BTK 5D, E) views were taken. The upper RAO showed three tibial arteries and right antrotibial artery was occluded at proximal portion (Fig. BTK 5B). The lower RAO view showed right dorsal pedis was patent (Fig. BTK 5C). The upper LAO view showed only peroneal is patent t (Fig. BTK 5D). The lower LAO view revealed right antrotibial artery was occluded at the ankle and right planter artery is not well seen (Fig. BTK 5E). Based on these angiograms, right antrotibial artery occlusion was targeted. By using 2.5mmX10cm over the wire balloon system, occluded anteoritibial artery was recanalaized (Fig. BTK 6). Post angioplasty angiogram was shown in Fig. BTK 7. Post intervention angiography showed right anterotibial was successfully recanalaized.and (Fig. BTK 7A). Two right anterior oblique view(RAO) (Fig. BTK 7B,C) and two left anterior oblique(LAO) (Fig. BTK 7D,E) views were taken to confirm the recanalized right antrotibial artery. The upper RAO showed three tibial arteries and right antrotibial artery was recanalized(Fig. BTK 5B). The lower RAO view showed peroneal override with anterotibial artery and could not separate two vessels(Fig. BTK 7C). The upper LAO view showed opened antrotibial artery(Fig. BTK 7D). The lower LAO view showed continuity between antrotibial to dorsal pedis was established (Fig. BTK 7E).

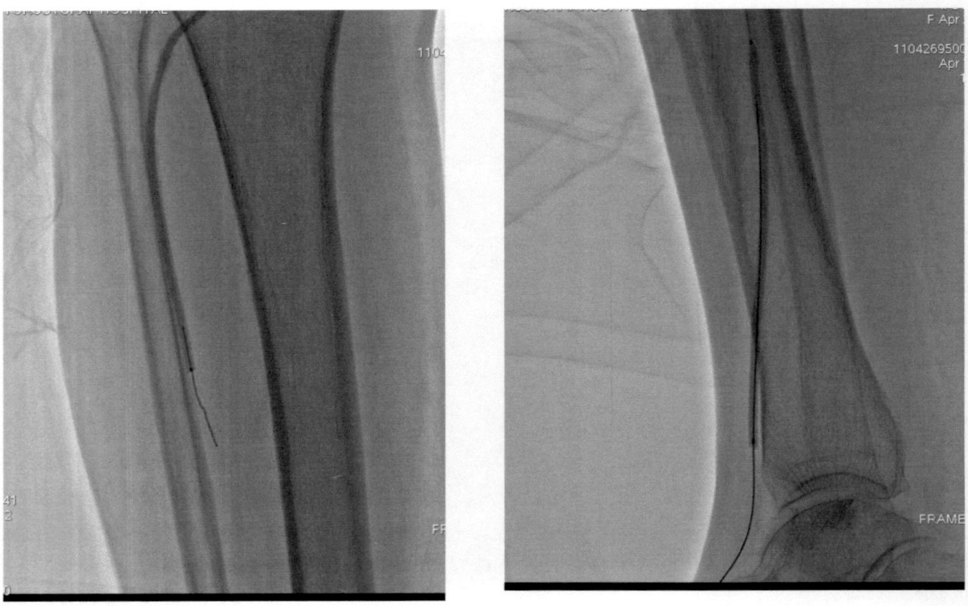

Fig. BTK 6: Balloon angioplasty to occluded anterotibial artery
Based on these angiograms, right antrotibial artery occlusion was targeted.
A: By using 2.5mmX10cm over the wire balloon system, the occluded proximal anteoritibila artery was recanalaized
B: The wire advanced to dorsal pedis and succeeded to recanalization

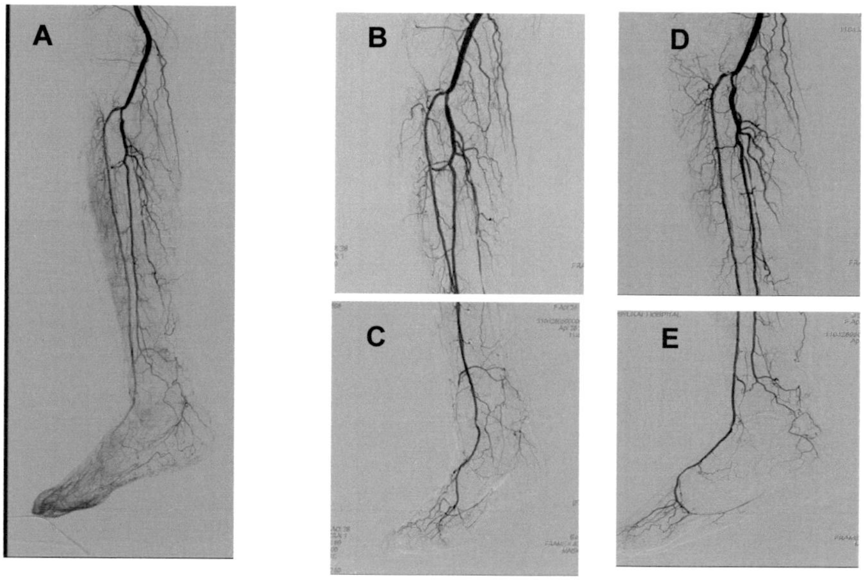

Fig. BTK 7: Post interventional BTK angiography for critical limb ischemia
A: Bolus chase
Right anterotibial artery was recanalized and straight line to dorsal pedis artery was established.
B: The upper RAO view
Right anterotibial artery was patent but midportion of anterotibial artery overrides with peroneal artery.
C: The lower RAO view
The continutity between anterotibial and dorsal pedis artery is confirmed.
D: The upper LAO view
Recanalized right anterotibial artey is well seen
E: The lower LAO view
Right anterotibial to dorsal pedis artey is shown.

8.6 Foot artery angiogram

In dealing with critical limb ischemia, precise knowledge of foot artery anatomy is needed. However, severe ischemic limb, foot artery angiogram is hard to obtain by the patient's leg movement. To minimize this problem, injection of small amount of contrast with inflow revascularization is mandatory. In Fig. BTK 8, typical ischemic foot artery is shown. Basically two views are good enough. One is antero-posterior view and the other is lateral view. In lateral view, complete occlusion of poterotibial artery is well seen and dorsal pedis show the short occlusion (Fig. BTK 8A). In anterior view, plantaris medial and lateralis are well separated (Fig. BTK 8B). And in anterior view, dorsalis pedis is well seen and suited for Retrograde dorsal pedis puncture (Fig. BTK 8B).

8.7 Summary

The effectiveness of BTK angioplasty for revascularization is well known **(18).** However, BTK angiography is one of the most difficult vessel for angiogram. Tibial arteries are small

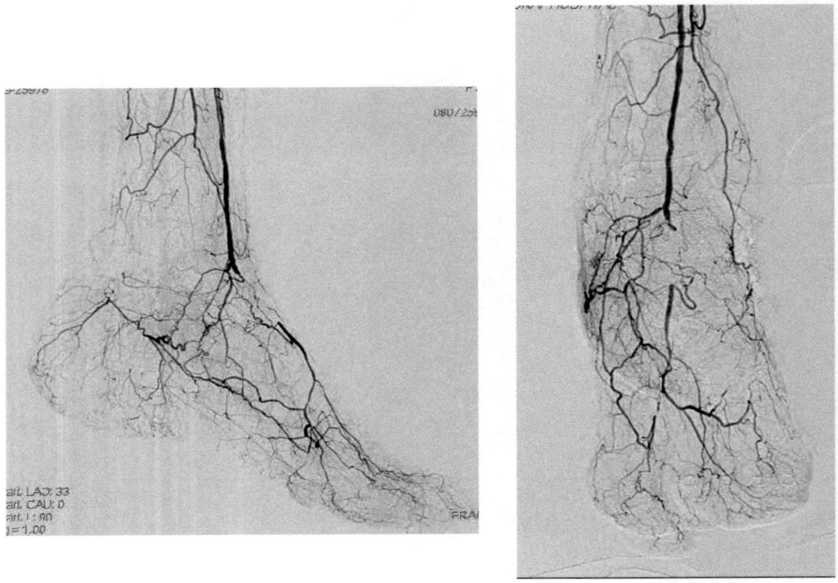

Fig. BTK 8: Foot artery angiogram:
A: Lateral view of left foot
Complete occlusion of poterotibial artery is well seen and dorsal pedis show the short occlusion
B: Anteroposterior view
Plantaris medial and lateralis artery are well separated. In anterior view, occluded dorsalis pedis artery is well seen

sized vessels with complicated anatomy. The amount of dye for injection is limited by patient's leg movement. However, angiogram is the only way to get the correct information BTK. The meticulous approach for BTK angiography should be taken.

9. Reference

[1] Wakhloo AK, Lieber BB, Seong J, Sadasivan C, Gounis MJ, Miskolczi L, Sandhu JS.Hemodynamics of carotid artery atherosclerotic occlusive disease. J Vasc Interv Radiol. 2004 ;15(1 Pt 2):S111-21.

[2] Sacco RL , Adams R, Albers G, et al; American Heart Association/American Stroke Association Council on Stroke; Council on Cardiovascular Radiology and Intervention; American Academy of Neurology. Guideline for prevention of stroke in patients with ischemic stroke or transient ischemic attack: a statement for healthcare professionals from the American Heart Association/American Stroke Association Council onStroke: co-sponsored by the Council on Cardiovascular Radiology and Intervention: the American Academy of Neurology affirms the value of this guideline. Circulation. 2006; 113:e409–e449.

[3] Nedeltchev K, Pattynama PM, Biaminoo G, Diehm N, Jaff MR, Hopkins LN, Ramee S, van Sambeek M, Talen A, Vermassen F, Cremonesi A; DEFINE Group. Standardized definitions and clinical endpoints in carotid artery and supra-aortic trunk revascularization trials. Catheter Cardiovasc Interv. 2010 Sep 1;76(3):333-44.

[4] Saba L, Mallarini G. MDCTA of carotid plaque degree of stenosis: evaluation of interobserver agreement. AJR Am J Roentgenol. 2008 Jan;190(1):W41-6.

[5] North American Symptomatic Carotid Endarterectomy Trial Collaborators. Beneficial effect of carotid endarterectomy in symptomatic patients with high-grade stenosis. N Engl J Med 1991;325:445-53.

[6] Peeters P, Verbist J, Deloose K, Bosiers M. Endovascular treatment strategies for supra-aortic arterial occlusive disease. J Cardiovasc Surg (Torino). 2005 Jun;46(3):193-200.

[7] Donmez H, Mavili E, Kaya MG, Soylu SO, Toker B. Endovascular treatment of coronary steal. Cardiovasc Revasc Med. 2011 Jan-Feb;12(1):67.e1-3. Epub 2010 Oct 20.

[8] Textor SC, Lerman L, McKusick M. The uncertain value of renal artery interventions: Where are we now? JACC Cardiovasc Interv 2009;2:175–182

[9] Kalra PA, Guo H, Kausz AT, Gilbertson DT, Liu J, Chen SC, Ishani A, Collins AJ, Foley RN. Atherosclerotic renovascular disease in United States patients aged 67 years or older: risk factors, revascularization, and prognosis. Kidney Int. 2005 Jul;68(1):293-301.

[10] ASTRAL Investigators, Wheatley K, Ives N, Gray R, Kalra PA, Moss JG, Baigent C, Carr S, Chalmers N, Eadington D, Hamilton G, Lipkin G, Nicholson A, Scoble J. Revascularization versus medical therapy for renal-artery stenosis. N Engl J Med. 2009;361:1953–1962.

[11] Cicuto KP, McLean GK, Oleaga JA, Freiman DB, Grossman RA, Ring EJ. Renal artery stenosis: anatomic classification for percutaneous transluminal angioplasty. AJR Am J Roentgenol. 1981 Sep;137(3):599-601.

[12] Lederman RJ, Mendelsohn FO, Santos R, Phillips HR, Stack RS, Crowley JJ.Primary renal artery stenting: characteristics and outcomes after 363 procedures. Am Heart J. 2001 Aug;142(2):314-23.

[13] Norgren L, Hiatt WR, Dormandy JA, Nehler MR, Harris KA, Fowkes FG; TASC II Working Group. Inter-Society Consensus for the Management of Peripheral Arterial Disease (TASCII). J Vasc Surg. 2007 Jan;45 Suppl S:S5-67.

[14] Jaff M, Dake M, Pompa J, Ansel G, Yoder T. Standardized evaluation and reporting of stent fractures in clinical trials of noncoronary devices. Catheter Cardiovasc Interv. 2007 Sep;70(3):460-2.

[15] Mewissen MW. Primary nitinol stenting for femoropopliteal disease. J Endovasc Ther. 2009 Apr;16(2 Suppl 2):II63-81.

[16] Laird JR. Limitations of percutaneous transluminal angioplasty and stenting for the treatment of disease of the superficial femoral and popliteal arteries. J Endovasc Ther. 2006 Feb;13 Suppl 2:II30-40.

[17] Day CP, Orme R. Popliteal artery branching patterns -- an angiographic study. Clin Radiol. 2006 Aug;61(8):696-9.

[18] Bosiers M, Deloose K, Verbist J, Peeters P. Update management below knee intervention. Minerva Cardioangiol. 2009 Feb;57(1):117-29.

8

Arterial Angioplasty in Congential Heart Disease

Thomas J. Forbes, Srinath Gowda and Daniel R. Turner
Wayne State University/Children's Hospital of Michigan, Detroit, MI
USA

1. Introduction

This chapter will describe the historical background, technical issues, outcomes, and future considerations of angioplasty to treat various congenital heart lesions in both the systemic and pulmonary arteries. Intravascular stent placement will be mentioned briefly, but the primary focus will be balloon angioplasty of arterial stenosis. Peripheral stenoses secondary to acquired arterial lesions will not be discussed.

2. Coarctation of the aorta

2.1 Historical background

Coarctation of the aorta is a condition where the aorta is narrowed in the area where the ductus arteriosus inserts (Figure 1). Coarctation represents 5-10% of all congenital heart disease. Coarctation is more common in Caucasian than Asian individuals and is less common among Native Americans. Males are affected 1.6-1.8 times as often as females. The overall incidence of coarctation in the United States is 64 per 100,000. The presentation can range from shock in infancy after closure of the ductus arteriosus to systemic hypertension in early childhood to adulthood.

The three treatment modalities for coarctation of the aorta are surgery, stent placement, and balloon angioplasty (BA). Candidates for BA will be discussed in detail below. In native coarctation of the aorta, the anatomy most suitable for BA is discrete, rather than diffuse, stenosis (Figures 2a and 2b). This is not necessarily the case in recurrent coarctation, where discrete or diffuse lesions secondary to surgical scarring are each amenable to BA. [1-3]

2.2 Neonates/infants

Balloon angioplasty of coarctation of the aorta in neonates/infants can typically be performed with low-profile balloon angioplasty catheters due to the smaller final inflation diameter required in this age group. The most common diameter used in this age group is 6-8 mm, although as the patient approaches 12 months of age, the diameter shifts to the 8-10 mm range. The most commonly used balloons are the TyShak II balloons (NuMed Corp, Hopkington, New York). Up to 8 mm diameter balloons take an 0.021" wire, can be introduced through 4-Fr sheaths, and have a rated burst pressure (RBP) of at least 4 atmospheres (ATMs). The 9-12 mm diameter balloons take an 0.025" (9-10 mm) or 0.035" (12 mm) wire, can be introduced through 5-Fr sheaths, and have a RBP of 3.5 ATMs. TyShak Mini balloons (NuMed), with diameters from 4-10 mm, are even lower profile, using 3-Fr

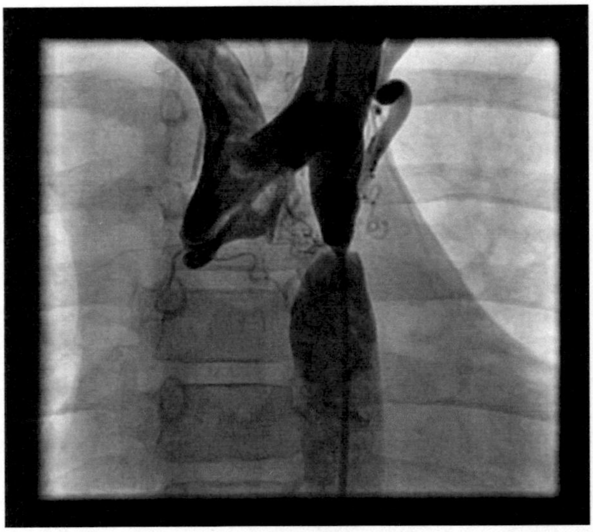

Fig. 1. Coarctation

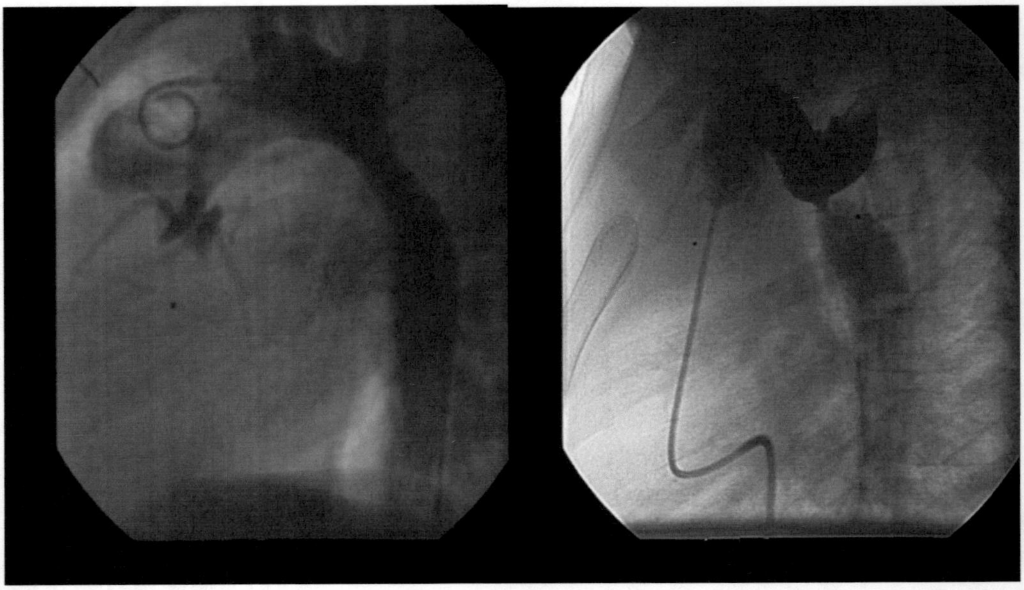

Fig. 2. a-b.

sheaths up to 8 mm diameter and 4-Fr sheaths for the 9-10 mm sizes. They take an 0.014" wire and can reach RBP of at least 3.5 ATMs. Most coarctations require 3 ATMs to obtain adequate dilation of the narrowed segment.

On occasion, high-profile, non-compliant balloon angioplasty catheters may be required to adequately dilate the coarctation segment. There are numerous balloon angioplasty catheters available: PowerFlex series (4-12 mm diameter, Cordis Corp, Warren, New Jersey), Z-Med II balloons (4-30 mm diameter, NuMed), and Cook ATB (4-10 mm diameter, Cook

Corp, Bloomington, IN). Each are similar, although certain sizes of PowerFlex and ATB balloons can be advanced through sheaths that are 1-Fr size smaller than Z-Med II. Rarely, cutting balloons (CB) may be required for coarctation angioplasty.[4] More specific information on CB will be given in the pulmonary angioplasty section.

The standard approach for native or recurrent coarctation of the aorta is retrograde via femoral- or umbilical-arterial access. This approach offers the most direct route to treat the coarctation site. In very small infants (< 1.5 kg), alternative approaches have been reported (Figures 3a, 3b, and 3c).[5] Angiograms of the coarctation and transverse aortic arch are performed prior to balloon angioplasty. In over 20% of patients, most commonly in cases of symptomatic neonatal/infant coarctation of the aorta, transverse aortic arch hypoplasia may be present. The definition of transverse aortic arch hypoplasia is a transverse arch-to-descending aortic ratio of < 0.60.[6-8] Measurements at the transverse aortic arch and descending aorta at the level of the diaphragm are made. The smaller of these diameters determines the size of the balloon catheter used to perform coarctation angioplasty. It is particularly important that the balloon be de-aired prior to inflation, as balloon rupture may cause air emboli into the brachiocephalic vessels. On initial inflation, one tries not to exceed a balloon-to-coarctation ratio of > 4:1.[7] Pre- and immediately post-pressure measurements are obtained. After the angioplasty, it is extremely important to obtain standard and orthogonal angiographic views of the coarctation area to exclude a small dissection or aneurysm. If high pressure or cutting balloon catheters are required for adequate dilation of the coarctation segment, a covered stent should be available in the catheterization lab in case one encounters aneurysm formation, an acute dissection, or vessel tear.

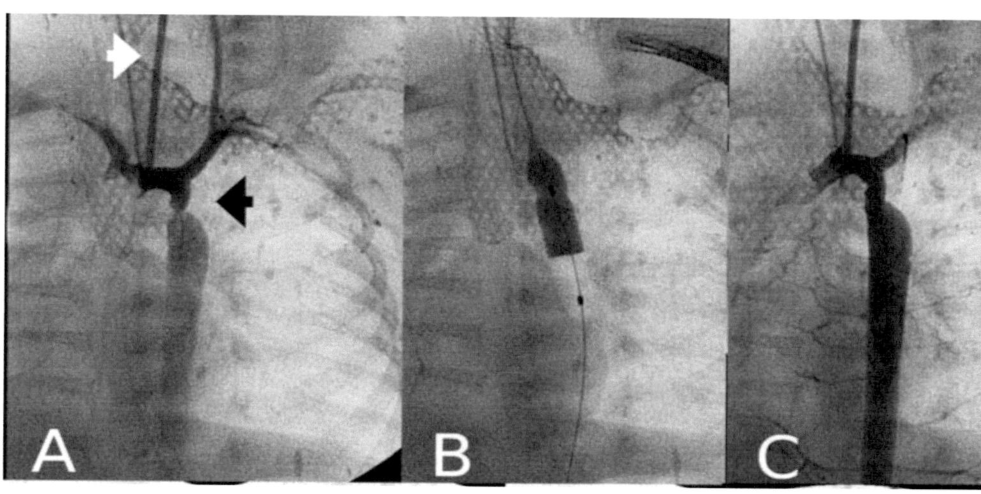

Courtesy of Prada F, et al. Rev Esp Cardiol. *2010 Jun;63(6):741-3.*

Fig. 3. a-c. Balloon angioplasty of a critical coarcation in a 1200 gram premature infant per the left carotid artery via a 3 Fr sheath using the Seldinger technique. A 4 mm TyShak Mini balloon was used with the coarctation segment increasing from 1.5 to 3.2 mm and a decrease in the systolic gradient from 35 to 7 mmHg. The infant developed recoarctation 2 months later and at 2200 grams underwent repeat balloon angioplasty from the femoral arterial system. At 6 months out from the procedure (5600 grams) the infant continues to do well with no evidence of recoarctation.

2.3 Outcomes

Infantile coarctation of the aorta typically occurs in conjunction with severe heart failure or shock. In this setting, coarctation is frequently associated with other congenital heart lesions (bicuspid aortic valve in 60-70%, ventricular septal defect in 40%, and other left-sided lesions, i.e. mitral valve stenosis, subaortic valve stenosis, and hypoplastic left ventricle 3% of the time). Performance of coarctation angioplasty is not recommended in patients with associated congenital lesions requiring surgery. The predominant treatment for isolated native coarctation of the aorta presenting in infancy is surgical repair with extended end-to-end anastomoses. Although many believe that surgical repair is the standard of care, some have advocated that BA in high-risk patients is a reasonable initial procedure to improve their surgical candidacy.[9] The overall outcome of BA is poor in infants presenting in heart failure or shock. Liang et al. performed a recent study where they evaluated 18 infants with native coarctation of the aorta and congestive heart failure who underwent balloon angioplasty. The mean age was just less than three months and the mean body weight was 4 kg. Congestive heart failure symptoms improved markedly in all patients immediately after BA. The incidence of re-coarctation was high in infants, requiring surgery if the systolic pressure gradient > 10 mmHg from ascending to descending aorta or if the coarctation diameter measured < 3 mm. The recurrent coarctation rate was 44% (8/18 patients) and the conclusion was that balloon angioplasty, in this setting, was ineffective and not recommended as a primary treatment alternative.[9]

In another recent study by Rau, et al., 51 infants less than 3 months of age who presented with heart failure underwent balloon coarctation angioplasty from the umbilical artery (16/51), femoral artery (26/51) and femoral venous antegrade across the inter-atrial communication (9/51). Findings included acute reduction in the peak gradient across the coarctation segment, increase in the diameter of the coarctation segment, and improved symptomatology following BA. Effective palliation was achieved in 47/51 infants (92%). At intermediate follow-up, 22/51 (43%) developed re-coarctation withn three months after balloon angioplasty, requiring either repeat BA (14/22) or surgical (8/22) intervention. Using avoidance of surgery for four weeks as the definition of success, the authors concluded that BA is an excellent alternative to surgical intervention for the management of native coarctation in the neonatal period. With > 50% of patients requiring reintervention within 10 months of initial BA, we believe that surgical treatment of this condition remains the standard of care in this subgroup of patients. [10]

2.4 Challenges for the future

The development of bioabsorable stents could potentially change this treatment paradigm. There are two current challenges with bioabsorable stent technology: (1) to reliably make a stent that can reach 6-7 mm diameter with adequate radial strength to overcome the coarctation; and (2) to be able to deliver the stent though a low profile sheath (4-5-Fr if performed retrograde and up to 7-Fr if performed antegrade from the venous route). There are currently two bioabsorbable stents being evaluated with the potential to enter clinical use in Europe within the next several years.

3. Aortic coarctation in children and adults

3.1 Historical overview

Balloon angioplasty for the treatment of native or recurrent coarctation of the aorta has been performed since the mid 1980s.[11] There is excellent data to support BA to treat recurrent coarctation of the aorta in this age group. Although BA is considered the treatment of choice for this lesion in children and adults,[12] controversy surrounds the use of BA for native coarctation of the aorta in these patients presenting with hypertension.

3.2 Technique

BA is performed from the retrograde femoral arterial route in the majority of children and adults undergoing BA for either recurrent or native coarctation. Recently, there have been reports of using radial access for recognition and treatment of potential complications, some advocating for BA though we, and others, feel radial access is more appropriate for stent treatment of coarctation of the aorta. [13] After a complete right and left heart catheterization is performed, the coarctation segment is approached retrograde from the descending to ascending aorta. It is important to rule out any potential left-sided lesions, including mitral valve stenosis, subaortic valve stenosis, or aortic valve stenosis, as these lesions can be also associated with coarctation of the aorta. Furthermore, significant diastolic dysfunction and increased diastolic pressures can be encountered in this patient group. For severe or nearly atretic coarctation of the aorta, crossing the narrowed segment retrograde may be quite difficult. Under those circumstances, transseptal technique is used to enter the left heart antegrade and the coarctation can then be crossed more easily from the ascending to descending aorta. Typically, either an angled 0.035" glide wire (Cook Corp, Bloomington, Indiana) or Wholey wire (Covidian Inc. Mansfield, MA) are used. The wire is then snared retrograde from the distal descending aorta and an arterial-venous loop is created, then allowing retrograde delivery of the balloon to the coarctation segment.

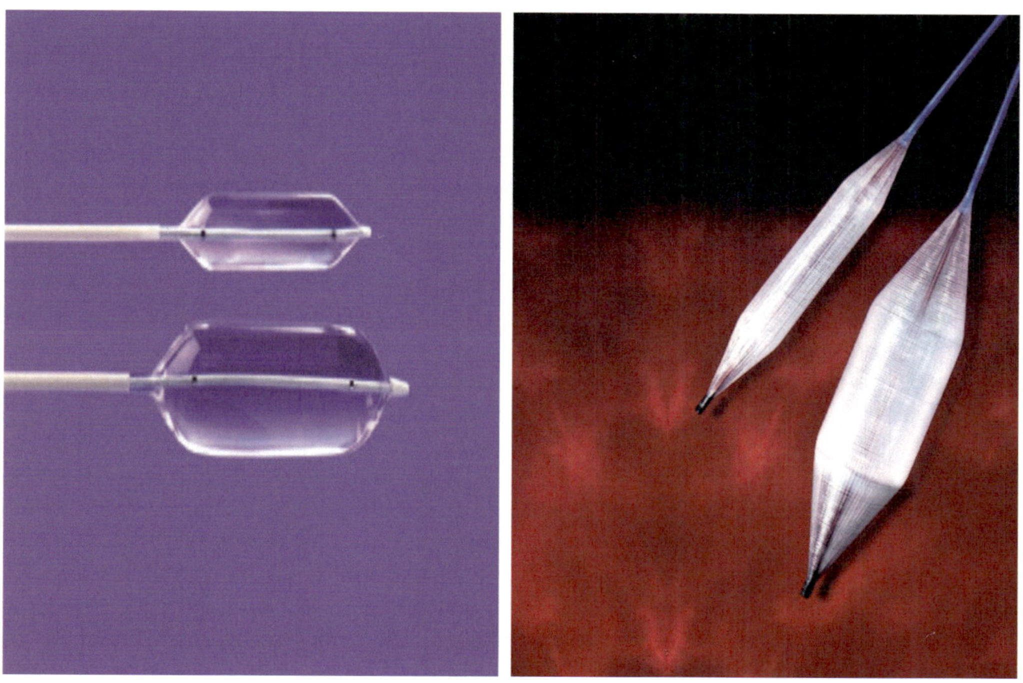

Fig. 4. a-b. Comparison between the Atlas and Z Med II balloon catheters. The tapered shoulder on the Atlas balloon significantly increases the actual balloon length as well as inflation/deflation time in comparison to the shorter Z Med II balloon.

Higher RBP for coarctation BA is more important as patients age. Although lower profile (TyShak II) balloons may be used, less compliant, higher profile balloon angioplasty catheters are usually required. PowerFlex, Maxi-Plus (Cordis corp, Warren, NJ), Z-Med II, Mullins (NuMed corp., Hopkington, NY), and Atlas (Bard Medical, Tempe, AZ) balloon angioplasty catheters have all been used. The Atlas balloon catheter has enhanced low profile (2-3 Fr sizes less than the others) and high RBP. The tapered shoulders of the Atlas balloon makes the balloon quite long and longer inflation/deflation times are required, making it more difficult to adequately position this balloon catheter across the coarctation segment (Figures 4a-b).

As one exceeds 5-6 atmospheres of pressure to achieve successful dilation of the coarctation segment, there is an increased likelihood of creating an acute dissection, aneurysm, or in rare cases, rupture of the aorta.[7] It has been recommended that one not exceed four times the narrowest coarctation segment during dilation in the initial setting. Patients with extremely tight coarctation segments therefore require a staged approach.

3.3 Outcomes

Balloon angioplasty of native coarctation of the aorta is part of the treatment paradigm in children and adults. In the Congenital Cardiovascular Interventional Study Consortium (CCISC) registry comparing surgical vs. stent vs. balloon angioplasty treatment of native coarctation of the aorta in children and adults, BA appeared to have an increased risk of aneurysm formation and dissection at short-term and intermediate follow-up (Tables 1 and 2) (Journal American College of Cardiology, *in press*). The overall hemodynamic outcome related to blood pressure management and upper to lower extremity blood pressure gradient appear to be equal between the three groups at short-term and intermediate follow-up. In the subgroup of patients undergoing balloon angioplasty, the incidence of aneurysm formation was as high as 43% at intermediate follow-up, some patients requiring placement of a covered stent (Figures 5a-b). Cowley et al., in comparing surgery with balloon angioplasty for native coarctation of the aorta, showed that aneurysm formation and the need for re-intervention was significantly higher in the balloon angioplasty group compared to the surgical group.[14] Hassan, et.al., looked at balloon angioplasty in the older adolescent and young adult populations only, age range from 14-54 years. In this age group, the aneurysm rate was much lower (7%) at intermediate follow-up.[15, 16] The difference between these studies may be related to the age group of patients treated with balloon angioplasty. In the Forbes study, the mean age was 6.8 years vs. 22 years in Hassan's study. Perhaps older patients are more likely to have successful outcomes and less likely to have aneurysm formation following BA.

The most severe complication, aortic rupture or large dissection, is rare, but occurs with increased incidence in older patients. As expected, it is the non compliant, adult aorta where this is more likely to occur. Aortic rupture or large aneurysm formation does not appear to be related to exceeding the balloon:coarctation ratios of 4:1, but may be related to exceeding 6 ATMs during initial balloon inflation. In one case, a 43 yo lady with moderate hypertension and coarctation of the aorta presented for transcatheter treatment of the coarctation segment. BA was unsuccessful in relieving the gradient. Stent placement was performed using a high pressure balloon angioplasty catheter. At the end of the procedure, a small amount of contrast was observed outside of the stent posteriorly. CT scan revealed near complete transection of the aorta. One month and one year follow-up CT imaging noted complete resolution of the peri-aortic hematoma with no evidence of dissection or aneurysm formation (Figures 6a-d).

Outcomes	Surgery (n = 26)	Balloon (n = 28)	Stent (n = 97)	p-value (2-sided)
Any Complications1	23.1%	32.1%	8.3%	0.003*
Aortic Wall Injury (%)	11.5%	21.4%	3.1%	0.004*
Dissection / Intimal Tear (%)	0.0%	7.1%	0.0%	0.062
Aneurysm (%)	11.5%	14.3%	3.1%	0.040*
Coarct / Dao ratio (mean)	0.91	0.73	0.82	0.003*
Coarct / Dao ≥ 0.6	87%	79%	90%	0.247
Any Re-obstruction	19.2%	32.1%	15.4%	0.057
Mild2	7.7%	17.9%	11.3%	
Moderate	7.7%	3.6%	4.1%	
Severe	3.9%	10.7%	0%	

[1]Defined as any moderate to severe reobstruction, aortic wall injury (aneurysm, dissection, intimal tear) or stent fracture.
[2]Mild reobstruction was not considered as a complication in our analysis.
* P- value < 0.05

Table 1. Short-Term Follow-up Outcomes by Integrated Imaging

Outcomes	Surgery (n = 16)	Balloon (n = 16)	Stent (n = 56)	p-value (2-sided)
Any Complications[1]	25.0%	43.8%	12.5%	0.020*
Aortic Wall Injury (%)	12.5%	43.8%	7.1%	0.003*
Dissection / Intimal Tear (%)	0.0%	6.3%	1.8%	0.598
Aneurysm (%)	12.5%	43.8%	5.4%	<0.001
Coarct / Dao ratio (mean)	0.98	0.79	0.80	0.011*
Coarct / Dao ≥ 0.6	88%	93%	89%	1.000
Any Re-obstruction	18.8%	18.8%	14.3%	0.923
Mild[2]	6.3%	18.8%	12.5%	
Moderate	6.3%	0%	1.8%	
Severe	6.3%	0%	0%	

[1]Defined as any moderate to severe reobstruction, aortic wall injury (aneurysm, dissection, intimal tear) or stent fracture.
[2]Mild reobstruction was not considered as a complication in our analysis.
* P- value < 0.05

Table 2. Intermediate Follow-up Outcomes by Integrated Imaging

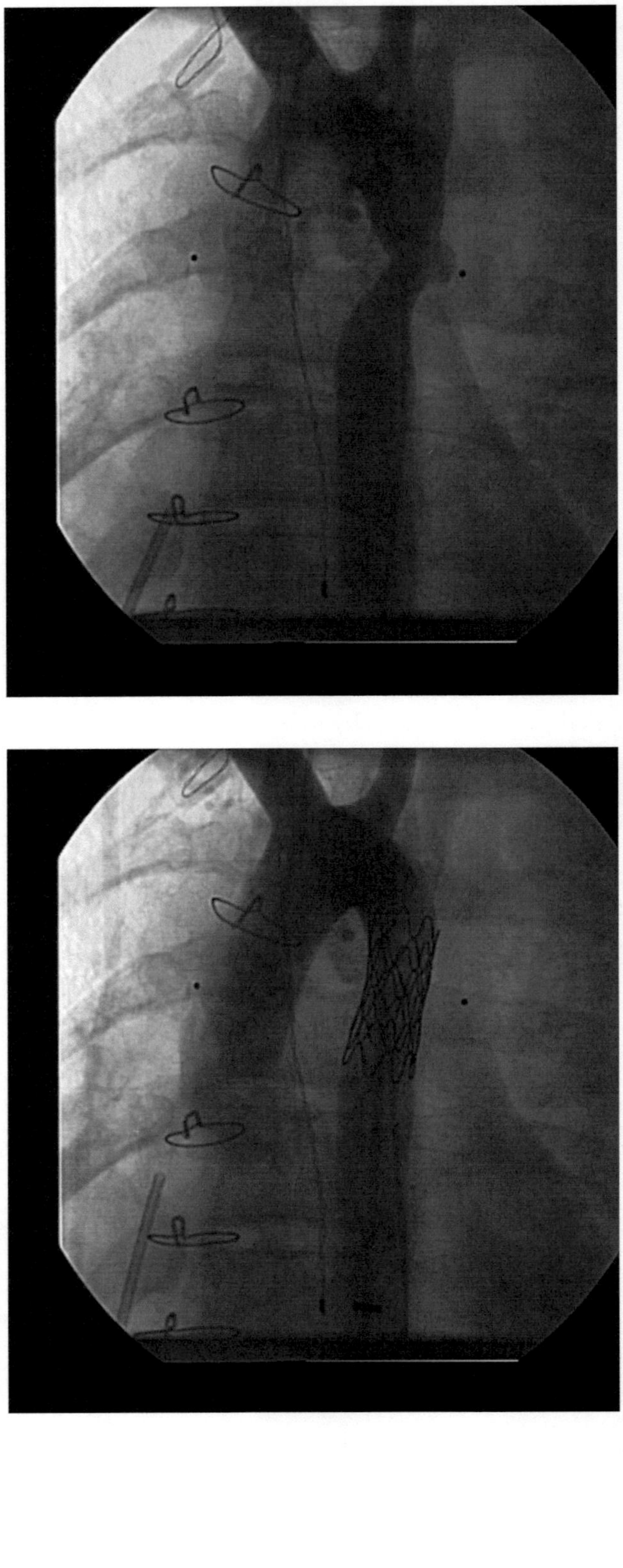

Fig. 5. a-b.

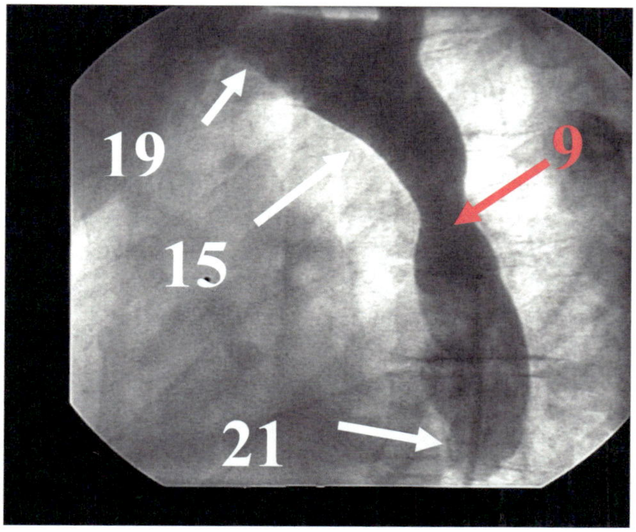

Fig. 6. a.

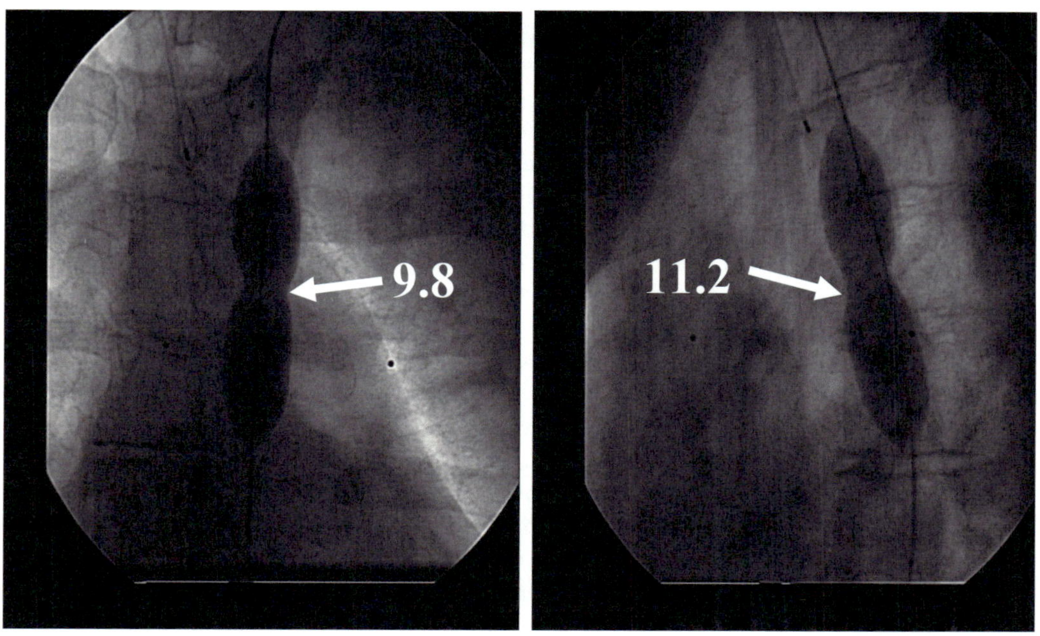

Fig. 6. b-c.

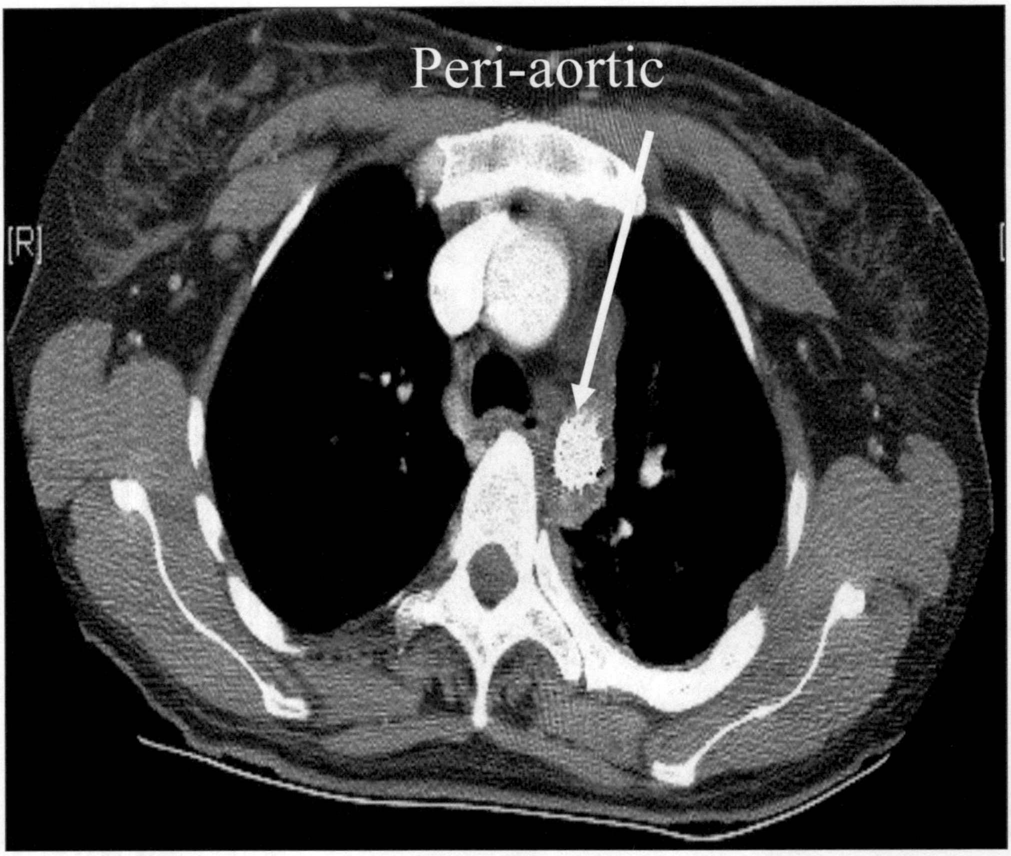

Fig. 6. d.

Re-obstruction, as defined as an upper to lower blood pressure gradient > 20 mmHg or narrowed segment > 50% of the native vessel diameter, appears to be less common as the age at the time of initial treatment increases. Re-obstruction frequency ranges from 3-20% in older children/adults undergoing primary BA of native coarctation compared to the nearly 50% re-obstruction rate seen in infant balloon angioplasty of their native coarctation. [9, 10, 15]

3.4 Challenges for the future

Stent treatment, particularly in older children and adults, appears to be the treatment of choice in treatment of native and recurrent coarctation of the aorta.[7, 8, 13, 17] Permeating balloons, where a drug is injected into the vessel wall during angioplasty to prevent the development of re-stenosis, have not been successful for adequate drug delivery in animal studies. The primary challenge involves unintentional delivery of the drug directly into the blood stream, and not into the vessel wall. Placement of markers 5 mm apart, marking the permeating holes within the balloon catheter may assist us in delivering the treatment drug directly into the vessel wall, though this remains to be seen. The length of time for inflation required to deliver the medication (1-3 minutes) would require adequate collateralization around the coactation lesion to decrease the likelihood of encountering lower extremity/bowel ischemia. The current medications that may have a role in this are similar to the current medications being placed on drug eluting stents. These can be broken down into cytotoxic/cytostatic drugs, which have recently been undergoing head-to-head trials in applications to coronary stenting [18, 19 20] or "pro-healing" drugs such as endogenous growth factors or endothelial progenotor cells.[21] What role, if any, in this approach to coarctation of the aorta, remains to be seen.

4. Pulmonary artery stenosis

4.1 Historical background

Balloon angioplasty, first described for use in pulmonary valve stenosis in 1983,[22] has become the treatment of choice for balloon angioplasty of branch pulmonary artery stenosis in most pediatric cardiology centers. [23, 24] Surgical repair of branch pulmonary artery stenosis has been sub-optimal, associated with increased morbidity, especially in young infants and children.

4.2 Technique

As with any interventional procedure, the first step in evaluating a pulmonary artery for BA is to understand the anatomy and pathophysiology of the stenotic lesion to be addressed. Generally, as in coarctation of the aorta, discrete lesions tend to be more amenable to BA compared to long segmental lesions. In Figures 7a-c, a patient with Tetralogy of Fallot with pulmonary valve atresia has multiple discrete and long segment stenosis of the right upper lobe segment. BA is performed both in the distal discrete stenosis and the more proximal long segment stenosis. Follow up imaging noted resolution of the distal discrete stenosis with persistence of the proximal stenosis, which required stent placement. In another patient with RPA stenosis following the arterial switch procedure (Figure 8), MRI imaging shows the RPA stenosis to be secondary to posterior compression from the aorta. Therefore stent placement, not BA, was necessary to treat this mechanical RPA stenosis.

Performance of branch pulmonary artery BA is relatively straightforward and can be through a short sheath. The most difficult part of the procedure is usually crossing the stenotic segment. Accurate angiographic imaging is essential. For proximal stenosis (prior to the takeoff of the upper lobe branch), the lesion is crossed with either a 0.025 or 0.035" wire where, depending on patient size, a 4-5 Fr pigtail or multipurpose catheter is advanced over the wire into the stenosed pulmonary artery. Hand or power angiography is performed. For distal branch stenosis, the stenotic lesion is usually crossed with a glide wire and then a 4-Fr JB-1 or similar glide catheter (Cook Corp, Bloomington, IN) is advanced over the wire distal to the lesion. Hand injections can be performed through the catheter with the wire remaining in place. BA is usually carried out over that same wire. If multiple lobar segments are involved, the BA catheter is pulled back into the proximal pulmonary arterial segment and the soft tipped 0.018" wire is used to cross other stenoses. Stent treatment of multiple branch PA stenosis is usually not recommended, as many of the affected branch vessels would be "jailed off" by the stent (Figure 9a-b).

The balloons typically required for branch pulmonary artery BA are the higher-pressure, non-compliant balloon catheters. Typically, the more distal or peripheral the stenosis, the greater the need for higher atmosphere balloons or cutting balloons (or both) to achieve adequate BA of the stenotic segment.

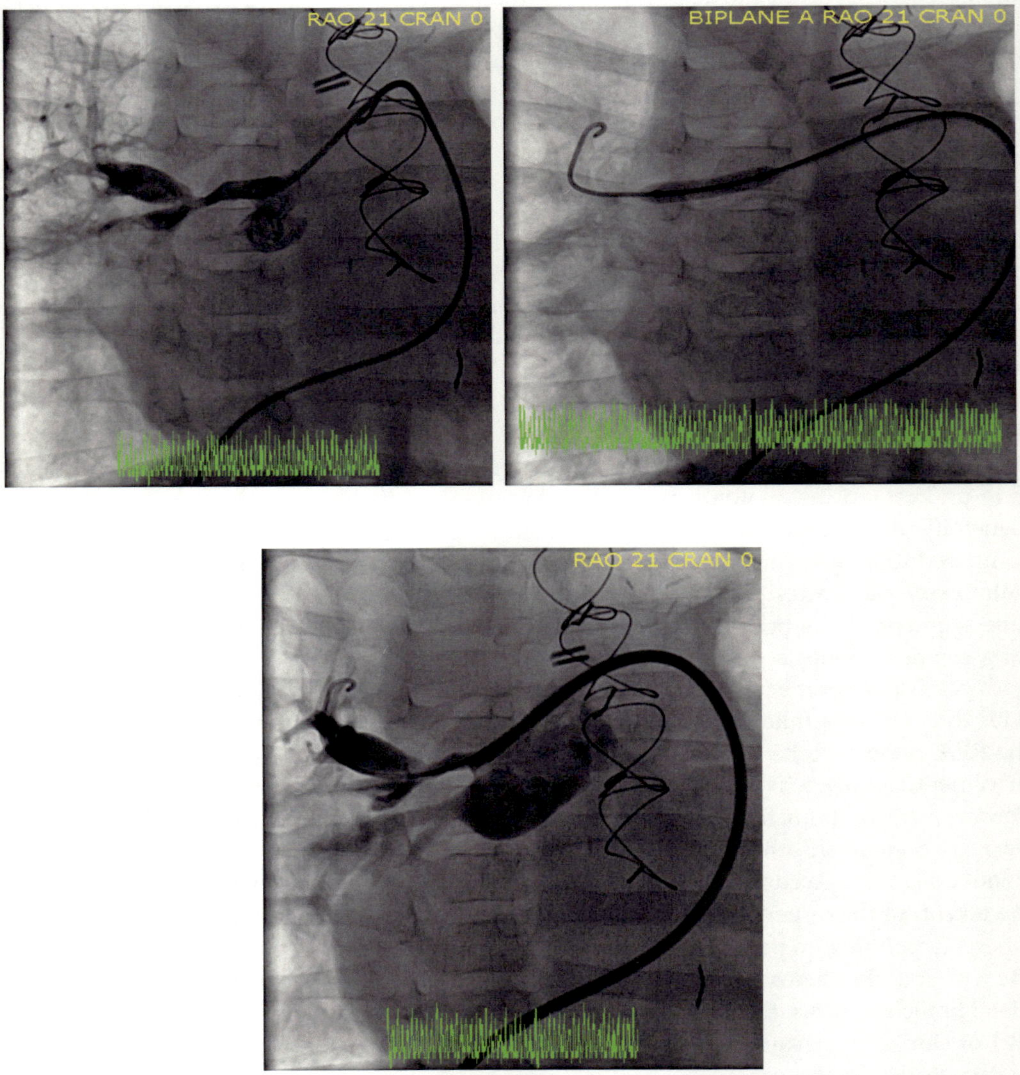

Fig. 7. a-c. Patient with Pulmonary Atresia and Ventricular Septal Defect with multiple distal stenosis of the RPA segment. BA is performed up to 19 ATMs with a 4 mm balloon angioplasty catheter. Left lower panel notes resolution of the distal discrete stenosis, though persistence of the proximal stenosis.

The cutting balloon (CB) is a dilation balloon made of noncompliant modified polyethylene terephthalate with available balloon diameters from 2-8 mm and lengths 10, 15, and 20 mm (Boston Scientific Corp., Natick, Massachusetts, Figure 10 a-b). The incremental increase in balloon size is 0.25 mm from 2-4 mm and 1 mm from 5-8 mm. Depending on the balloon diameter, 3 or 4 microsurgical blades are attached every 90 or 120 degrees, each blade with a working height of 0.11-0.18 mm. Prior to dilation, the folds of the balloon cover the microsurgical blades and following dilation, the blades wrap into the folds of the balloon with deflation. Use of the CB requires a long sheath, 4-Fr for a 4 mm CB, 6-Fr for a 5 mm CB, and 7-Fr for a 6-8 mm CB. Wires are 0.014" up to 4 mm diameter and 0.018" from 5-8 mm diameter. These balloons reach full inflation at 6 ATMs with burst pressure at 10 ATMs. Aggressive balloon angioplasty of the vessel (up to 22 ATM pressure) with a standard balloon angioplasty catheter is usually performed prior to performing CB. (Figure 11a-d). The CB is usually dilated 1-2 mm larger than the narrowest segment of the stenosis. Following this, standard BA is performed up to the native vessel size. The balloons may undergo repeat dilation, but it is recommended that no more than 10 inflation/deflation cycles be used for one balloon catheter. Rapid inflation and deflation of CB should not be performed; rather slowly inflating and deflating these balloons over a one minute period of time is recommended. Finally, exceeding the burst pressure of these balloons should never be undertaken. Balloon rupture, which typically is longitudinal, prevents the proper folding of the balloon and subsequent coverage of the microblades, thereby making it more likely to strip a blade off the balloon catheter during removal of the CB. CB angioplasty is performed via either long flexor sheaths (Cook Flexor, Cook corp, Bloominton, IN) or various guiding sheaths.

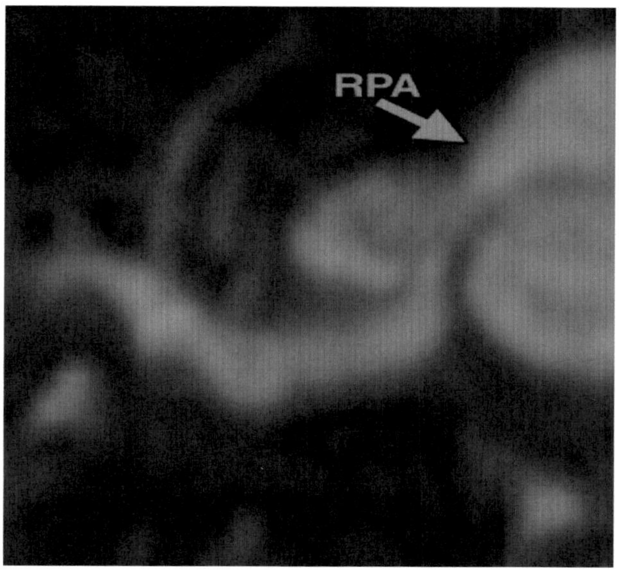

Fig. 8.

Patients with multiple bilateral peripheral pulmonary artery stenoses can suffer from re-perfusion injury following dilation of multiple affected lung segments. This situation can be life threatening in patients who are already compromised with severe elevation of the right ventricular pressure. Multiple techniques have been addressed in an attempt to avoid this circumstance. One is to dilate one segment or pulmonary arterial side with no treatment of the contralateral side at the same cath procedure. Another is selectively ventilating the contralateral lung segment during the BA procedure, thereby decreasing blood flow to the treated lung and theoretically decreasing the likelihood of encountering re-perfusion injury of those involved segments. [25]

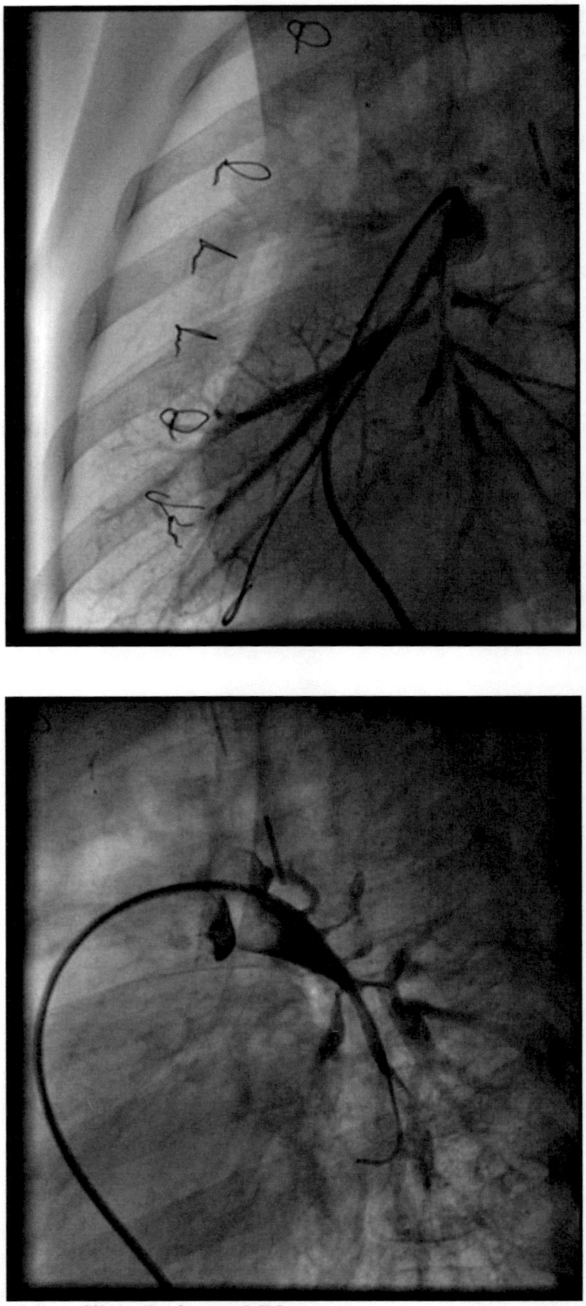

Courtesy Allison Cabalka, Mayo Clinic, Rochester, MN

Fig. 9. a-b. Multiple right and left pulmonary artery stenosis of the distal branches. Patient has systemic right sided pressures and is planning on undergoing multiple balloon angioplasty dilations. One can see discrete as well as diffuse stenosis of the distal branch vessels.

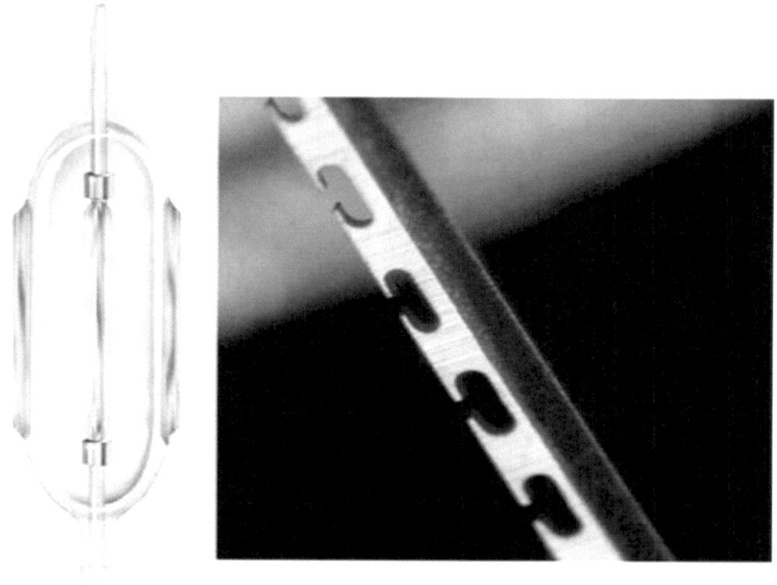

Fig. 10. a-b.

4.3 Outcomes

The performance of pulmonary balloon valvuloplasty to treat pulmonary valve stenosis has been an extremely effective procedure. Unfortunately, balloon dilation of stenoses of the pulmonary arteries distal to the pulmonary valve has not been as satisfactory.[23, 26] Although the stenotic vessels often can be dilated with angioplasty balloons, even to three or four times the original size, the stenoses frequently recur immediately after balloon deflation. The recurrence of obstruction following dilation is thought to be due to the natural elastic recoil of the tissue in native pulmonary arterial stenosis or to resilience and resistance of scar tissue in postoperative cases. Rothman, et al. reported the only large series of balloon pulmonary artery dilations in 135 patients. [27] They noted that previous reports of surgery for the direct relief of pulmonary artery lesions was difficult and often ineffective.[28] The mean diameter of the lesion increased from 3.8 +/- 1.7 to 5.5 +/- 2.1 mm with dilation ($p = 0.001$). The overall success rate was 58% (127/218 dilations), assessed by the following criteria: an increase greater than or equal to 50% of predilation diameter, an increase greater than 20% in flow to the affected lung, or a decrease greater than 20% in systolic right ventricular to aortic pressure ratio. A pulmonary artery aneurysm occurred in 5% of the pulmonary arteries dilated. Two patients died at angioplasty. Restenosis occurred in 16% of the restudied patients with initial successful dilation. They concluded that balloon angioplasty was an established, highly useful procedure in the management of branch pulmonary artery stenosis. [27]

The use of cutting balloons (CB) has increased the success rate of pulmonary artery BA from 50-60% to 80%, irrespective of whether CB were used de novo or following failure of standard balloon angioplasty.[26] One area where CB have been particularly effective is in severe, multiple discrete stenosis of the distal pulmonary arterial branches (Figure 9a-b). [29, 30]

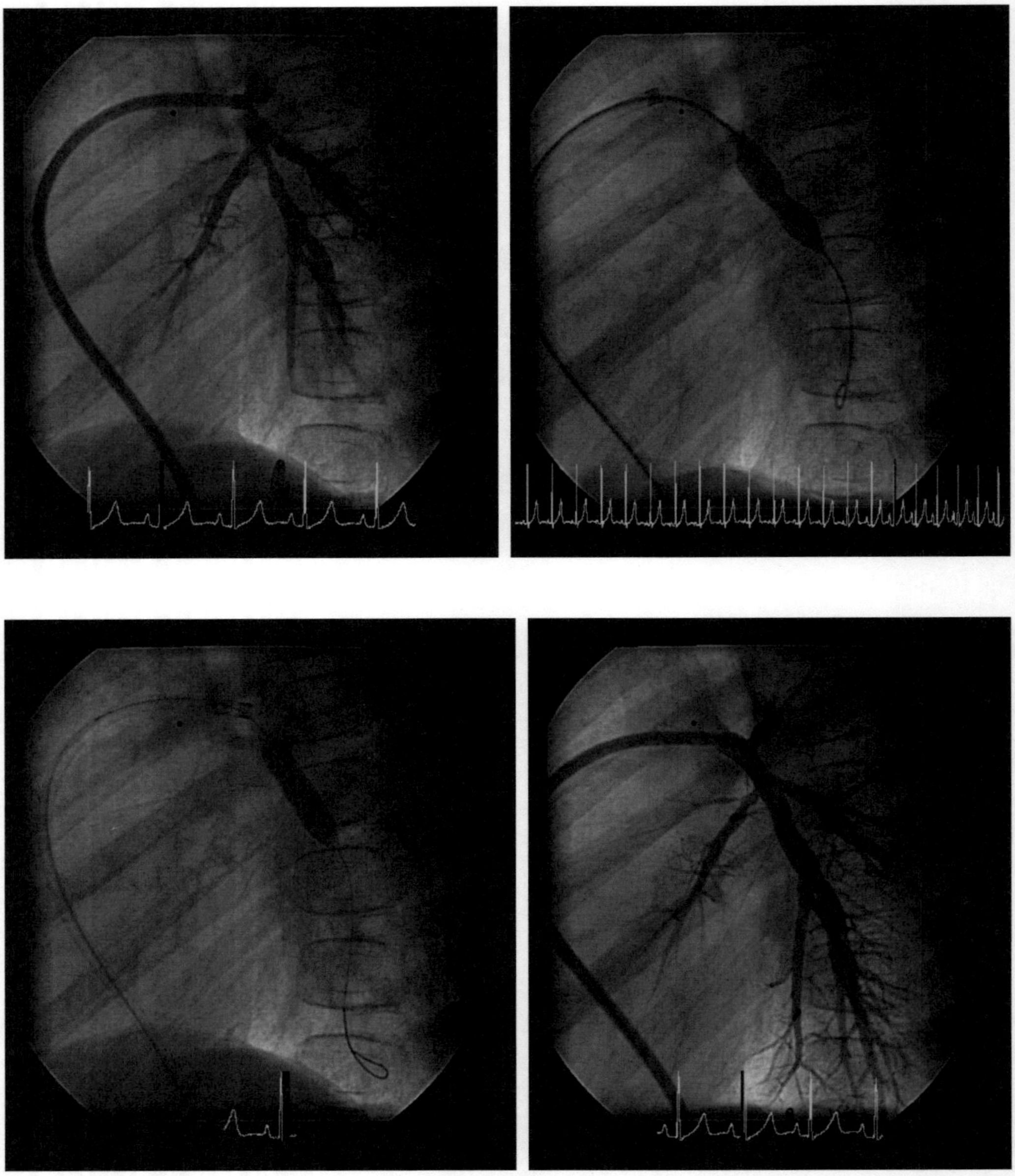

Courtesy Jaqueline Kreutzer, Children's Hospital of Pittsburgh, Pittsburgh, PA

Fig. 11. a-d. Cutting balloon angioplasty of distal branch left lower lobe pulmonary artery stenosis. Upper left panel notes the stenotic segments of the left lower lobe branches. Right upper panel notes failed aggressive balloon angioplasty at 18 ATMs. Left lower panel, successful cutting balloon dilation of the stenotic segment. Right lower panel, resolution of the left lower lobe stenosis following cutting balloon angioplasty.

This is a rare condition that can be idiopathic or associated with William's/Alagille syndrome. [29, 31] Primary stenting is generally not recommended for these lesions due to the likelihood of jailing off adjacent pulmonary arterial branches. Balloon angioplasty of these lesions almost always requires high-pressure balloons and in many cases is resistant to standard BA. [23] Aneurysm, dissection, and vessel perforation have been associated with BA of pulmonary artery stenosis, with one patient having a late rupture of an aneurysm with subsequent death. [32] These procedures can be tedious but the outcomes, over time, can be dramatic.

Surgical repair of pulmonary arterial stenosis has also been ineffective and carries considerably greater morbidity and probably greater mortality. [28] Surgical problems with these lesions relate to the location of the narrowings, often in the distal branch pulmonary arteries, an area difficult to reach from a standard midline sternotomy or lateral thoracotomy. Recurrent stenosis has been reported in up to 31% of patients who had surgical repair of the right pulmonary artery after Waterston shunt placement.[28]

4.4 Challenges for the future

Although BA has its limitations, it remains a very important treatment modality for pulmonary and systemic arterial stenosis. CBs have improved the treatment of resistant lesions. The improvement of balloon technology has significantly decreased the number of vascular complications over the past 15 years. Drug delivery through permeable balloons (see section under Challenges for the Future in Coarctation) has significant potential application for the treatment of stenosis in the pulmonary arterial system. The tolerance of longer inflation times and smaller vessel size observed in the pulmonary arterial system makes this a technically easier undertaking in comparison to attempting drug delivery in the systemic arterial system.

5. Conclusion

Balloon angioplasty has proven to be successful in the treatment of pulmonary artery stenosis and coactation of the aorta. Significant challenges remain, primarily in the prevention of recurrent stenosis. The development of biodegradable stents and permeable balloon catheters will undoubtedly improve outcomes for both pulmonary artery and aortic coarctation angioplasty, most importantly in the area of restenoses.

6. References

Yetman AT, Nykanen D, McCrindle BW, Sunnegardh J, Adatia I, Freedom RM, Benson L. Balloon angioplasty of recurrent coarctation: a 12-year review. *J Am Coll Cardiol.* 1997;30(3):811-816.

Li F, Zhou A, Gao W, Wang R, Yu Z, Huang M, Yang J. Percutaneous balloon angioplasty of coarctation of the aorta in children: 12-year follow-up results. *Chin Med J (Engl).* 2001;114(5):459-461.

McCrindle BW, Jones TK, Morrow WR, Hagler DJ, Lloyd TR, Nouri S, Latson LA. Acute results of balloon angioplasty of native coarctation versus recurrent aortic obstruction are equivalent. Valvuloplasty and Angioplasty of Congenital Anomalies (VACA) Registry Investigators. *J Am Coll Cardiol.* 1996;28(7):1810-1817.

Ozawa A, Predescu D, Chaturvedi R, Lee KJ, Benson LN. Cutting balloon angioplasty for aortic coarctation. *J Invasive Cardiol.* 2009;21(6):295-299.

Prada F, Carretero J, Mortera C, Velasco D. Balloon angioplasty in a 1200-gram premature infant with critical aortic coarctation. *Rev Esp Cardiol.*63(6):741-743.

Hamdan MA, Maheshwari S, Fahey JT, Hellenbrand WE. Endovascular stents for coarctation of the aorta: initial results and intermediate-term follow-up. *J Am Coll Cardiol.* 2001;38(5):1518-1523.

Forbes TJ, Garekar S, Amin Z, Zahn EM, Nykanen D, Moore P, Qureshi SA, Cheatham JP, Ebeid MR, Hijazi ZM, Sandhu S, Hagler DJ, Sievert H, Fagan TE, Ringewald J, Du W, Tang L, Wax DF, Rhodes J, Johnston TA, Jones TK, Turner DR, Pedra CA, Hellenbrand WE. Procedural results and acute complications in stenting native and recurrent coarctation of the aorta in patients over 4 years of age: a multi-institutional study. *Catheter Cardiovasc Interv.* 2007;70(2):276-285.

Forbes TJ, Moore P, Pedra CA, Zahn EM, Nykanen D, Amin Z, Garekar S, Teitel D, Qureshi SA, Cheatham JP, Ebeid MR, Hijazi ZM, Sandhu S, Hagler DJ, Sievert H, Fagan TE, Ringwald J, Du W, Tang L, Wax DF, Rhodes J, Johnston TA, Jones TK, Turner DR, Pass R, Torres A, Hellenbrand WE. Intermediate follow-up following intravascular stenting for treatment of coarctation of the aorta. *Catheter Cardiovasc Interv.* 2007;70(4):569-577.

Liang CD, Su WJ, Chung HT, Hwang MS, Huang CF, Lin YJ, Chien SJ, Lin IC, Ko SF. Balloon angioplasty for native coarctation of the aorta in neonates and infants with congestive heart failure. *Pediatr Neonatol.* 2009;50(4):152-157.

Rao PS, Jureidini SB, Balfour IC, Singh GK, Chen SC. Severe aortic coarctation in infants less than 3 months: successful palliation by balloon angioplasty. *J Invasive Cardiol.* 2003;15(4):202-208.

Lock JE, Bass JL, Amplatz K, Fuhrman BP, Castaneda-Zuniga W. Balloon dilation angioplasty of aortic coarctations in infants and children. *Circulation.* 1983;68(1):109-116.

Reich O, Tax P, Bartakova H, Tomek V, Gilik J, Lisy J, Radvansky J, Matejka T, Tlaskal T, Svobodova I, Chaloupecky V, Skovranek J. Long-term (up to 20 years) results of percutaneous balloon angioplasty of recurrent aortic coarctation without use of stents. *Eur Heart J.* 2008;29(16):2042-2048.

Dehghani P, Collins N, Benson L, Horlick E. Role of routine radial artery access during aortic coarctation interventions. *Catheter Cardiovasc Interv.* 2007;70(4):622-623.

Cowley CG, Orsmond GS, Feola P, McQuillan L, Shaddy RE. Long-term, randomized comparison of balloon angioplasty and surgery for native coarctation of the aorta in childhood. *Circulation.* 2005;111(25):3453-3456.

Hassan W, Awad M, Fawzy ME, Omrani AA, Malik S, Akhras N, Shoukri M. Long-term effects of balloon angioplasty on left ventricular hypertrophy in adolescent and adult patients with native coarctation of the aorta. Up to 18 years follow-up results. *Catheter Cardiovasc Interv.* 2007;70(6):881-886.

Hassan W, Malik S, Akhras N, Amri MA, Shoukri M, Fawzy ME. Long-term results (up to 18 years) of balloon angioplasty on systemic hypertension in adolescent and adult patients with coarctation of the aorta. *Clin Cardiol.* 2007;30(2):75-80.

Golden AB, Hellenbrand WE. Coarctation of the aorta: stenting in children and adults. *Catheter Cardiovasc Interv.* 2007;69(2):289-299.

Kim JS, Shin DH, Kim BK, Ko YG, Choi D, Jang Y, Hong MK. Optical coherence tomographic comparison of neointimal coverage between sirolimus- and resolute zotarolimus-eluting stents at 9 months after stent implantation. *Int J Cardiovasc Imaging.*

Klauss V, Serruys PW, Pilgrim T, Buszman P, Linke A, Ischinger T, Eberli F, Corti R, Wijns W, Morice MC, di Mario C, van Geuns RJ, van Es GA, Kalesan B, Wenaweser P, Juni P, Windecker S. 2-year clinical follow-up from the randomized comparison of biolimus-eluting stents with biodegradable polymer and sirolimus-eluting stents with durable polymer in routine clinical practice. *JACC Cardiovasc Interv.*4(8):887-895.

Simsek C, Magro M, Boersma E, Onuma Y, Nauta S, Daemen J, Gaspersz M, van Geuns RJ, van der Giessen W, van Domburg R, Serruys P. Comparison of Six-Year Clinical Outcome of Sirolimus- and Paclitaxel-Eluting Stents to Bare-Metal Stents in Patients with ST-Segment Elevation Myocardial Infarction: An Analysis of the RESEARCH (Rapamycin-Eluting Stent Evaluated at Rotterdam Cardiology Hospital) and T-SEARCH (Taxus Stent Evaluated at Rotterdam Cardiology Hospital) Registries. *J Invasive Cardiol.*23(8):336-341.

Klomp M, Beijk MA, Varma C, Koolen JJ, Teiger E, Richardt G, Bea F, van Geloven N, Verouden NJ, Chan YK, Woudstra P, Damman P, Tijssen JG, de Winter RJ. 1-Year Outcome of TRIAS HR (TRI-Stent Adjudication Study-High Risk of Restenosis) A Multicenter, Randomized Trial Comparing Genous Endothelial Progenitor Cell Capturing Stents With Drug-Eluting Stents. *JACC Cardiovasc Interv.*4(8):896-904.

Lock JE, Castaneda-Zuniga WR, Fuhrman BP, Bass JL. Balloon dilation angioplasty of hypoplastic and stenotic pulmonary arteries. *Circulation.* 1983;67(5):962-967. Hosking MC, Thomaidis C, Hamilton R, Burrows PE, Freedom RM, Benson LN. Clinical impact of balloon angioplasty for branch pulmonary arterial stenosis. *Am J Cardiol.* 1992;69(17):1467-1470.

Kan JS, Marvin WJ, Jr., Bass JL, Muster AJ, Murphy J. Balloon angioplasty--branch pulmonary artery stenosis: results from the Valvuloplasty and Angioplasty of Congenital Anomalies Registry. *Am J Cardiol.* 1990;65(11):798-801.

De Giovanni JV. Balloon angioplasty for branch pulmonary artery stenosis--cutting balloons. *Catheter Cardiovasc Interv.* 2007;69(3):459-467.

Gentles TL, Lock JE, Perry SB. High pressure balloon angioplasty for branch pulmonary artery stenosis: early experience. *J Am Coll Cardiol.* 1993;22(3):867-872.

Rothman A, Levy DJ, Sklansky MS, Grossfeld PD, Auger WR, Ajami GH, Behling CA. Balloon angioplasty and stenting of multiple intralobar pulmonary arterial stenoses in adult patients. *Catheter Cardiovasc Interv.* 2003;58(2):252-260.

Wilson JM, Mack JW, Turley K, Ebert PA. Persistent stenosis and deformity of the right pulmonary artery after correction of the Waterston anastomosis. *J Thorac Cardiovasc Surg.* 1981;82(2):169-175.

Gandy KL, Tweddell JS, Pelech AN. How we approach peripheral pulmonary stenosis in Williams-Beuren syndrome. *Semin Thorac Cardiovasc Surg Pediatr Card Surg Annu.* 2009:118-121.

Sugiyama H, Veldtman GR, Norgard G, Lee KJ, Chaturvedi R, Benson LN. Bladed balloon angioplasty for peripheral pulmonary artery stenosis. *Catheter Cardiovasc Interv.* 2004;62(1):71-77.

Zalzstein E, Moes CA, Musewe NN, Freedom RM. Spectrum of cardiovascular anomalies in Williams-Beuren syndrome. *Pediatr Cardiol.* 1991;12(4):219-223.

Zeevi B, Berant M, Blieden LC. Late death from aneurysm rupture following balloon angioplasty for branch pulmonary artery stenosis. *Cathet Cardiovasc Diagn.* 1996;39(3):284-286.

9

Carotid Angioplasty

Parth Shah and Michael Dahn
Department of Surgery, Section of Vascular Surgery
University of Connecticut Health Center, Farmington, CT
USA

1. Introduction

Carotid intervention for the amelioration of symptoms due to carotid stenosis has been a controversial therapeutic concept for much of its history. Operative carotid surgery (carotid endarterectomy) underwent considerable turmoil and challenge during the late 20th century, eventually becoming a generally accepted approach in the management of symptomatic critical carotid artery stenosis. A similar circumstance currently confronts carotid angioplasty. Carotid endarterectomy (CEA) now represents the clinical standard against which any carotid intervention is compared and carotid angioplasty must "measure up" to this reference procedure. However, it must be recognized that the time line for acceptance of CEA measured approximately 40 years suggesting that the clinical community must exercise patience in the evaluation of carotid angioplasty which enjoys a relatively short history. Conversely, there is considerable vested interest by several specialties for carotid angioplasty to be accepted (cardiology, radiology) or rejected (vascular surgery) indicating the need for critical analysis of this procedure's efficacy. This process of procedure assessment remains a difficult task in view of the constantly changing technological advances that surround this field. This chapter focuses on the key elements of technique and clinical experience which represent the status of carotid angioplasty today.

2. History

The association of carotid artery blood flow to the brain as a vital element to sustain neurologic function dates back to Hippocrates (Figure). As a corollary, it has become accepted that atherosclerotic disease of the carotid artery is associated with stroke. This concept was first described by Ramsay Hunt in 1914 and subsequently popularized as one of the most significant risk factors for developing stroke. It wasn't until the 1950's, when durable reconstructive carotid surgery was described and further refined and popularized by Debakey, Eastcott, Rob, Thompson, Moore, Baker and Wylie, that the field of carotid intervention was popularized. Some of the landmark large randomized controlled trials like North American Symptomatic Carotid Endarterectomy (NASCET)[1], Asymptomatic Carotid Atherosclerosis Study (ACAS)[2] and European Carotid Surgery Trial (ECST)[3] showed statistically significant reductions in stroke in the patients undergoing carotid endarterectomy versus medical treatment alone.

Currently, there are approximately 165,000 carotid endarterectomy (CEA) procedures performed across United States annually and this procedure is considered the "gold standard" for revascularization of the internal carotid artery due to atherosclerotic stenosis.

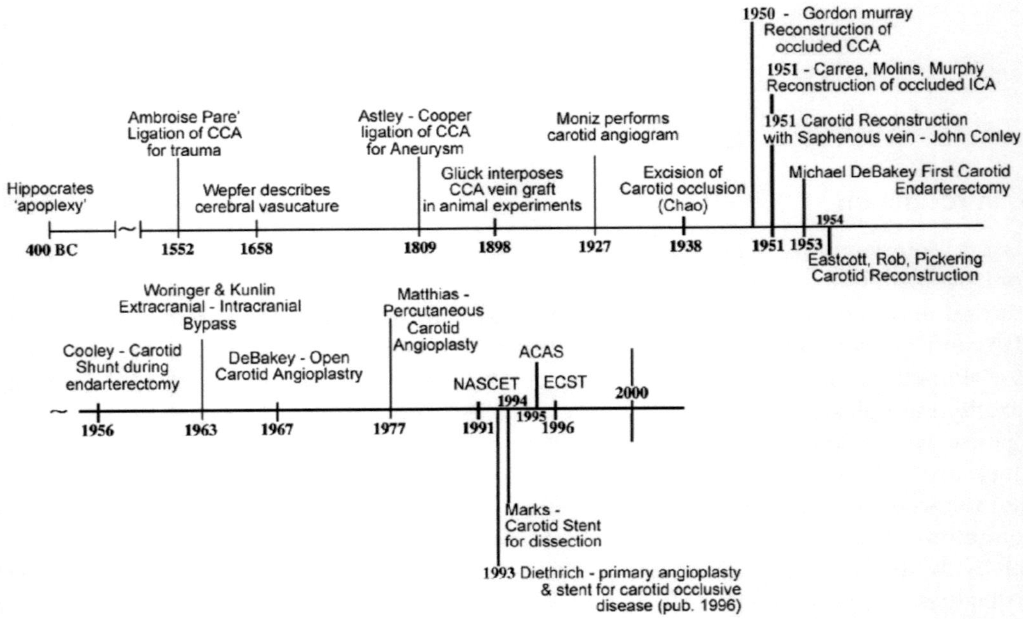

Adapted From Hippocrates to Palmaz-Schatz, the history of carotid surgery. [4]
Robicsek F, Roush TS, Cook JW, Reames MK. Eur J Vasc Endovasc Surg. 2004 Apr;27(4): 389-97.

Moniz described carotid and cerebral angiography in 1927 and thereafter, further improvements in the extracranial carotid imaging facilitated more patients being diagnosed with occlusive carotid diseases and hence treatment advancement. Debakey and his coworkers described intraluminal angioplasty of the internal carotid artery in 1968 for fibromuscular dysplasia.[5] Percutaneous transluminal angioplasty of carotid artery was described in 1977 by Mathias[6] and subsequently Diethrich[7] reported the first large series of carotid angioplasty and stenting in 1995, although the risk of neurological complication was as high as 10.7% in his report. Subsequently, multiple technical advances have taken place in percutaneous carotid artery interventions including stent augmentation of carotid angioplasty, routine use of cerebral embolic protection and improved patient selection.

Carotid angioplasty and stenting (CAS) provides a few advantages over traditional CEA including avoidance of a neck incision, general anesthesia and freedom from cranial nerve injuries. These benefits have sustained the evolution of CAS over the last 20-30 years.

3. Technical aspects of carotid angioplasty and stenting

Key for successful endoluminal intervention is patient evaluation and proper patient selection, choice of optimum vascular access site, a thorough evaluation of the access route, any anatomic or morphologic anomalies, appropriate selection of devices and accurate sizing of the target lesion and vessels.

Pre-procedural assessment of carotid artery disease is obtained by duplex ultrasound (DU). DU allows an assessment of the degrees of stenosis and extent of calcification. Highly calcified lesions may be more embologenic or unyielding to balloon angioplasty resulting in a suboptimal dilatation. Further information on the target lesion may be obtained by magnetic resonance (MR) or computed tomographic (CT) arteriography. These two imaging modalities are useful confirmatory studies following duplex imaging and offer an assessment of unsuspected occlusive disease outside the DU imaging window. Furthermore, these non-invasive means evaluate access site, aortic arch morphology and any incidental pathology in the access route which are invaluable in the planning of a procedure.

4. Aortic arch configuration

Initially, a 4 or 5 Fr sheath access is obtained in the common femoral artery. A flush pigtail catheter may be positioned in the ascending aorta for the initial arch aortogram which is performed in left anterior oblique (LAO) position. Depending on the degree of tortuosity and configuration of the aortic arch, we like to have between 30 degrees to as much as 60 degrees of LAO projection. The performance of the arch angiogram is useful to identify the target vessel origin. In difficult anatomic arrangements, the aortogram is very helpful but it may also increase procedure morbidity. Utilizing diffusion weighted MRI imaging, silent microembolic lesions are detectable in up to two-thirds of patients undergoing CAS[8]. At least half of these lesions can be identified in the cerebral hemisphere contralateral to the target lesion. This suggests that manipulation of devices, including diagnostic catheters used for arch angiography, are a substantial source of embolic events during CAS.

The aortic arch configuration varies due to multiple patient factors. Probably the dominant factor is age since the aorta tends to elongate with increasing age contributing to a worsening of the arch type. There are mainly three arch types depending on the radiographic morphology (Figure).

5. Diagnostic catheters

Safe selective cannulation of the great vessels is the rate-limiting step. Usually the appropriate diagnostic catheters are available in 100 cm to 125 cm lengths. The longer lengths are required should one use the telescoping technique (*vida infra*).

For the Type I aortic arch, the standard angled catheters like the angle taper Glidecath® (Terumo Medical Corporation, Somerset, NJ, USA) or a Berenstein catheter (Boston Scientific, Natick, MA, USA) or Headhunter or JB 1 (Cook Medical, Bloomington, IN, USA) are usually successful.

For more challenging aortic arch morphology, with types II and III configuration, reverse-curve catheters like Simmons type catheters (I or II), JB 2 or the VTK catheter (Cook Medical, Bloomington, IN, USA) may be used.

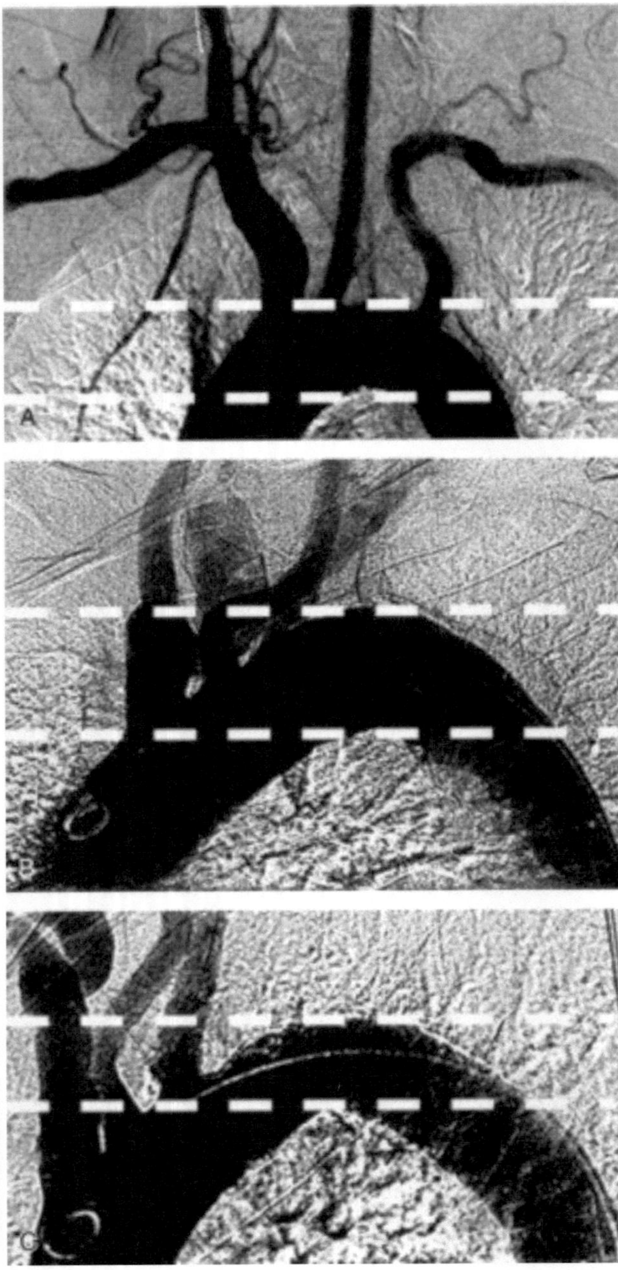

Type I - The great vessels originate from the same horizontal plane of the outer curvature of the arch

Type II - Innominate artery originates between the horizontal planes of outer and inner curvature of the arch

Type III - Innominate artery originates below the horizontal plane of inner curvature of the arch

A Type IV arch is a term that may be applied to an exaggerated Type III arch with severe angulation of the great vessels.

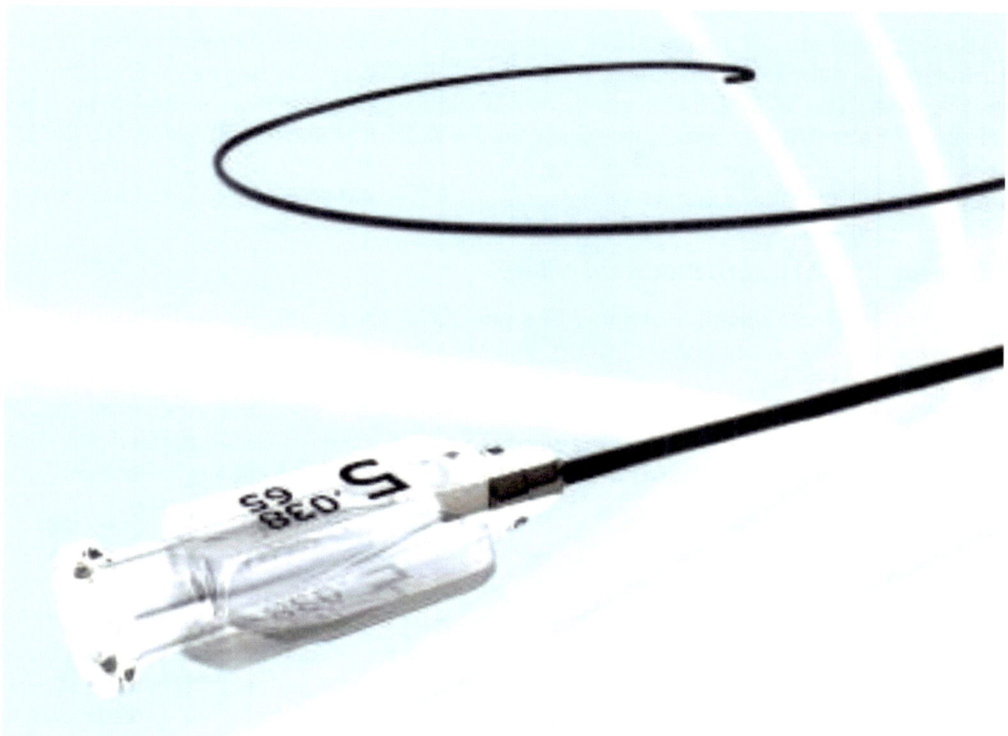

Glidecath®

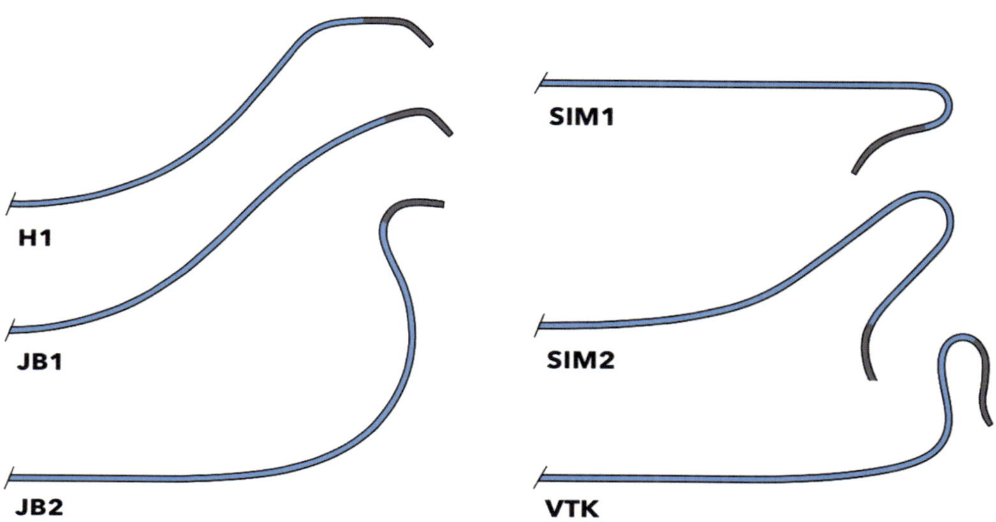

These are the configurations of some of the catheters commonly used in the carotid angioplasty procedure.

6. Sheath access

Positioning of a sheath in the CCA is a prerequisite to CAS. Typically, this requires placement of a diagnostic catheter into the CCA followed by advancement of a glide-wire into the ECA. This allows introduction of the catheter into the ECA followed by a wire exchange for a stiff wire forming the guide for a 6 Fr Shuttle sheath. Occasionally, the ECA is occluded or severely diseased requiring the use of a stable stiff wire access into common carotid artery (CCA) alone and a 6 Fr sheath is advanced and parked into proximal CCA.

7. Cannulation of internal carotid artery

After obtaining stable sheath access into proximal CCA, the embolic protection device (EPD) is deployed into the appropriate position. The pros and cons of different cerebral EPDs are discussed in next section.

The different approches of obtaining ICA access depend upon the degree of stenosis, amount of tortuosity and type of EPD used. Usual access to the ICA is obtained with a standard 0.014" wire or EPD dedicated wire followed by delivery of the balloon and stent system.

8. Telescoping catheter technique

Positioning of the Shuttle sheath system into the CCA is a prerequisite for the CAS procedure. Typically, this is performed over a stiff wire anchored in the ECA. However, advancement of the stiff wire into the CCA through a diagnostic catheter may be a challenge. If tortuous anatomy prevents this maneuver, a softer, 125 cm 6 or 6.5 Fr catheter is used to replace the obturator of the Shuttle sheath. The additional 35 cm lead portion of this catheter which is telescoped into the 90 cm Shuttle serves as a sufficient support over which to slide the sheath once the catheter tip is introduced into the CCA. Thus, the inner catheter effectively serves as a "stiff guide".

9. Right brachial/axillary artery access technique (double wire technique)

Access to the right carotid system can be achieved under essentially all anatomically difficult circumstances with this technique. This approach has been successful even with an exaggerated Type III aortic arch configuration (effectively a Type IV arch). The technique requires gaining access to the brachial or axillary artery on the right with passage of an exchange length glide wire retrograde into the thoracic aorta. The wire is snared from a femoral access point for through and through wire control. A 7 or 8 Fr sheath is now advanced into the innominate artery. The wire may be changed out for a smaller wire to reduce occupied space within the sheath while stabilizing it. This is then followed by the transfemoral advancement of a second steerable 0.014" wire into the CCA. The second wire now permits the delivery of a cerebral protection system and completion of the CAS procedure.

10. Transtemporal technique

Access to the CCA can be quite difficult if the carotid anatomy is tortuous or the aortic arch type is unfavorable. The transtemporal approach may be used on either side but it has its greatest utility on the left since the right CCA can be cannulated using the double wire technique noted above. The transtemporal approach involves ultrasound guided access or direct dissection of the superficial temporal artery followed by retrograde placement of a coronary wire into the aorta where it is snared from the femoral artery. This provides through and through access permitting advancement of a Shuttle sheath into proper position for the CAS procedure. The remainder of the procedure is then performed in the usual fashion.

11. Ultra-critical stenosis

Sometimes the standard 0.014" wire is not successful in traversing an ultra-critical stenosis, in which case a 0.012" Headliner® Glidewire® (45 degrees, 200 cm) (Terumo Medical Corporation, Somerset, NJ, USA), supported by 1.9 Fr (0.026") Prowler® microcatheter (Cordis, Miami Lakes, FL, USA) may be successful. Following traversal of the lesion with the microcatheter, the 0.012" wire is replaced with a more supportive 0.014" wire which can be parked in the treatment area. The new wire may now be used to deliver a balloon, EPD or a flow arrest/reversal system (*vida infra*) for completion of the CAS. [9]

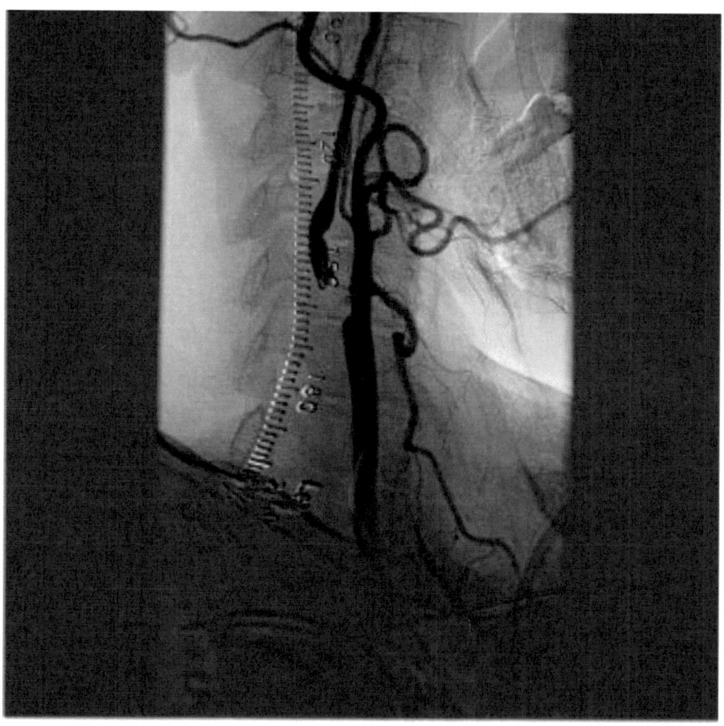

This figure shows a pre-occlusive lesion of the right internal carotid artery which would not accept a 0.014" wire.

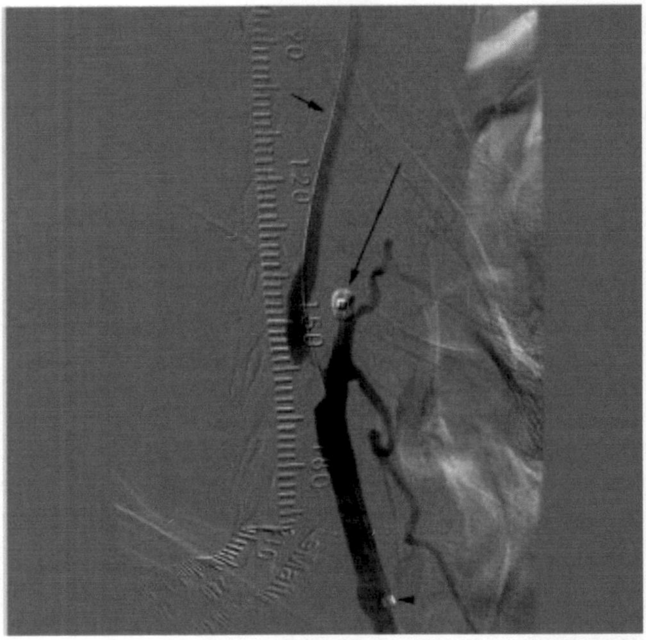

The lesion has been passed using an 0.012″ wire followed by replacement with an 0.014″ wire and placement of a MOMA flow arrest device within the external carotid artery balloon inflated (long arrow).

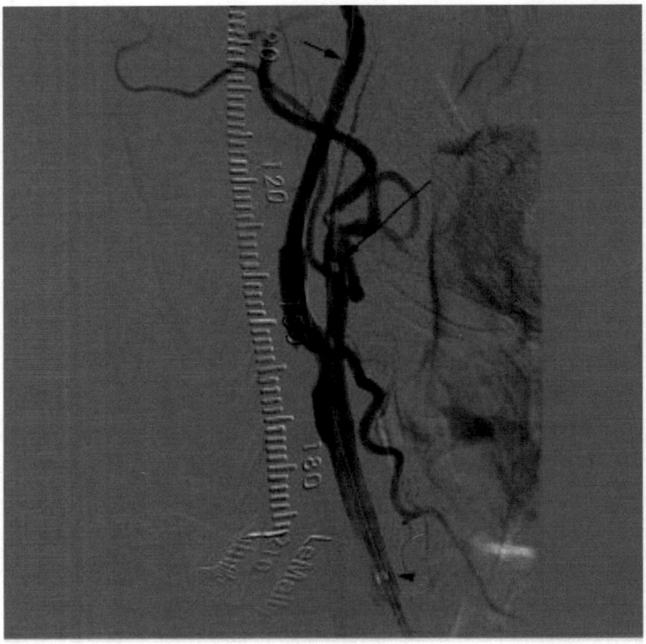

The ICA angioplasty is complete. The MOMA flow arrest device is still in place with the ECA and CCA balloons deflated and flow re-established to the brain.

12. Transcervical occlusion and protective shunting technique

This technique uses a partially open operative approach. The procedure is performed under local anesthesia utilizing a small incision just above the clavicle. A large (9 Fr) and medium (6 Fr) sheath are introduced into the CCA directed in a cephalad orientation through the incision. Additionally, a 6 Fr sheath is introduced into the jugular vein directed caudally. An over-the-wire fogerty catheter is used to occlude the external carotid artery and the proximal CCA is clamped following anticoagulation. Flow reversal in the carotid system is established by connecting the sideports of the 9 Fr arterial and 6 Fr venous sheaths and flow direction is verified using a small injection of contrast. Now, the angioplasty is performed through the 9 Fr sheath and any loose debris that results is carried into the venous system or trapped by any interposed filter. The arterial puncture sites are sutured at the time of final sheath removal. This approach appears fairly labor intensive within a small field and the use of a partially open portion of the angioplasty procedure seems to defeat the minimally invasive nature of CAS. Nonetheless, it has been suggested as a reliable means of controlling embolization.

13. Review of literature

Mathias first described the percutaneous carotid artery angioplasty (CA) technique in 1977.[10] Subsequently he reported a case series of 3 high surgical risk patients undergoing percutaneous carotid angioplasty.[11] During this time, percutaneous carotid intervention was limited to fibromuscular dysplasia and was not applied to atherosclerotic diseases due to risk of embolic events and secondly, CEA was considered a very safe procedure and its utilization was widespread. There were occasional case reports of CA, but it wasn't until 1990's when this technique was more systematically studied for its feasibility, safety and outcomes. The summary of early clinical studies is shown in Table 1. The most feared complication of CA is embolic phenomenon and evidence of early and delayed embolization after percutaneous CA was reported by Markus et al. [12]

	Study number (Follow-up)	Technical success	Stroke	Overall complications (MI/Stroke/Death)
Diethrich EB[13] (1996)	110 (7.6 months)	99%	12 (10.9%)	12 (10.9%)
Roubin GS[14] (1996)	146 (6 months)	99%	9 (6%)	11(7.5%)
Gil-Peralta A[15] (1996)	85 (18.7 months)	91.8%	7 (8.6%)	7 (8.6%)
Yadav JS[16] (1997)	107 (6 months)	100%	9 (8.4%)	10(9.3%)
Jordan WD, Jr[17] (1997)	107 (6 months)	NA	9 (8.4%)	10 (9.3%)
Vozzi CR[18] (1997)	22 (10 months)	NA	2 (9%)	2 (9%)
Teitelbaum GP[19] (1998)	25 (6 months)	96.2%	2 (7.7%)	6 (27%)

Table 1.

In 1992, Brown[20] reviewed approximately 100 cases reported in the literature with stroke rate of 4%. In May 1998, Wholey[21] published a review of 2,048 cases of carotid stents across 24 centers world-wide and reported a 98.6% technical success rate. Also the complication rates were 3.08% for minor strokes, 1.32% major strokes and 1.37% peri-procedural mortality. The 6-month re-stenosis rate was 4.8% by duplex-ultrasound or angiographic method. The stents being utilized for carotid stenting at the time were Palmaz (Cordis) or

Palmaz-Schatz (Johnson and Johnson) balloon expandable stents (53%), followed by Wallstent (Schneider, Minneapolis, MN) (39%), Strecker (8%) and Inegra (1%) (Medi-Tech) stents. Subsequently, he reported updated data for 5,210 cases across 36 centers in June 2000. This showed a rapid rise in global popularity of this procedure. The incidence of major and minor stroke remained 1.49% and 2.72%. This review observed lower stroke rates in the centers with more than 50 procedures performed indicating the importance of a learning curve. Overall procedure-related complication rates declined from 5.72% in 1998 to 4.75% in 2000. Since the cerebral protection technology had not yet evolved, these results derived from "unprotected" procedures.

Theron et al[22] first reported the use of cerebral embolic protection in carotid artery angioplasty and stenting procedures. There were no procedure related complications in 136 cases of carotid artery stenting with use of the cerebral embolic protection for atherosclerotic stenosis.

The Carotid Revascularization using Endarterectomy or Stenting Systems (CaRESS)[23] was a non-randomized prospective trial designed for high-risk patients with or without symptoms. Total of 397 patients were studied and the outcomes at 4-years showed a stroke incidence of 9.6% in CAS group versus 8.6% in CEA group (p=0.444) and an overall complication (death/stroke) rate of 26.5% in CEA versus 21.8% (p=0.361) in CAS. However, at the long-term follow-up, there were significantly higher re-stenosis and re-intervention rates in the CAS arm.

14. Randomized controlled trials

14.1 CAVATAS

In 1996, the European Carotid Angioplasty trial group reported the rationale, design and protocol of the first multicenter randomized trial, the Carotid and Vertebral Artery Transluminal Angioplasty Study (CAVATAS).[24] Preceding this trial, a single center trial in the UK was stopped after enrolling 20 patients due to unacceptable rate of stroke in the carotid angioplasty arm (7/10 patients).[25] The CAVATAS trial involved 22 centers across Europe, Canada and Australia and the patient enrollment was between March 1992 and July 1997. Five hundred and four patients were randomized to either CEA or CAS. The majority of patients (90%) in both arms had symptoms within 6 months of randomization and exhibited >70% carotid stenosis. Because the stents suitable for CAS were developed during the course of this study, all the patients before 1994 had primary balloon angioplasty alone versus the cases thereafter, which utilized stenting with Wallstent (Schneider, Minneapolis, MN), Streker (Medi-Tech, USA) and Palmaz (Johnson and Johnson, USA) stents. High-risk patients were excluded from the study. The major stroke and death rates were not statistically significantly different between two groups (30-day: 10% for CAS versus 10% for CEA; 3-years: 14.3% in CAS versus 14.2% in CEA). The primary limitation of this study is that very low number of patients (26%) who underwent carotid artery stenting and that the stroke and death rates were unusually high. However, subgroup analysis showed the incidence of stroke was only 2% in the stented patients, which lead to more widespread use of stent application after balloon angioplasty of a carotid artery stenosis.

15. WALLSTENT[26]

The Carotid WALLSTENT trial enrolled 223 patients with symptomatic carotid artery stenosis > 60%. No cerebral embolic protection was used. The trial was stopped due to unacceptably high risk of stroke in CAS group (12.1 %) versus CEA (4.5%, P=0.022).

16. Stenting and Angioplasty with Protection of the Patients at High Risk for Endarterectomy (SAPPHIRE)[27]

This multicenter, industry-supported randomized trial enrolled 747 patients from 29 centers between 2000 and 2002. The major "high-risk"criteria were significant cardiac or pulmonary disease, contralateral carotid occlusion, prior neck radiation or radical neck surgery, recurrent stenosis, contralateral recurrent laryngeal nerve palsy or age greater than 80 years. The study showed that CAS was non-inferior to CEA when evaluating the cumulative incidence of major stroke, MI or death in 30-day period and at 1-year.

17. Stent-supported Percutaneous Angioplasty of the Carotid artery versus Endarterectomy (SPACE)[28]

The SPACE trial was designed as non-inferiority trial for CAS versus CEA. 1214 patients with symptomatic high grade stenosis of carotid artery (>70%) were randomized into CAS or CEA between March 2001 and February 2006. The primary end-point of ipsilateral stroke or death rate was 6.45% in CEA group versus 6.92% in CAS group which did not reach the statistical significance level (p=0.09) for non-inferiority for CAS. At 2-year follow-up, the overall mortality was 6.3% in CAS versus 5% in CEA (p=0.68), and the ipsilateral ischemic stroke rate was 2.2% vs 1.9%. However, recurrent stenosis (>70% by ultrasound criteria) was 10.7% in CAS versus 4.6% in CEA group (p=0.0009). The subgroup analysis showed patients greater than 68 years of age had higher event rates with CAS compared to CEA, whereas the younger patients did better with CAS compared to CEA.

18. Endarterectomy Versus Angioplasty in patients with Symptomatic Severe Carotid Stenosis (EVA-3S) trial[29]

This trial was a French multicenter, prospective randomized non-inferiority trial. The patient enrollment started in November 2000 and ended in September 2005. A total of 527 patients were enrolled and randomized into two arms. All the CAS cases after January 2003 were done with approved EPDs at the time, which left initial 73 cases being done without any cerebral protection. The 30-day risk of stroke or death was 3.9% in CEA group versus 9.6% in CAS group, and risk of any peri-procedural disabling stroke or death was 1.5% in CEA group versus 3.4% in CAS group. The 4-year hazard ratio (HR) of any disabling or fatal stroke or death was 2.0 (p=0.17) slightly favoring endarterectomy. Although the peri-procedural risk was unusually higher in the stenting group, overall long-term secondary prevention of stroke was similar in both arms. The major criticism of this study was that despite a requirement of a minimum procedure volume performed prior to enrollment in the study as an operator, overall operator experience was too limited and may have influenced the outcomes.

19. The International Carotid Stenting Study (ICSS)[30]

The ICSS study, also known as CAVATAS-2, was designed. A meta-analysis of 3 trials, EVA-3S (2008), SPACE (2008) and the ICSS (2010) showed significantly lower event rate in the CEA group (OR 1.73, 95% CI: 1.29 - 2.32)[20]. Age, greater than 70 years, was a risk factor for poorer outcomes with CAS (12%) compared to CEA (5.9%), RR = 2.04. However, the patients younger than 70 years had no difference in outcomes.[31]

20. Carotid Revascularization Endarterectomy versus Stenting Trial (CREST)[32]

This North American prospective randomized controlled trial enrolled 2502 patients from 117 centers (symptomatic and asymptomatic). The primary end-points of any stroke, MI or death were similar in both groups of CEA (6.8%) and CAS (7.2%). Although there was a lower incidence of MI in the CAS group versus lower stroke rate in the CEA group, these rates did not reach statistical significance. Also the younger patients had slightly better outcomes with CAS whereas the older patients did slightly better after CEA. At one year, subgroup analysis revealed that stroke had a lasting effect on quality of life as opposed to the effects of MI. Nonetheless, overall, both procedures were safe when done by a skilled operator.

21. Cerebral embolic protection devices

The first safety and feasibility study of the ICA filter devices for cerebral embolic protection was done by Reimers et al.[33] The 3-types of the filter devices used in that study are shown below.

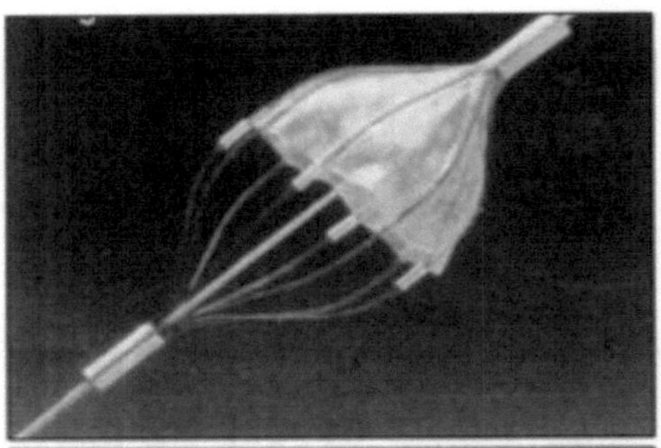

Angioguard

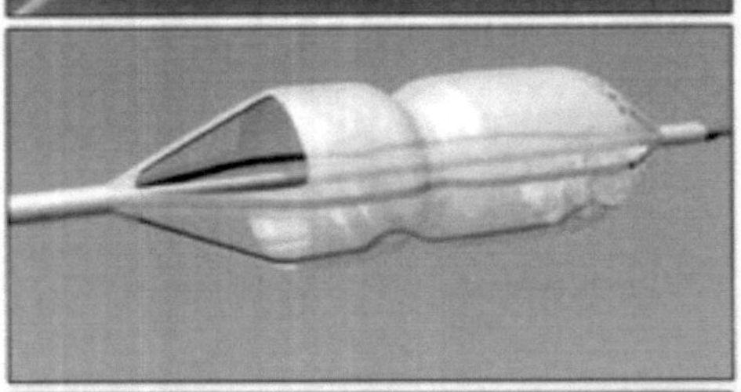

Neuroshield / Emboshield

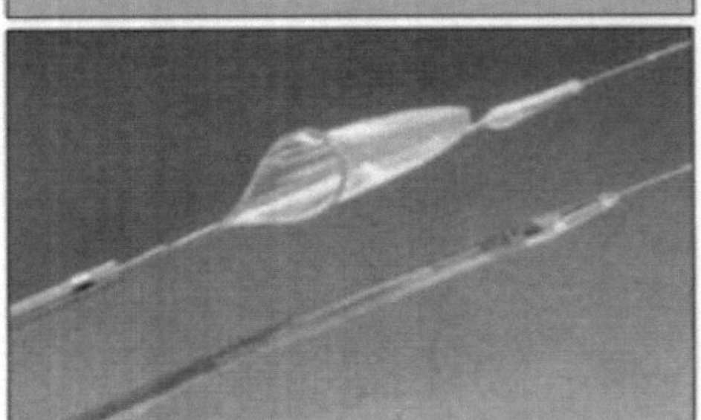

FilterWire EX

Subsequently, the EPD field has expanded with the addition of other filtration systems such as those shown below. All of these devices are based upon a similar principal of flow-through filtration.

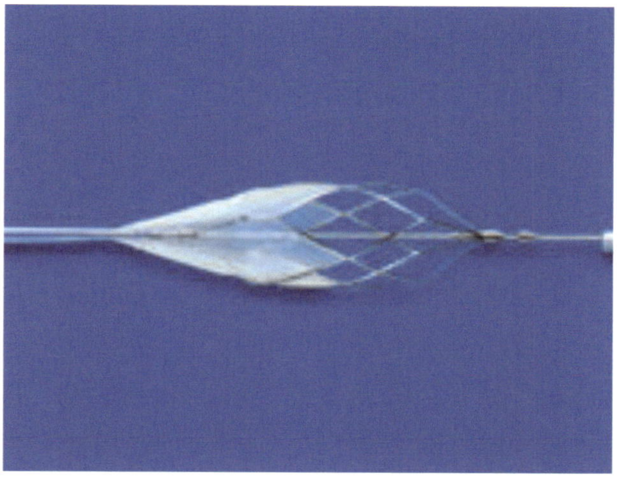

Rx Accunet

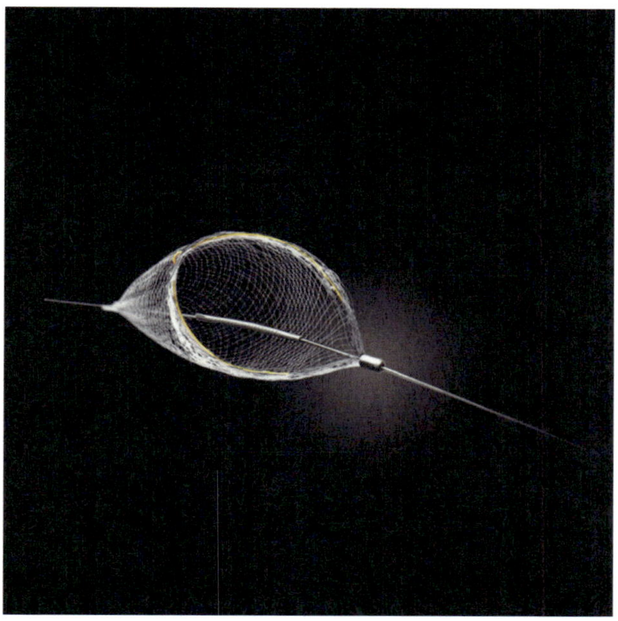

Spider

Overall, there are three major functional principles upon which all EPDs are based. (1) Distal ICA balloon occlusion with flow arrest (2) filtration with continuous flow through (as noted in the above figures), and (3) proximal balloon occlusion with flow stagnation or flow reversal. The pros and cons of these devices are enumerated in Table 2.

Type	Pros	Cons	Currently available in Market in the US
Filter	Maintains flow throughout the procedure Can perform angiogram during the procedure	Risk of embolism while traversing the lesion Technically difficult in tortuous vessels Risk of microembolism (smaller than pore size of the filter) Risk of filter thrombosis	• Rx Accunet • Filter-wire • Angioguard • Emboshield • Spider
Distal ICA occlusion	Offers complete distal embolic protection	Risk of embolism while traversing the lesion Potential for arterial injury by balloon Inability of some patients to tolerate ICA occlusion Inability to perform angiogram during the procedure	• GuardWire
Proximal occlusion	Does not require traversing the lesion unprotected Offers complete distal embolic protection	Complete flow arrest or reversal during the procedure Potential for arterial injury by balloon Cerebral Intolerance	• MO.MA • PAES (Parodi antiembolism system)

Table 2.

22. Filter protection

All filter devices have similar design. The filter is mounted on a 0.014″ wire with floppy tip. The filter is made up from nitinol (nickel-titanium alloy) covered with polyurethane membrane. The porous size of the filter ranges from 30 to 140 microns. Each filter comes in with its own deployment and retrieval sheaths. The filter basket and the sheath are flushed carefully with heparinized saline with particular attention to avoid any air-bubbles. Once the filter is deployed in the distal straight portion of the ICA, the more proximal diseased area is treated over the 0.014″ wire. The size of the filter is chosen considering the luminal diameter of the distal ICA. At the conclusion of the procedure, the filter is retrieved and then the entire system is removed. The currently available filter-devices have a crossing profile between 3Fr and 4Fr and accommodate the vessels from 3mm to 7mm diameter.

23. Flow arrest or flow reversal technique

Embolic protection during CAS can be accomplished with carotid flow arrest or reversal. The MOMA device is a 9 Fr sheath incorporating a small compliant balloon introduced into the ECA and a larger balloon located on the distal main body of the device used for CCA occlusion. Intubation of the ECA is performed using a 0.035" wire placed during a standard initial approach. The ECA wire serves as a guide for initial device placement. Following anticoagulation, the ECA and CCA balloons are inflated providing for carotid flow arrest. Any standard 0.014" wire may now be used to deliver angioplasty balloons and stents to the target lesion. An advantage to this system is that the working wire does not need to be advanced deep into the ICA territory thereby making this a favorable method when there is severe tortuosity to the ICA which will not accept distally placed filtration EPDs. Debris in the carotid bulb and ICA is aspirated at the conclusion of the procedure prior to balloon deflation.
Initial data in a multicenter, intention-to-treat trial, ARMOUR Trial(Proximal Protection with the MO.MA Device During Carotid Stenting), showed that the major 30-day event rate (major cardiac and cerebrovascular) was 2.7% and 30-day major stroke rate was 0.9% in the patients undergoing CAS with MO.MA cerebral protection device.[34]

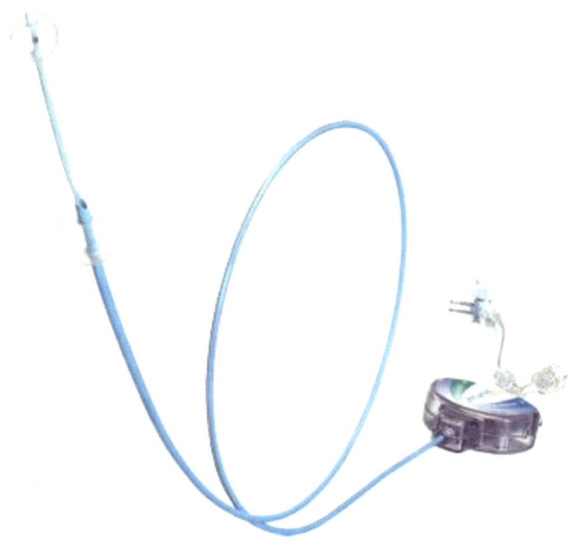

MO.MA device. (Source: Invatec Inc., Italy)

Flow reversal uses a similar principal of ECA and CCA occlusion during the angioplasty procedure but with dynamic flow reversal of blood from the carotid bulb into the femoral vein via a system side port. The flow reversal is encouraged by the higher arterial back pressure from the ICA compared to the venous system once the balloon system is inflated. This device is called the Parodi antiembolism system (PAES). Both devices serve the role of EPD as well as access sheath.

24. Neurorescue during carotid artery stenting

24.1 Procedural embolization

Embolization can occur during the carotid artery stenting procedure and that can be in the form of micro- or macro-embolization. However, the risk of embolization is particularly high during the diagnostic phase, deployment of EPD period and during retrieval of the EPD. Most cases with micro-embolization are asymptomatic at the time of the procedure and in the immediate post-procedural phase, but their impact on long-term functional outcome (eg., cognitive function) is largely unknown.

The risk of embolization can be minimized by peri-procedural antiplatelet therapy (oral or intravenous GPIIB-IIIA inhibitors) and anticoagulation. These agents reduce platelet aggregation when subintimal tissue or stent material is exposed to the blood system during CAS. However, should macro-embolization occur, mainly due to technical error or failure of EPD, one should be prepared with mechanical retrieval/aspiration systems or catheter-directed thrombolysis.

24.2 Thrombosis

Thrombosis during the CAS procedure is associated with the use of EPDs. This is usually treated with direct aspiration of thrombus and/or direct administration of a thrombolytic (ie. Alteplase) or GPIIb-IIIa inhibitor intra-arterially, if possible. Also, distal embolization can be prevented by adopting an incomplete filter-retrieval technique in which case the filter retrieval system is not closed completely upon removal in order to prevent thrombus from being squeezed out of the system.

Acute stent thrombosis is rare (< 2%) and can be further minimized by appropriate periprocedural antiplatelet and anticoagulation strategy. The treatment consists of direct infusion of thrombolytic agent and/or GPIIb-IIIa inhibitor. This latter maneuver must be weighed against the risk of precipitating embolization during the lysis of an established ICA clot. In rare circumstances, when endoluminal techniques fail, the patient should immediately be taken to operating room and thrombectomy should be performed after appropriate anticoagulation and obtaining distal control to prevent progression of thrombosis and distal embolization.

24.3 Dissection

Dissection is fortunately a rare phenomenon and is usually related to stent insertion and/or balloon dilation. If the dissection does not limit the flow-lumen significantly, "wait-and-observe" strategy can be employed with or without use of continued anticoagulation. In case of significant flow-limiting dissection, the deployment of second stent may be advocated versus open surgical repair.

25. CAS surveillance

25.1 Carotid restenosis

The need for post-procedure surveillance is typically recommended by physicians who perform CAS. Surveillance options include duplex ultrasound (DU), MRA and CTA. MRA suffers from signal degradation due to the presence of a metallic stent and CTA involves significant ionizing radiation and the use of iodinated contrast, which may cause nephrotoxicity and allergic reactions[35]. Consequently, because of the absence of risk, DU surveillance after CAS has become the standard.

Post-procedure sonography is performed in order to (1) identify undetected procedural faults associated with residual stenosis, (2) evaluate the occurrence of neointimal hyperplasia at the stented site, and (3) monitor the progression of contralateral disease. The incidence of significant contralateral disease ranges 25-50% making this the most compelling reason for ongoing duplex surveillance. Assessment of restenosis at the angioplasty site represents the second most frequent need for longitudinal surveillance.

Risk factors for restenosis after CAS largely remain undefined. When various factors are analyzed, a history of head and neck cancer and prior carotid endarterectomy (CEA) were found to be marginally significant for the development of early in-stent restenosis (ISR).[36,37] The time line for the occurrence of ISR is somewhat variable but the majority (>70%) of these cases are identified within 12 months following the index procedure[3]. However, this disease process may be ongoing as evidenced by an increasing incidence over a five year follow-up. Lal et al[38], reported ISR rates of 2.7% and 6.4% at 1 and 5 years, respectively. These data utilize 80% stenosis as a measure of disease with this frequency rising if lower degrees of restenosis criteria are selected. Interestingly, ISR may regress over time but the temporal profile of this process as well as factors predictive of regression remain undefined.

25.2 Duplex ultrasound criteria

The baseline post-procedural duplex velocities for stented vessels tend to exhibit higher values than unstented vessels of normal luminal caliber. This may result from either under dilatation of the ICA during CAS or a change in the mechanical properties of the ICA. A common notion is that the purpose of balloon dilatation is to ensure an adequate ICA lumen and not an anatomically cosmetic perfect result. This conservative approach may predispose to a minor residual stenosis exemplified by a peak systolic velocity (PSV) higher than normal. Alternatively, some authorities have reported that the introduction of a stent into the carotid bulb and ICA alters the biomechanical properties of the vessel resulting in a stent-arterial complex with decreased compliance. This translates into an elevated PSV because energy normally applied to dilate the artery is now expended as increased flow velocity[39]. Consequently, recommendations have been advocated for the increase of velocity criteria corresponding to higher degrees of stenosis following CAS. Table 3 shows current recommendations by several clinical laboratories.

The variability of the recommended criteria values depends upon the balance between sensitivity and specificity desired by the laboratory performing the studies. Surveillance is usually performed every six months following CAS for at least two years. If the patient exhibits contralateral disease, this surveillance may be continued indefinitely.

Stenosis	PSV (cm/sec)	EDV (cm/sec)	ICA/CCA ratio
>50%	>225	-	>2.5[40]
	>240	-	>2.45[42]
>70%	>170	>120[41]	-
	>350	-	>4.75[40]
	>450	-	>4.3[42]
>80%	>340	-	>4.15[38]
	>325	>119	>4.53[39]

PSV=peak systolic velocity; EDV=end diastolic velocity

Table 3. Recommended Velocity Criteria for Restenosis of the ICA following CAS

26. Conclusion

Carotid angioplasty and stenting is very slowly increasing in popularity. Currently, approximately 12% of carotid interventions in the United States involve CAS. The major limitation in its adaption is the reimbursement climate. Presently, the Center for Medicare Services restricts reimbursement for CAS to high risk, symptomatic patients (stenosis > 50%) and high risk asymptomatic patients (stenosis >80%) who are on a clinical trial or registry. At least one private insurance carrier has elected to support payment for high risk asymptomatic patients (>80%) indicating that reimbursement restrictions are gradually relaxing. Furthermore, the FDA has approved the use of the Acculink/Accunet carotid stent system in asymptomatic patients. These changes in regulatory requirements for CAS suggest that eventually, in the not too distant future, this procedure will be approved for all patients exhibiting carotid stenosis. Whether CAS should be performed in asymptomatic patients remains a controversial issue and will remain a topic in evolution as pharmaceutical therapy and life-style changes become increasingly aggressive.

27. References

[1] North American Symptomatic Carotid Endarterectomy Trial Collaborators, Beneficial effect of carotid endarterectomy in symptomatic patients with high grade carotid stenosis. N Engl J Med. 1991 Aug 15;325(7):445-53

[2] Endarterectomy for asymptomatic carotid artery stenosis. Executive Committee for the Asymptomatic Carotid Atherosclerosis Study. JAMA. 1995 May 10;273(18):1421-8.

[3] European Carotid Surgery Trialists' Collaborative Group, Ran-domised trial of endarterectomy for recently symptomatic carotid stenosis: final results of the MRC European Carotid Surgery Trial (ECST). Lancet. 1998 May 9;351(9113):1379-87.

[4] Robicsek F, Roush TS, Cook JW, Reames MK. From Hippocrates to Palmaz-Schatz, the history of carotid surgery. Eur J Vasc Endovasc Surg. 2004 Apr;27(4):389-97.

[5] Morris GC Jr, Lechter A, DeBakey ME. Surgical treatment of fibromuscular disease of the carotid arteries. Arch Surg. 1968 Apr;96(4):636-43.

[6] Mathias K. [A new catheter system for percutaneous transluminal angioplasty (PTA) of carotid artery stenoses]. Fortschr Med. 1977 Apr 21;95(15):1007-11. German.

[7] Diethrich EB, Ndiaye M, Reid DB. Stenting in the Carotid artery. Initial experience in 110 patients. J Endovasc Surg. 1996 Feb;3(1):42-62.

[8] Hammer FD, Lacroix V, Duprez T, et al: Cerebral microembolization after protected carotid artery stenting in surgical high-risk patients: Results of a 2-year prospective study. J Vasc Surg 2005;42:847-53.

[9] Dahn M, Cheema M, Bozeman P, Divinagracia T. Crossing an ultracritical carotid stenosis for carotid angioplasty. Vasc Endovascular Surg. 2009 Dec;43(6):589-91. Epub 2009 Oct 14.

[10] Mathias K. [A new catheter system for percutaneous transluminal angioplasty (PTA) of carotid artery stenoses]. Fortschr Med. 1977 Apr 21;95(15):1007-11. German.

[11] Bockenheimer SA, Mathias K. Percutaneous transluminal angioplasty in arteriosclerotic internal carotid artery stenosis. AJNR Am J Neuroradiol. 1983 May-Jun;4(3):791-2.

[12] Markus HS, Clifton A, Buckenham T, Brown MM. Carotid angioplasty. Detection of embolic signals during and after the procedure. Stroke. 1994 Dec;25(12):2403-6.

[13] Diethrich EB, Ndiaye M, Reid DB. Stenting in the Carotid artery. Initial experience in 110 patients. J Endovasc Surg. 1996 Feb;3(1):42-62.

[14] Roubin GS, Yadav S, Iyer SS, Vitek J. Carotid stent-supported angioplasty: a neurovascular intervention to prevent stroke. Am J Cardiol. 1996 Aug 14;78(3A):8-12.
[15] Gil-Peralta A, Mayol A, Marcos JR, Gonzalez A, Ruano J, Boza F, Duran F. Percutaneous transluminal angioplasty of the symptomatic atherosclerotic carotid arteries. Results, complications, and follow-up. Stroke. 1996 Dec;27(12):2271-3.
[16] Yadav JS, Roubin GS, King P, Iyer S, Vitek J. Angioplasty and stenting for restenosis after carotid endarterectomy. Initial experience. Stroke. 1996 Nov;27(11):2075-9.
[17] Jordan WD Jr, Schroeder PT, Fisher WS, McDowell HA. A comparison of angioplasty with stenting versus endarterectomy for treatment of carotid artery stenosis. Ann Vasc Surg. 1997 Jan;11(1):2-8.
[18] Vozzi CR, Rodriguez AO, Paolantonio D, Smith JA, Wholey MH. Extracranial carotid angioplasty and stenting. Initial results and short term follow-up. Tex Heart Inst J. 1997;24(3):167-72.
[19] Teitelbaum GP, Lefkowitz MA, Giannotta SL Carotid angioplasty and stenting in high-risk patients. Surg Neurol. 1998 Oct;50(4):300-11; discussion 311-2.
[20] Brown MM. Balloon angioplasty for cerebrovascular disease. Neurol Res 1992; 14(suppl): 159-173
[21] Wholey MH, Wholey M, Bergeron P, Diethrich EB, Henry M, Laborde JC, Mathias K, Myla S, Roubin GS, Shawl F, Theron JG, Yadav JS, Dorros G, Guimaraens J, Higashida R, Kumar V, Leon M, Lim M, Londero H, Mesa J, Ramee S, Rodriguez A, Rosenfield K, Teitelbaum G, Vozzi C. Current global status of carotid artery stent placement. Cathet Cardiovasc Diagn. 1998 May;44(1):1-6.
[22] Theron JG, Payelle GG, Coskun O, Huet HF, Guimaraens L. Carotid artery stenosis: treatment with protected balloon angioplasty and stent placement. Radiology. 1996 Dec;201(3):627-36.
[23] Zarins CK, White RA, Diethrich EB, Shackelton RJ, Siami FS; CaRESS Steering Committee and CaRESS Investigators. Carotid revascularization using endarterectomy or stenting systems (CaRESS): 4-year outcomes. J Endovasc Ther. 2009 Aug;16(4):397-409.
[24] Sivaguru A, Venables GS, Beard JD, Gaines PA. European Carotid Angioplasty Trial. J Endovasc Surg. 1996 Feb;3(1):16-20.
[25] Naylor AR, Bolia A, Abbott RJ, Pye IF, Smith J, Lennard N, Lloyd AJ, London NJ, Bell PR. Randomized study of carotid angioplasty and stenting versus carotid endarterectomy: a stopped trial. J Vasc Surg. 1998 Aug;28(2):326-34.
[26] Alberts MJ. Results of a multicenter prospective randomized trial of carotid artery stenting vs. carotid endarterectomy. Stroke 2001.
[27] Yadav JS, Wholey MH, Kuntz RE, Fayad P, Katzen BT, Mishkel GJ, Bajwa TK, Whitlow P, Strickman NE, Jaff MR, Popma JJ, Snead DB, Cutlip DE, Firth BG, Ouriel K; Stenting and Angioplasty with Protection in Patients at High Risk for Endarterectomy Investigators. Protected carotid-artery stenting versus endarterectomy in high-risk patients. N Engl J Med. 2004 Oct 7;351(15):1493-501.
[28] Eckstein HH, Ringleb P, Allenberg JR, Berger J, Fraedrich G, Hacke W, Hennerici M, Stingele R, Fiehler J, Zeumer H, Jansen O. Results of the Stent-Protected Angioplasty versus Carotid Endarterectomy (SPACE) study to treat symptomatic stenoses at 2 years: a multinational, prospective, randomised trial. Lancet Neurol. 2008 Oct;7(10):893-902. Epub 2008 Sep 5. Erratum in: Lancet Neurol. 2009 Feb;8(2):135.
[29] Mas JL, Trinquart L, Leys D, Albucher JF, Rousseau H, Viguier A, Bossavy JP, Denis B, Piquet P, Garnier P, Viader F, Touzé E, Julia P, Giroud M, Krause D, Hosseini H, Becquemin JP, Hinzelin G, Houdart E, Hénon H, Neau JP, Bracard S, Onnient Y,

Padovani R, Chatellier G; EVA-3S investigators. Endarterectomy Versus Angioplasty in Patients with Symptomatic Severe Carotid Stenosis (EVA-3S) trial: results up to 4 years from a randomised, multicentre trial. Lancet Neurol. 2008 Oct;7(10):885-92. Epub 2008 Sep 5.

[30] International Carotid Stenting Study investigators, Ederle J, Dobson J, Featherstone RL, Bonati LH, van der Worp HB, de Borst GJ, Lo TH, Gaines P, Dorman PJ, Macdonald S, Lyrer PA, Hendriks JM, McCollum C, Nederkoorn PJ, Brown MM. Carotid artery stenting compared with endarterectomy in patients with symptomatic carotid stenosis (International Carotid Stenting Study): an interim analysis of a randomised controlled trial. Lancet. 2010 Mar 20;375(9719):985-97. Epub 2010 Feb 25.

[31] Bonati LH, Fraedrich G; Carotid Stenting Trialists' Collaboration. Age modifies the relative risk of stenting versus endarterectomy for symptomatic carotid stenosis--a pooled analysis of EVA-3S, SPACE and ICSS. Eur J Vasc Endovasc Surg. 2011 Feb;41(2):153-8. Epub 2011 Jan 26.

[32] Brott TG, Hobson RW, Howard G, Roubin GS, Clark WM, Brooks W, et al: Stenting versus endarterectomy for treatment of carotid artery stenosis. N Engl J Med 2010;363:11-23.

[33] Reimers B, Corvaja N, Moshiri S, Saccà S, Albiero R, Di Mario C, Pascotto P, Colombo A. Cerebral protection with filter devices during carotid artery stenting. Circulation. 2001 Jul 3;104(1):12-5.

[34] Ansel GM, Hopkins LN, Jaff MR, Rubino P, Bacharach JM, Scheinert D, Myla S, Das T, Cremonesi A; Investigators for the ARMOUR Pivotal Trial. Safety and effectiveness of the INVATEC MO.MA proximal cerebral protection device during carotid artery stenting: results from the ARMOUR pivotal trial. Catheter Cardiovasc Interv. 2010 Jul 1;76(1):1-8.

[35] Rizzo JA, Dodge A, White P, Martin ED. Magnetic resonance angiography in the evaluation of carotid stent patency. Perspect Vasc Surg Endovasc Ther 2010;22:261-3.

[36] Skelly CL, et al. Risk factors for restenosis after carotid artery angioplasty and stenting. J Vasc Surg 2006;44:1010-5.

[37] Zhou W, et al. Management of in-stent restenosis after carotid artery stenting in high risk patients. J Vasc Surg 2006;43:305-12.

[38] Lal BK, et al. In-stent recurrent stenosis after carotid artery stenting: Life table analysis and clinical relevance. J Vasc Surg 2003;38:1162-9.

[39] Abu Rahma AF, et al. Optimal carotid duplex velocity criteria for defining the severity of carotid in-stent restenosis. J Vasc Surg 2008;48:589-94.

[40] Stanziale SF, et al. Determining in-stent restenosis of carotid arteries by duplex ultrasound criteria. J Endovasc Ther 2005;12:346-53.

[41] Peterson BG, et al. Duplex ultrasound remains a reliable test even after carotid stenting. Ann Vasc Surg 2005;19:793-7.

[42] Chi YN, White CJ, Woods TC, Goldman CK. Ultrasound velocity criteria for carotid in-stent restenosis. Catheter Cardiovasc Interv 2006;69:349-54.

10

Revascularization of Tibial and Foot Arteries: Below the Knee Angioplasty for Limb Salvage

Marco Manzi, Luis Mariano Palena and Giacomo Cester
Interventional Radiology Unit -Policlinico Abano Terme, Padua
Italy

1. Introduction

Advanced atherosclerosis with extended tibial arteries lesions is a common concern, especially in diabetic patients having critical-limb ischemia (CLI) and skin wounds. Chronic critical limb ischemia is a major worldwide cause of morbidity and, especially when threatening the limb, mortality (Faglia E. et al. 2006). Certainly, major and minor amputations are associated with significant increases in mortality risk, and every efforts should be pursued to minimize amputations and ensure limb salvage (Norgen L. et al. 2007).

Infragenicular atherosclerotic is the most common cause of CLI, usually due to multilevel and diffuse arterial disease with compromised foot arteries run-off. Vascular disease is very often associated with arterial wall calcifications, that are usually severe and diffuse. The combination of severe peripheral arterial occlusion with the increased blood flow requirement necessary to achieve the healing of the skin wounds or surgical incisions, makes this population very challenging. Additionally, diabetics and CLI population have a high rate of comorbidities (Bargelini I, et al. 2008).

Clinical manifestations range from Intermittent claudication to limb-threatening ischemia, with rest pain, non healing ulcers and gangrene.

Despite the benefits of pharmacologic therapy (e.g. Angiotensin-converting enzyme inhibitors, antidiabetic drugs, antiplatelet agents and statins), arterial revascularization remains a mainstay in the management of CLI, with restoration of arterial blood flow to the foot, achieving a relief of rest pain and improving wound healing.

In the last decade surgical revascularization has been adopted as the elective treatment option in patients with suitable anatomical conditions, however surgical by-pass is not always feasible due to the involvement of the foot arteries by the atherosclerotic disease, or recommended because of high surgical risk or contraindications in several cases, lack of venous conduits or poor vessels run-off, that compromise surgical by-pass patency (HerstenNR, et al. 2007; Norgen L, et al. 2007; Walsh Db, et al. 1991).

In recent years, related to good technical and clinical results, endovascular treatment options growing acceptance as the primary therapeutic strategy, especially in subjects with significant risk factors for surgical by-pass. In fact, since its initial applications, endovascular recanalization of tibial vessels and foot arteries has proven to be feasible and safe. Actually it is an established treatment option for limb salvage, avoiding amputations in lot of cases and improving wound healing(Adam DJ, et al. 2005; Balmer H, et al. 2002; Dorros G, et al. 2001; Faglia E, et al. 2005, 2006; Ferraresi R, et al. 2009; Romiti M, et al. 2008; Soder HR, et al 2000; Wack C, et al. 1994).

The development of new technologies, such as dedicated guide-wire or low profile catheter balloons helps the interventionists to achieve technical and clinical results. Nevertheless, the knowledge of the most important techniques should be indispensable to obtain the procedural success and clinical outcome. In fact, the advances in distal lower extremity revascularization have revolutionized salvage of the ischemic limb.

2. Epidemiology of peripheral arterial disease

The management of the patient with peripheral arterial disease (PAD) has to be planned in the context of the epidemiology of the disease, its natural history and, in particular, the modifiable risk factors for the systemic disease as well as those that predict deterioration of the circulation to the limb (Norgen L, et al. 2007).

2.1 Incidence of peripheral arterial disease

Total disease prevalence based on objective testing has been evaluated in several epidemiologic studies and is in the range of 3-10%, increasing to 15% to 20% in persons over 70 years (Criqui MH et al. 1985; Hiatt WR, et al. 1995; Norgen et al. 2007; Selvin E, et al. 2004).

Intermittent claudication (IC) s usually diagnosed by a history of muscular leg pain on exercise that is relieved by a short rest. This symptom does not always predict the presence or absence of PAD. A patient with quite severe PAD may not have the symptom of IC because some other condition limits exercise or they are sedentary. In contrast, some patients with what seems to be IC may not have PAD. Likewise, patients with very mild PAD may develop symptoms of IC only when they become very physically active.

Black ethnicity increases the risk of PAD by over two-fold, and this risk is not explained by higher levels of other risk factors such as diabetes, hypertension or obesity (Criqui MH, et al. 2005). A high prevalence of arteritis affecting the distal arteries of young black South Africans has also been described.

3. Risk factors of peripheral arterial disease

Although the various factors described in this section are usually referred to as risk factors, in most cases the evidence is only for an association. The criteria used to support a risk factor require a prospective, controlled study showing that altering the factor alters the development or course of the PAD, such as has been shown for smoking cessation or treatment of dyslipidemia. Risk may be conferred by other metabolic or circulatory abnormalities associated with diabetes (Norgen L, et al. 2007).

3.1 Race, gender and age

The National Health and Nutrition Examination Survey in the United States found that an ABI ≤0.90 was more common in non-Hispanic Blacks (7.8%) than in Whites (4.4%). Such a difference in the prevalence of PAD was confirmed by the recent GENOA (Genetic Epidemiology Network of Arteriopathy) study (Kullo IJ, et al. 2003), which also showed that the difference was not explained by a difference in classical risk factors for atherosclerosis.

The prevalence of PAD, symptomatic or asymptomatic, is slightly greater in men than women, particularly in the younger age groups. In patients with IC, the ratio of men to women is between 1:1 and 2:1. This ratio increases in some studies to at least 3:1 in more severe stages of the disease, such as chronic CLI. Other studies have, however, shown a more equal distribution of PAD between genders and even a predominance of women with CLI.

The striking increase in both the incidence and prevalence of PAD with increasing age is apparent from the earlier discussion of epidemiology (Norgen L, et al. 2007).

3.2 Smoking

The relationship between smoking and PAD has been recognized since 1911, when Erb reported that IC was three-times more common among smokers than among non-smokers. It has been suggested that the association between smoking and PAD may be even stronger than that between smoking and coronary artery disease (CAD). Furthermore, a diagnosis of PAD is made approximately a decade earlier in smokers than in non-smokers. The severity of PAD tends to increase with the number of cigarettes smoked. Heavy smokers have a four-fold higher risk of developing IC compared with non-smokers. Smoking cessation is associated with a decline in the incidence of IC (Norgen L, et al. 2007).

Results from the Edinburgh Artery Study found that the relative risk of IC was 3.7 in 7 smokers compared with 3.0 in ex-smokers (who had discontinued smoking for less than 5 years).

3.3 Diabetes mellitus

Many studies have shown an association between diabetes mellitus and the development of PAD. Overall, IC is about twice as common among diabetic patients than among non-diabetic patients. In patients with diabetes, for every 1% increase in hemoglobin A1c there is a corresponding 26% increased risk of PAD (Selvin E, et al. 2004).

Over the last decade, mounting evidence has suggested that insulin resistance plays a key role in a clustering of cardiometabolic risk factors which include hyperglycemia, dyslipidemia, hypertension and obesity. Insulin resistance is a risk factor for PAD even in subjects without diabetes, raising the risk approximately 40% to 50%. PAD in patients with diabetes is more aggressive compared to non-diabetics, with early large vessel involvement coupled with distal symmetrical neuropathy. The need for a major amputation is five- to ten-times higher in diabetics than non-diabetics. This is contributed to by sensory neuropathy and decreased resistance to infection. Based on these observations, a consensus statement from the American Diabetes Association recommends PAD screening with an ABI every 5 years in patients with diabetes (Norgen L, et al. 2007).

3.4 Hypertension

Hypertension is associated with all forms of cardiovascular disease, including PAD. However, the relative risk for developing PAD is less for hypertension than diabetes or smoking (Norgen L, et al. 2007).

3.5 Dyslipidemia

In the Framingham study, a fasting cholesterol level greater than 7 mmol/L (270 mg/dL) was associated with a doubling of the incidence of IC but the ratio of total to high-density lipoprotein (HDL) cholesterol was the best predictor of occurrence of PAD. In another study, patients with PAD had significantly higher levels of serum triglycerides, very low-density lipoprotein (VLDL) cholesterol, VLDL triglycerides, VLDL proteins, intermediate

density lipoprotein (IDL) cholesterol, and IDL triglycerides and lower levels of HDL than controls (Attinder CE, et al. 2001; Criqui MH, et al. 1985; Fowkes FG, et al. 2004; Norgen L, et al. 2007; Selvin E, et al. 2004; Senti M, et al. 1992).
Although some studies have also shown that total cholesterol is a powerful independent risk factor for PAD, others have failed to confirm this association. It has been suggested that cigarette smoking may enhance the effect of hypercholesterolemia. There is evidence that treatment of hyperlipidemia reduces both the progression of PAD and the incidence of IC. An association between PAD and hypertriglyceridemia has also been reported and has been shown to be associated with the progression and systemic complications of PAD. Lipoprotein(a) is a significant independent risk factor for PAD.

3.6 Hyperviscosity and hypercoagulable states

Raised hematocrit levels and hyperviscosity have been reported in patients with PAD, possibly as a consequence of smoking. Increased plasma levels of fibrinogen, which is also a risk factor for thrombosis, have been associated with PAD in several studies. Both hyperviscosity and hypercoagulability have also been shown to be markers or risk factors for a poor prognosis (Norgen L, et al. 2007).

3.7 Hyperhomocysteinemia

The prevalence of hyperhomocysteinemia is as high in the vascular disease population, compared with 1% in the general population. It is reported that hyperhomocysteinemia is detected in about 30% of young patients with PAD. The suggestion that hyperhomocysteinemia may be an independent risk factor for atherosclerosis has now been substantiated by several studies. It may be a stronger risk factor for PAD than for CAD (Norgen L, et al. 2007).

3.8 Chronic renal insufficiency

There is an association of renal insufficiency with PAD, with some recent evidence suggesting it may be causal. In the HERS study (Heart and Estrogen/Progestin Replacement Study), renal insufficiency was independently associated with future PAD events in postmenopausal women (O'Hare AM, et al. 2004; Norgen L, et al. 2007).

4. Vascular anatomy and angiosome concept - The first step toward pedal recanalization

Knowledge of vascular anatomy of the leg, ankle and foot, and an understanding of the dynamic nature of that vasculature are essential for limb salvage (Taylor G, et al. 1992).
The concept that divides the body into three-dimensional vascular territories supplied by specific source arteries, known as the angiosome principle, was introduced by Taylor and expanded for the clinical treatment of ischemic lesions at the foot and ankle level by Attinger (Attinger CE, et al. 2001). The foot and the ankle can be divided into six distinct angiosomes; each fed by a specific arterial branch. Recent data suggest a different clinical outcome of successful revascularization procedures based on the possibility of providing inline vascular supply to the specific angiosome of the ischemic wound.
By combining the anatomic and functional aspects of foot circulation, the angiosome theory can be useful in planning the endovascular revascularization strategy in cases of ischemic

wounds at foot and ankle level. In particular, the angiosome concept can help to select the target vessel for revascularization, that is, the artery which will yield the best local results.

4.1 Normal vascular anatomy and main variations

By definition the popliteal artery ends at the origin of the first tibial artery, which typically is the Anterior Tibial Artery. In about 4% of cases we find a so-called high origin of the Anterior tibial Artery at the level of the knee joint or even some centimetres more proximal. Similarly, in a small proportion of the population (1-2%) a high origin of the posterior tibial artery has been described. Normally, the direct continuation of the popliteal artery, after the branch of the anterior tibial artery, is the tibioperoneal trunk. This vascular segment splits into the posterior tibial artery and the peroneal artery (Fig. 1).

As a variation, a triforcation of the popliteal artery into all three lower leg arteries at the same point has been observed in 0.4% of patients. The posterior tibial artery may be missing completely in 1-5% of a normal adult population.

The vascular anatomy of the foot is composed of the anterior and posterior circulation, connected through the pedal arches. The anterior tibial artery continues into the dorsal pedal artery. The posterior tibial artery continues into the common plantar artery and then in the lateral and medial plantar arteries. The peroneal artery splits above the ankle joint into and anterior and posterior branch, the ramus perforans that anastomoses with the dorsal pedal artery, and the ramus communicans that anastomoses with the plantar arteries. The dorsalis pedis artery and the lateral plantar artery communicate via the plantar arch (Fig. 2 and Fig. 3).

The digital branches origin from the plantar arch and there are a dorsal and plantar branches for each toe. The plantar digital branch for first toe ususally origin from medial plantar artery.

Both tibial arteries, together with the peroneal artery, supply different portions of the foot and ankle. The plantar foot and the medial ankle are fed by the posterior tibial artery, the anterior ankle and the dorsum of the foot by the anterior tibial artery, and the antero-lateral ankle and rear foot by the peroneal artery.

As a anatomic variations of the foot dorsalis pedis artery may be absent in 6-12% of cases; in this patient the lateral tarsal artery often became predominant and develop anastomosis through the plantar arch to the plantar circulation.

In some cases the lateral plantar artery, through plantar arch, is the predominant artery for the I toe. In a few cases has been described the absence of plantar arch, in this situation the dorsalis pedis is the predominant artery for the I and II toe and the lateral plantar artery, is the predominant artery supplying the III, IV and V toe.

4.2 Angiosome and wound related artery concept

The angiosome principle was defined by Ian Taylor's landmark anatomic study and divides the body into individual angiosomes: three-dimensional blocks of tissue fed by "source" arteries. He defined an angiosome as a three-dimensional anatomic unit of tissue fed by a source artery and defined at least 40 angiosomes in the body, including six in the foot and ankle region. Adjacent angiosomes are bordered by choke vessels, which link neighboring angiosomes to one another and demarcate the border of each angiosome. In addition, these choke vessels are important safety conduits that allow a given angiosome to provide blood flow to an adjacent angiosome if the latter's source artery is damaged (Calligari PR, et al. 1992; Taylor GI, et al. 1992a, 1992b).

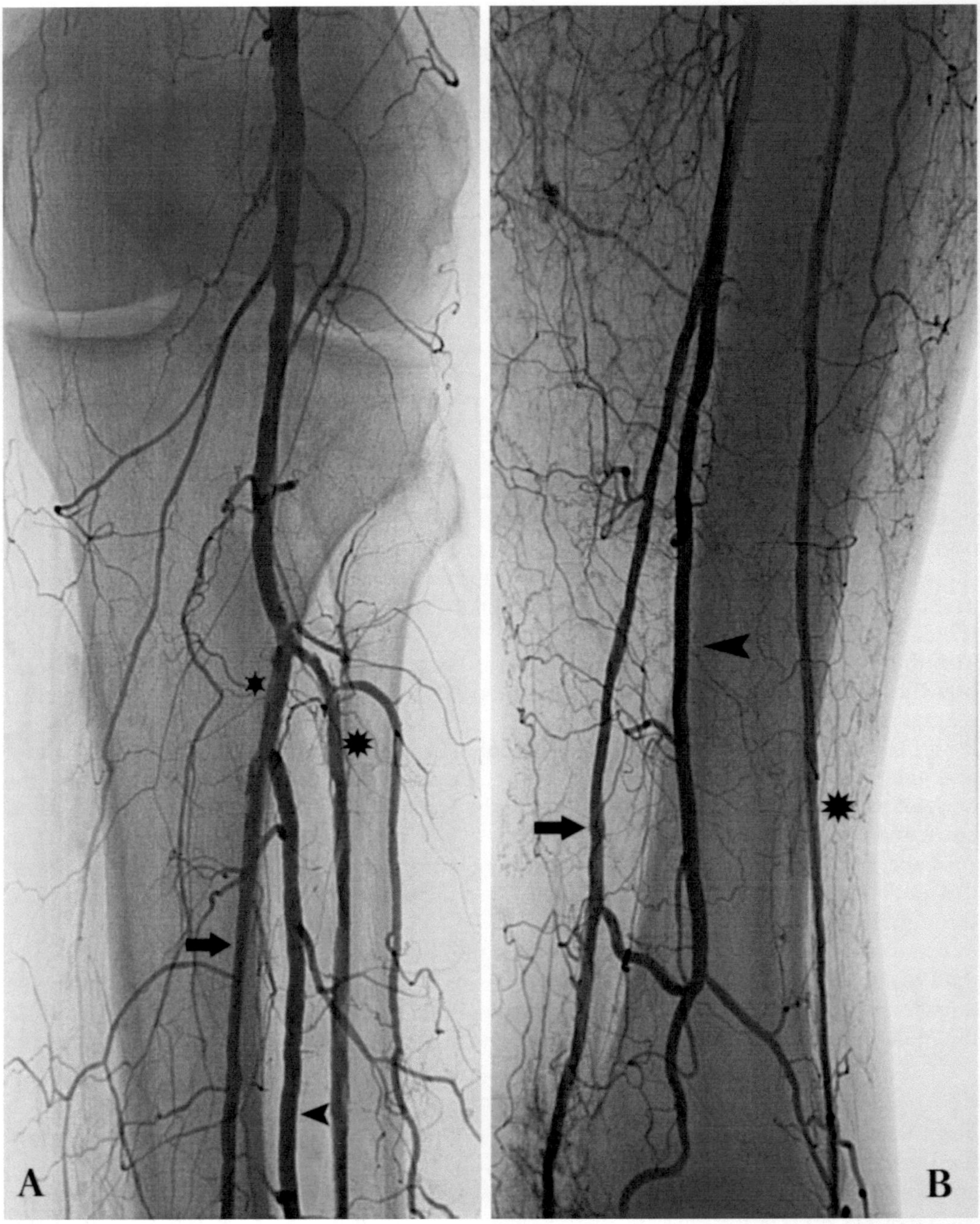

Fig. 1. A. Anteroposterior view of the tibial trifurcation show anterior tibial artery (✹), tibio-peroneal trunk (✶), peroneal artery (➤) and posterior tibial artery (➡). B. Lateral view at the distal leg and ankle level show the anterior (✹) and posterior (➡)tibial arteries and the peroneal artery (➤) with the collateral branches.

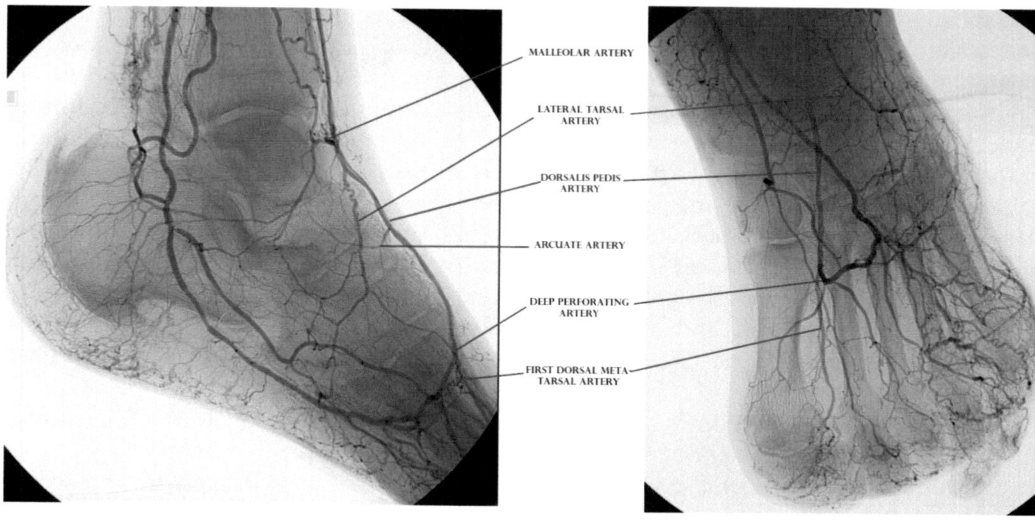

Fig. 2. Anterior and dorsal circulation. The major arteries are visualized in the lateral-oblique view (left side) and in the antero-posterior view (right side) angiographic projections.

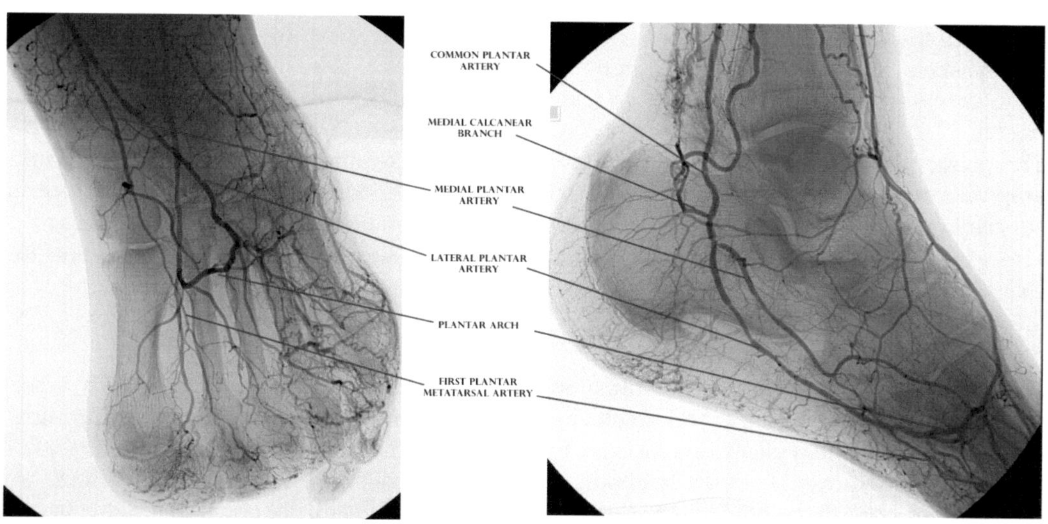

Fig. 3. Posterior and plantar circulation. The major arteries are visualized in antero-posterior view (left side) and in the lateral-oblique view (right side) angiographic projections.

The choke vessel system links the angiosomes to one another. A unified network is created so that one source artery can provide blood flow to multiple angiosomes beyond its immediate border.

While the choke vessels provide an indirect connection among angiosomes, there are also direct arterial-arterial connections that allow blood flow to immediately bypass local obstructions in the vascular tree.

The six angiosomes of the foot and ankle originate from the three main arteries to the foot and ankle. The posterior tibial artery supplies the medial ankle and the plantar foot, the anterior tibial artery supplies the dorsum of the foot, and the peroneal artery supplies the anterolateral ankle and the lateral rear foot. The large angiosomes of the foot can be further broken into angiosomes of the major branches of the above arteries. The three main branches of the posterior tibial artery each supply distinct portions of the plantar foot: the calcaneal branch (heel), the medial plantar artery (instep), and the lateral plantar artery (lateral midfoot and forefoot). The two branches of the peroneal artery supply the anterolateral portion of the ankle and rear foot, the anterior perforating branch (lateral anterior upper ankle) and the calcaneal branch (plantar heel). The anterior tibial artery supplies the anterior ankle and then becomes the dorsalis pedis artery that supplies the dorsum of the foot (Attinger CE, et al. 1997; Attinger CE, et al. 2001; Sarrafain SK. 1993; Taylor GI, et al. 1998).

The dorsalis pedis artery follows a curved pathway on the forefoot to join the first plantar space, where meets the posterior circulation through the perforating deep artery.

In according with angiosome concept, the foot lesion location is related to an specific angiosome and the revascularization of this specific angiosome is our target vessel or wound related artery.

5. Endovascular intervention

Endovascular recanalization of tibial vessels and foot arteries should be the first line treatment in patients with CLI, because of its good technical and clinical outcomes.

Endovascular treatment is possible in most cases, with the known low complication rate of PTA. In cases in which endovascular revascularization failed, all surgical options remain open.

The primary indications for tibial and foot arteries intervention is limb salvage, to avoid amputations. Patients with chronic leg ischemia face a gloomy future, in fact, long-term survival rate with CLI is significantly lower than that of a matched population.

Limb salvage is of more importance to these patients. The most plausible explanation for this is that healing the wounds and/or infection will reduce the oxygenation demand.

5.1 Vessel features

Calcified vessels are the most difficult situation in endovascular treatment, especially when calcifications are very dark and thick, in a visual evaluation. We propose intraluminal approach in very heavy calcified vessels, using dedicated 0.014' guide wire and short, low-profile OTW dedicated catheter balloons, like coronary balloons. OTW catheter balloon are necessary in order to be able to inject contrast material and check the position and to change the wire, when necessary.

Non calcified vessel allows different recanalization alternative, as endoluminal or subintimal approach. It the occluded tract is short, may be endoluminal approache could be the first alternative. In long occlusions, especially when there is a good distal re-entry, subintimal approach could be a good alternative.

In calcified vessel, when is imposible to cross the lesion trough the true lumen and vascular situation are dramatic and the indications to revascularization, related to wounds on the foot are present, a more aggressive strategy could be adopted. A subintimal attempt is justified in these cases and could bring to good result.

5.2 Technical strategies

Antegrade access in the common femoral artery is, in our experience, the best approach to perform tibial and foot arteries revascularization, with excellent guide-ability of the guide-wire and good push-ability of the catheter balloons due to this access is closer to the lesions. Contra-lateral approach is indicated in cases in which iliac treatment is required or is possible to treat contro-lateral common femoral artery or Superficial femoral artery. In cases of BTK interventions makes the procedure more difficult, require long shafts catheter balloons, limits some technical strategies and makes complications management considerably more complex.

In some selected cases antegrade access in the popliteal artery could be useful, because it is closer to the lesions and ensure more push-ability of the devices, but the prone position of the patient is required.

Previously to begging the procedure are injected, systematically, a intra-arterial bolus of 5.000 I.U of heparin. The patients are undergo to double anti-platelets therapy with ticlopidine, 250 mg daily and acetylsalicylic acid 100 mg daily, 3 days before the procedure. The double antiaggregation is continued for 6 weeks after the procedure and acetylsalicylic acid is prescribed quoad vitam.

5.2.1 Transluminal recanalization

Transluminal recanalization is the preferred techniques to treat stenotic lesions, very short occlusions (<1 cm) (Hauser H, et al. 1996) or lesions that involve the bifurcations. In our experience, is the best technical strategy to recanalize calcified vessels and it could be the first choice in CTO lesions with very heavy calcified arteries.

The classic approach to intraluminal recanalization use a guide-wire in conjunction with a support catheter to cross the lesion (Patel PJ, et al. 2010).

In our experience we prefer to use a 0.014"-in. guide-wire (Pilot®200 - Abbott) with an angulated tip (45° angle), that allows to guide the guide-wire, avoiding subintimal progression or vessel spills. A straight CTO dedicated guide-wire can also be used, with good results, in calcified and insuperable lesions.

The first step is to penetrate the proximal occlusion followed by negotiation the full extent of the occlusion, until the distal patent lumen. A drilling motion of the guide-wire is performed to properly penetrate and cross the lesion. Often times, a short and low profile coaxial catheter balloon can be used as a support catheter (Patel PJ, et al. 2010). Coaxial catheter balloon system is preferred to monorail system, because monorail system work well when the sheath tip can be placed close to the lesion. Coaxial system allows to remove the guide-wire, inject contrast media and check the position of the catheter and, if necessary, change the guide-wire .

When the recanalization is completed, we perform a pre-dilatation with the support catheter balloon. A definitive dilatation is performed with a long catheter balloon, and based in the authors experience, in a heavy calcified vessels we prefer to avoid dissections during PTA dilating the crural vessels to 2.5 mm and the foot arteries to 2 mm in diameter (Fig 4 and 5).

Diagnostic angiography. (A-B) Obstruction of the anterior and posterior arteries, patency of the tibio-peroneal trunk and peroneal artery. (C-D) patency of common plantar artery, dorsalis pedis artery and plantar arch, in a heavy calcified vessels.

(E-H) Intraluminale recanalization of the posterior tibial artery, lateral plantar artery, plantar arch and the digital branch for the first toe and angioplasty of the digital branch (1.5 x 20 mm catheter balloon). (I-J) Intraluminal PTA of the posterior and anterior tibial arteries (2.5 x 220 mm catheter balloon).

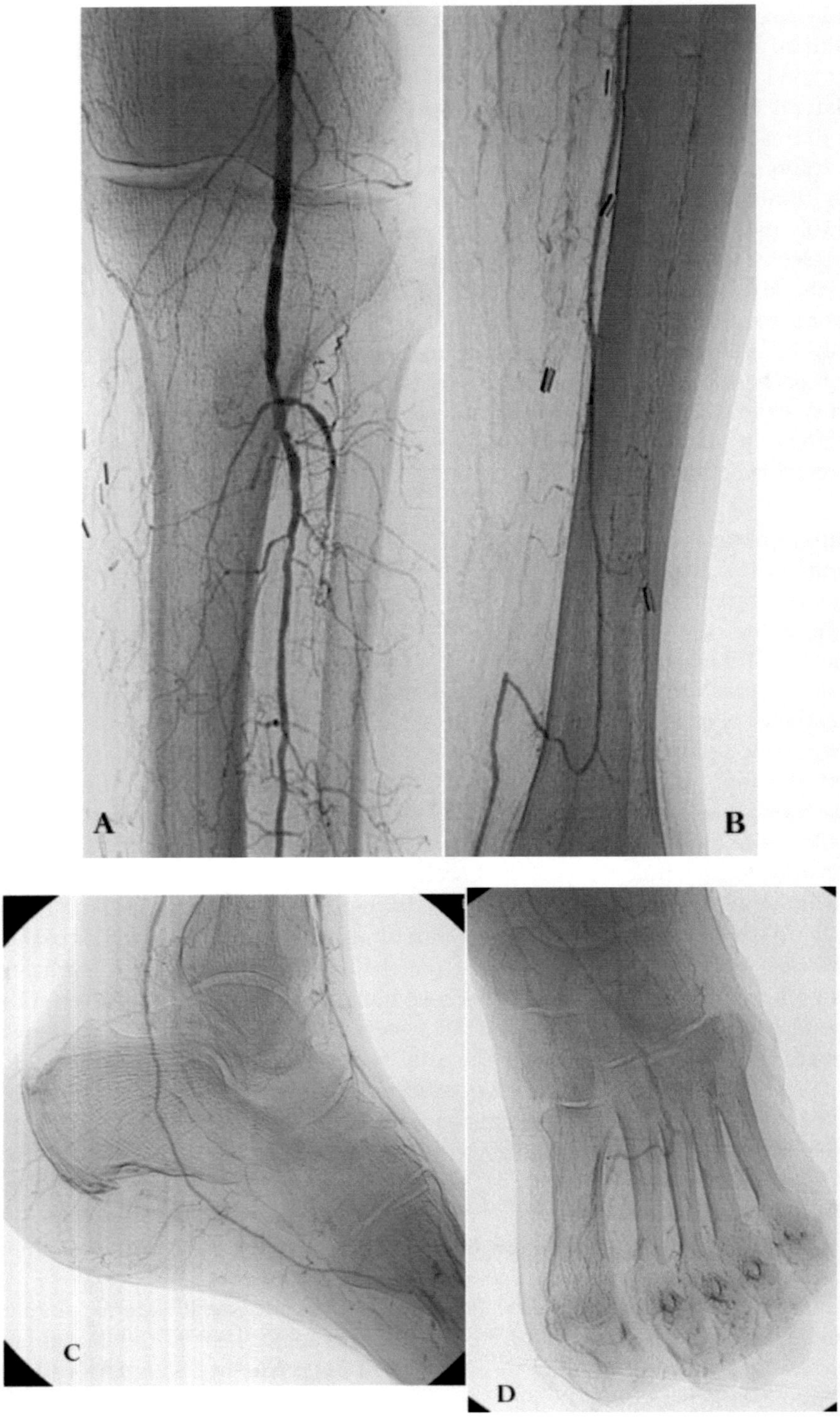
A
B
C
D

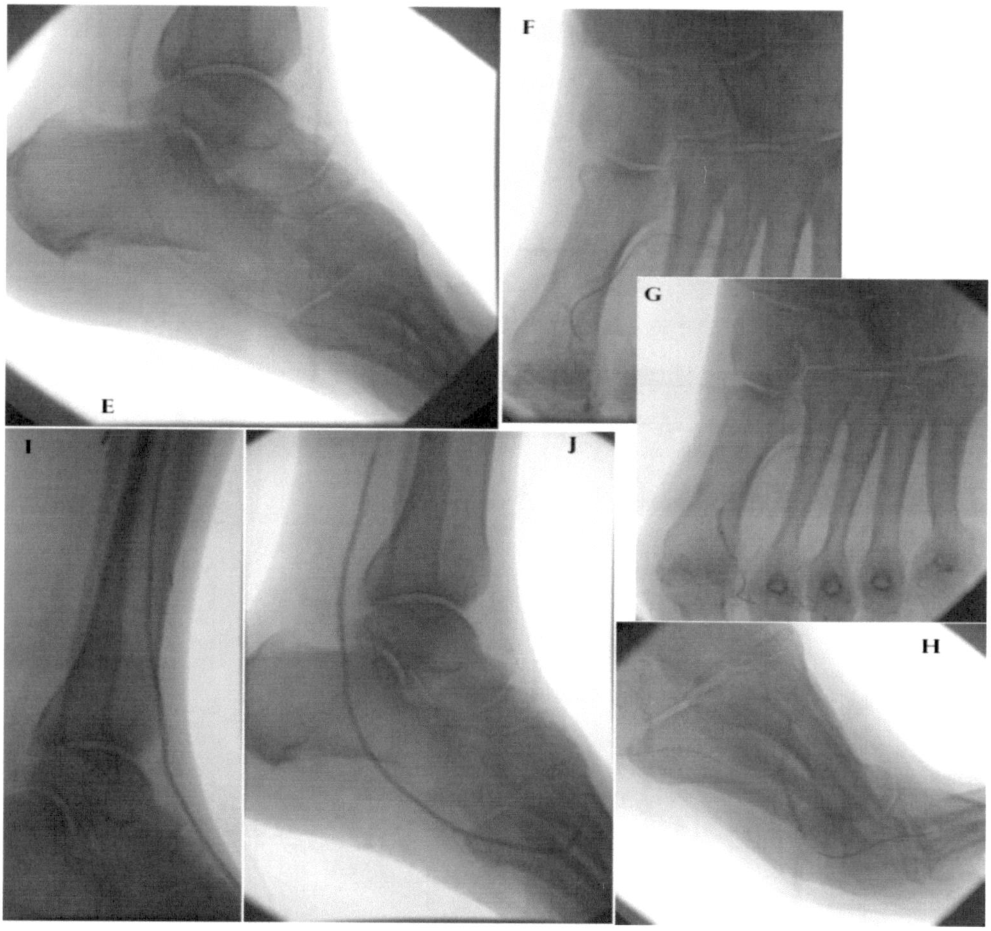

Fig. 4. Case 1. Diabetic patient with apical ulcer on the first toe, TcPO2: 13 mmHg.

Diagnostic angiography. (A-B) Obstruction of the anterior and posterior arteries, patency of the tibio-peroneal trunk and peroneal artery. (C-D) patency of common plantar artery, dorsalis pedis artery and plantar arch, in a heavy calcified vessels.
(E-H) Intraluminale recanalization of the posterior tibial artery, lateral plantar artery, plantar arch and the digital branch for the first toe and angioplasty of the digital branch (1.5 x 20 mm catheter balloon / FlexeCTO - Clearstream). (I-J) Intraluminal PTA of the posterior and anterior tibial arteries (2.5 x 220 mm catheter balloon / Bantamα - Clearstream).

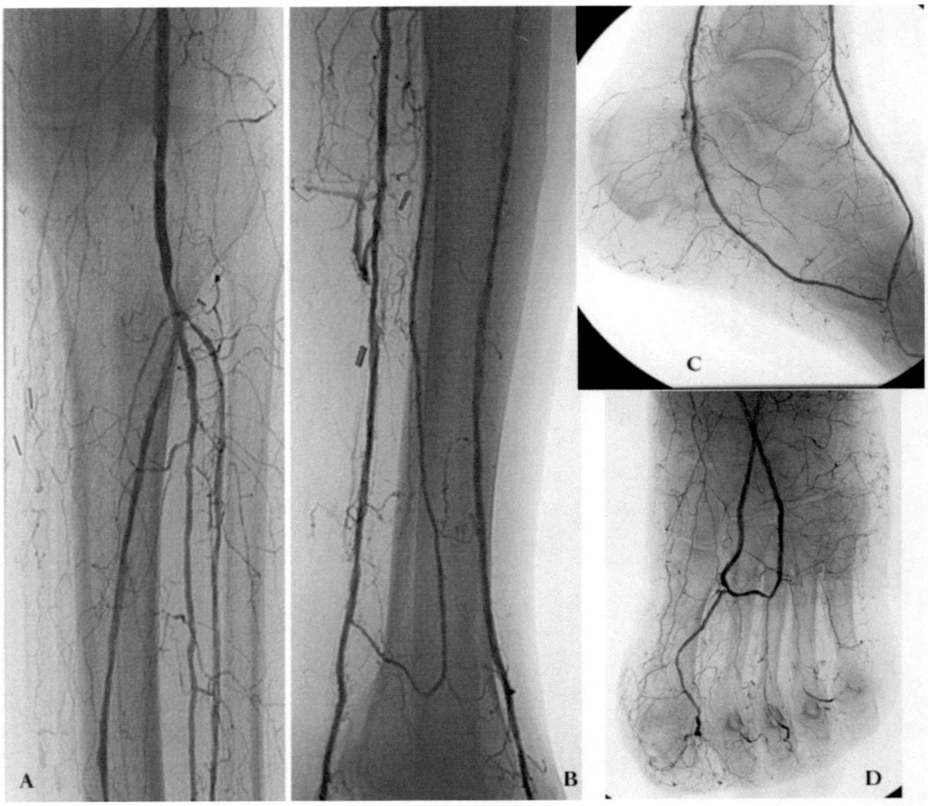

Fig. 5. Case 1. Technical and clinical results.

(A-D) Angiographic results of the intraluminal recanalization of the anterior and posterior tibial arteries; lateral plantar and dorsali pedis arteries, plantar arch and the first digital branch, with excellent blood flow in the target vessel.
Clinical follow up at 4 months show increased of the TcPO2 to 42 mmHg and ulcer healing, avoiding amputation.

5.2.2 Subintimal recanalization

On the other hand, when the arteries are not calcified or low and incomplete calcifications are observed, a subintimal recanalization is proposed as the first technical strategy. Subintimal angioplasty was first described by Bolia (Bolia A et al. 1990) and since them there have been a lot of publications confirming the value and assess the clinical results of this technique to treat tibial vessels (Alexandrescu V, et al. 2009; Bolia A, et al. 1994, Bown MJ, et al. 2009; Chun JY, et al. 2010; Ingle H, et al. 2002; Met R, et al. 2008; Reekers J, et al. 1994, Spinosa DJ, et al. 2004).
A subintimal recanalization in a heavy calcified crural vessels can also be considered, after failure of intraluminal attempts, with the impossibility to cross the lesion (Bolia A. 1998.)
This technical strategy could also be used in Pedal arteries and a published paper described this technical option to recanalize the Pedal arch (Fusaro M, et al. 2007).
The principal advantages of this technique are the ability to cross long chronic occlusions and the option of recanalization of more than one crural vessel. In our experience, the failure of this technical strategy is related to heavy calcified vessels, with fissuring the arterial wall

during the subintimal progression of the guide-wire, rupture of the arterial wall and failure of the recanalization.
We perform a subintimal recanalization in crural arteries with a 0.018"-in guide-wire (V18® - Boston Scientific) or, less frequent, with 0.014"-in guide-wire (Pilot®200 - Abbott).
The 0.014"-in guide-wire should be preferred to perform a subintimal recanalization in the Pedal arteries.
Is also possible to perform a subintimal dissection using a 0.035"-in hydrophilic guide-wire, but in our opinion this more aggressive approach in reserved for cases with heavy calcified vessel and is not indicated for Pedal arteries recanalization. A diagnostic catheter (Berenstain II® - Cordis) or a balloon catheter, is used to support the guide-wire during subintimal progression.
We prefer to avoid a pre-dilatations of the subintimal dissection before to reach the distal patent lumen and check the re-entry. This is just a modification of Bolia technique, in order to avoid the risk of potential bleeding secondary to vessel perforation or to prevent the dilatation of the subintimal dissection that could not re-entry and could need to change the subintimal way to obtain technical success. When the re-entry is achieve, we change a guide-wire with a new one, usually 0.014"-in to avoid spasm in the foot arteries and Pedal arch.
After pedal distal patent lumen recanalization, we deploy a low profile catheter balloon and perform a pre-dilatations of the crural vessel. After short balloon pre-dilatation, a longer one can be placed and a final dilatation performed. We usually dilate crural vessels with a 3 mm diameter balloon and Pedal arteries, including Pedal arch with 2.5 mm diameter balloon. When the result is still not satisfactory, dilatation can be repeated.
In a recent published study (Met R, et al. 2005) a systematic review showed that subintimal recanalization can be a useful option in the treatment of patients with CLI, with primary success rate of 80-90% and 1 year limb salvage rate as high as 90% and conclude that despite the moderate long-term patency rates of the revascularized segments, subintimal angioplasty may serve as a "temporary by-pass", providing wound healing and limb salvage.

5.3 Antegrade and retrograde recanalization

In our experience antegrade approach should be the first choice to treat tibial vessels and foot arteries and a retrograde recanalization should be seen as a support or problem solving strategy, in cases of antegrade failure, such as the inability to re-enter in the true patent distal lumen after subintimal recanalization.
In this context, the retrograde recanalization can be performed and there are different technical options, such as trans-collateral navigation and retrograde recanalization, Pedal-Plantar Loop technique or, retrograde distal access and recanalization.
In our opinion, perform a distal retrograde access is the last technical strategy in order to create a re-entry or resolve problems.

5.3.1 Trans-collateral recanalization

In many cases of extreme vascular intervention, it is not possible to perform regular antegrade recanalization of occluded tibial arteries, which makes even the most expert interventionist resort to unusual techniques (Bolia A, 2005; Fusaro M, et al. 2008; Graziani L, et al. 2008, 2011) to restore direct blood flow to the foot. Combined retrograde-antegrade arterial recanalization through collateral vessels, essentially combined retrograde and antegrade arterial recanalization using a single entry site.
This technical strategy, largely tested by the authors, has been described in published papers (Fusaro M, et al 2008, Graziani L, et al. 2011) and is intended as option to recanalize tibial arteries.

In our experience it could also be used to recanalize foot arteries, using a natural anastomoses in the foot, such as the so-called "Deep arch" of the foot, that communicate medial plantar artery with lateral tarsal branch and can be tracking in each other sense, to recanalize anterior or posterior tibial artery or in order to arrive to the Pedal arch, through the tarsal branch.

In the same way, there is a natural anastomoses between peroneal artery and the "Deep arch" of the foot (Palena LM, et al. 2011), through a perforating deep branch and tracking this way is possible to retrogradely racanalize the other tibial arteries, via peroneal artery, using a "Deep arch" of the foot.

The vessels are finally recanalized by antegrade PTA (Fig. 6 and 7).

There are another collateral ways or natural anastomoses between tibial and foot arteries that allows to perform retrograde-antegrade recanalization of the tibial and the foot arteries, and its represent an alternative option to recanalize the target vessel.

However, the use of this technique may be considered selectively, even in last-attempt efforts, when other options are not possible or are contraindicated. This technique may be of value specifically when a proximal occlusion stump is not evident, when a dissection flap or a perforation in the proximal tract of the target vessel impairs guide-wire advancement.

This technique may represent a feasible endovascular option to avoid more invasive, time-consuming or riskier procedures.

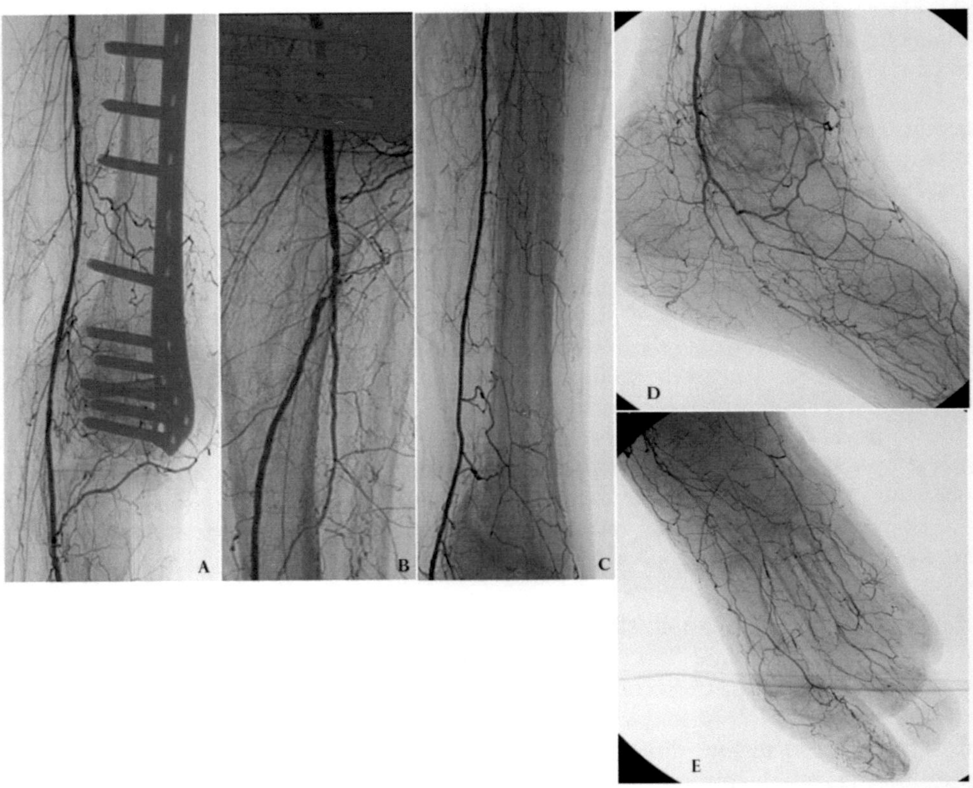

Fig. 6. Case 2. Diabetic patient with amputation of the II and V toes, previously undergone to endovascular treatment with poor outcome and guide-wire fracture at the origin of the dorsalis pedis artery with loss the rest of the wire in a subintimal lumen. TcPO2: 6 mmHg.

(A-D) Diagnostic angiography shown patency of the posterior tibial artery and obstruction of the peroneal and anterior tibial arteries. On the foot patency of the first tract of the medial plantar artery and tarsal branch, obstruction of the lateral plantar and dorsalis pedis arteries.

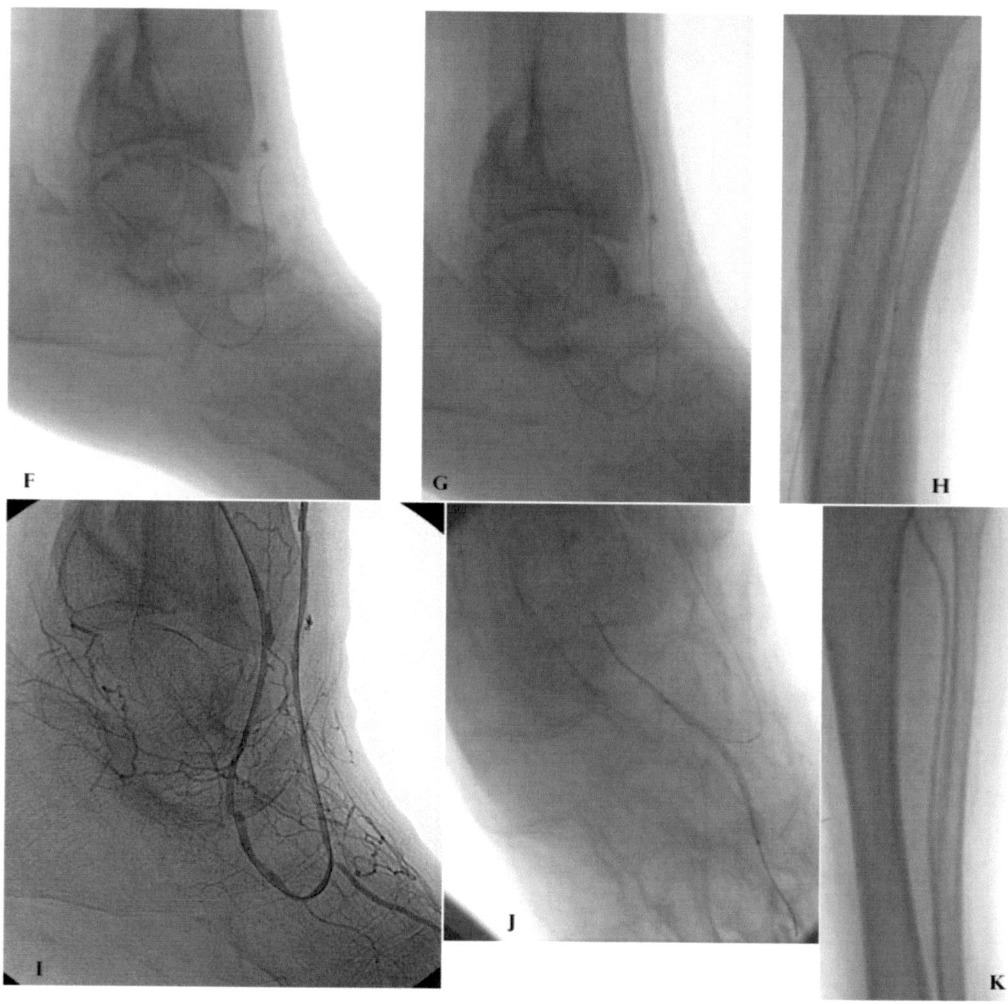

Fig. 6. (cont). (F-H) recanalization of the peroneal artery and, through the "deep arch", retrogradely recanalization of the anterior tibial artery. After antegrade catheterization of the anterior tibial artery, (I) injection of the contrast material shown patency of the lateral tarsal branch. (J-K) PTA of the lateral tarsal branch (2 x 40 mm / FlexeCTO - Clearstream) and PTA of the anterior tibial artery (2.5 x 220 mm catheter balloon / Bantamα - Clearstream).

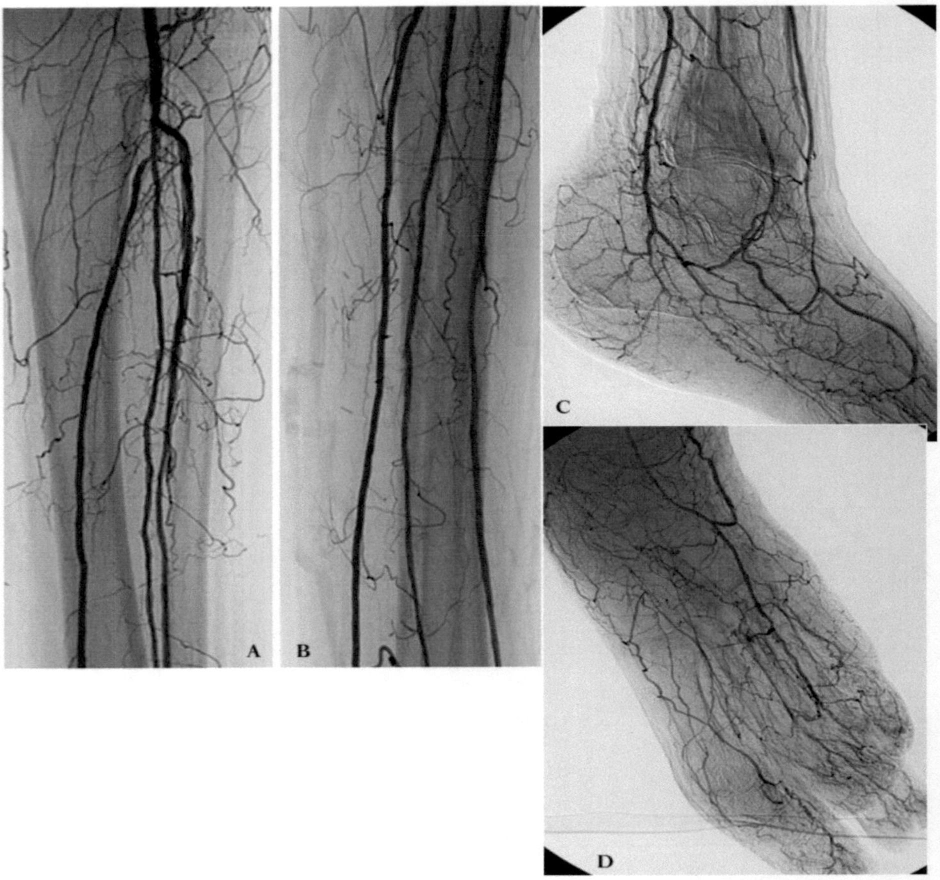

Fig. 7. Angiographic results. (A-B) Recanalization of the anterior and peroneal arteries, patency of the posterior tibial artery. (C-D) Recanalization of the lateral tarsal branch and plantar arch, with good blood flow for the foot and the toes.

Clinical follow up. TcPO2 increased to 37 mmHg with healing the surgical treatment.

5.3.2 Pedal-Plantar LOOP technique

In a high percentage of cases the success rate of PTA remains suboptimal, particularly when the atherosclerotic disease involving also the distal run-off. In these cases the support of Pedal-Plantar LOOP technique could be necessary.

This technical approach, intended for the recanalization of challenging below-the-knee and below-the-ankle lesions, has been already described (Fusaro M, et al 2007) and the clinical results of its application in revascularization of tibial and foot vessels has thoroughly been described in a recent paper (Manzi M, et al. 2009).

Specifically, this technique consist in either one or both the following two approaches: antegrade recanalization of the anterior tibial artery and the pedal artery, including the pedal arch, followed by retrograde recanalization of the lateral plantar artery and then of the posterior tibial artery; or antegrade recanalization of the posterior tibial artery and the lateral plantar artery, including pedal arch, followed by retrograde recanalization of the pedal artery and then of the anterior tibial artery. After successfully crossing the target lesion with the guide-wire, usually 0.014"-in (Pilot® 200 - Abbott), a dedicated low-profile over-the-wire catheter balloon should be deployed for PTA and the check to confirm the position of the tip of the catheter in the distal true lumen should be done, injecting contrast media through the catheter.

Pedal-Plantar LOOP technique is based on the creation of a loop with the guide-wire from the anterior tibial to the posterior tibial arteries (or vice versa) by means of guide-wire tracking through the pedal arch of the foot.

Clearly, this strategy can be adapted case by case and a combination of other technical possibilities, such as subintimal recanalization of the tibial vessel recanalized antegradely, followed by a re-entry on the foot artery or a subintimal recanalization of the foot and tibial artery recanalized retrogradely, followed by a re-entry at the origin of the tibial vessel, could help to reach both, technical and clinical success.

This technique may be of particular value whenever a proximal occlusion stump is unavailable, when dissection flap or a perforation in the proximal tract of the target vessel impairs the guide-wire advancement, as well as when distal disease makes retrograde percutaneous puncture impossible.

5.3.3 Retrograde percutaneous revascularization

In our opinion this should be the last technical strategy, considered when the possible solutions before described failed.

It is intended as a direct percutaneous retrograde puncture of the distal tract of the tibial vessel or foot arteries, in order to retrogradely recanalization of the target vessel (Fig. 8 and 9).

This approach has been described as a solution for the re-entry in a subintimal recanalization (Gandini R, et al. 2007; Spinosa DJ, et al 2003, 2005), that in a small percentage of patients in whom antegrade subintimal recanalization is unsuccessful or there is a limited distal target vessel "landing" zone, a retrograde distal puncture can be performed and a retrograde recanalization, following by antegrade PTA and haemostasis may be a solution.

The possible retrograde access site may be different, such as distal tract of the posterior tibial artery, pedal artery (Fusaro M, et al. 2006, 2007) or peroneal artery, but the difficulties to perform the puncture increase from each other site and the risk to damage the distal patent vessel, compromising the possibility to perform a distal by-pass, should be considered.

In our experience, in selected and very challenging cases in whom a distal by pass is contraindicated, antegrade revascularization attempts failed and retrograde percutaneous distal access on the target vessel is not possible or failed too, an antegrade percutaneous distal access on the Pedal artery or in the common plantar artery, followed by antegrade recanalization of the foot artery, pedal arch and retrograde recanalization of the target vessel, is possible, but should be considered as indication in cases in whom every other endovascular or surgical strategy failed or are contraindicated.

Endovascular recanalization of the tibial vessels and foot arteries, especially in diabetics with CLI is actually an excellent treatment option and, in our experience, should be considered as the first treatment option for revascularization. Different clinical studies and registries show that technical success rate is between 80% and 90% and clinical success rate, intended as limb salvage, is about 70% at 12 months. These technical and clinical outcomes are obtained in a dedicated centers, combining all technical strategies described before.

Stent deployment in the below-the-knee district, in our opinion, should be considered as the last treatment option, because in-stent re-stenosis and occlusion related to neo-intimal hyperplasia or struts fractures, is a frequent complication and the presence of occluded stent represent a foreign body that makes new endovascular treatment very difficult.

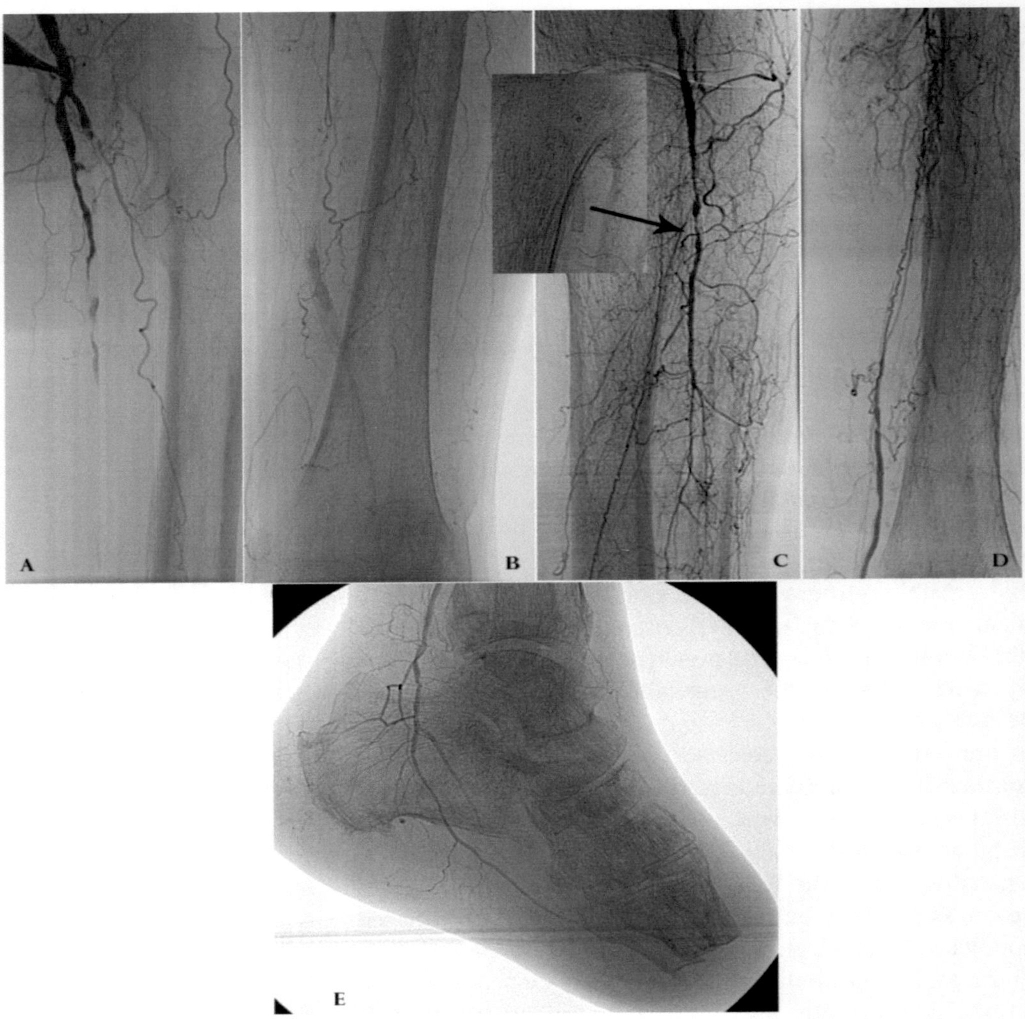

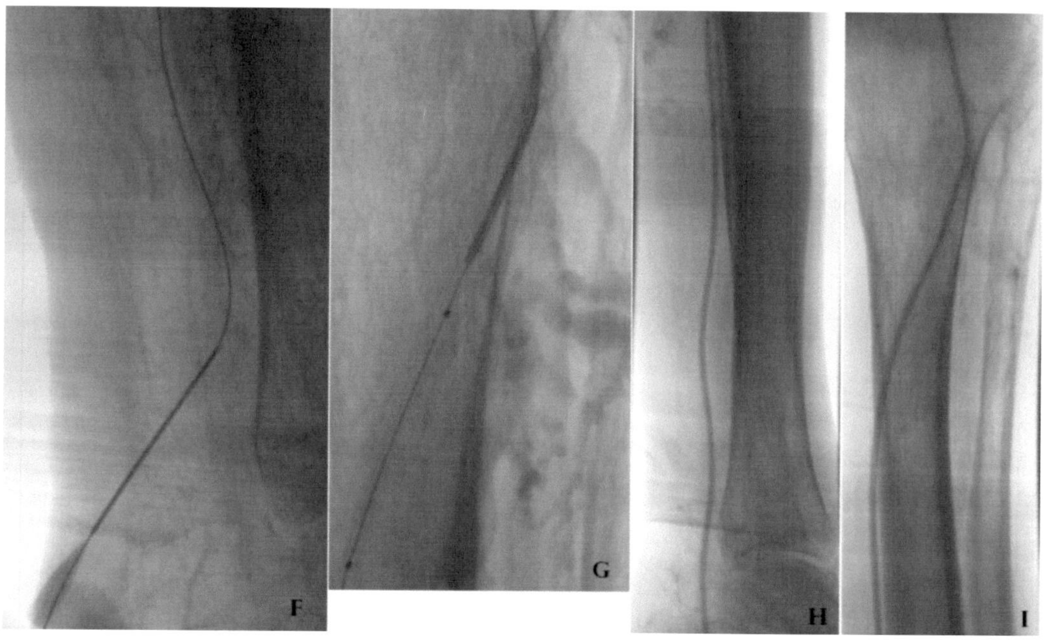

Fig. 8. Case 3. Diabetics patient, previously underwent to TMA, with apical ischemic wound. The patient was underwent to endovascular treatment and stenting in the tibio-peroneal trunk, without any stump of the posterior tibial artery origin. TcPO2: 4 mmHg. (A-E) Oclussione of the SFA with stent, occluded in the distal tract. Patency of the popliteal artery and the tibio-peronel trunk, with in-stent re-stenosis and patency of the peroneal artery and the distal truck of the posterior tibial artery. On the foot patency of the plantar arteries. (F-I) Retrograde puncture of the distal tract of the posterior tibial artery and retrograde recanalization. Antegrade long balloon PTA (2.5 x 220 mm catheter balloon / Bantamα - Clearstream).

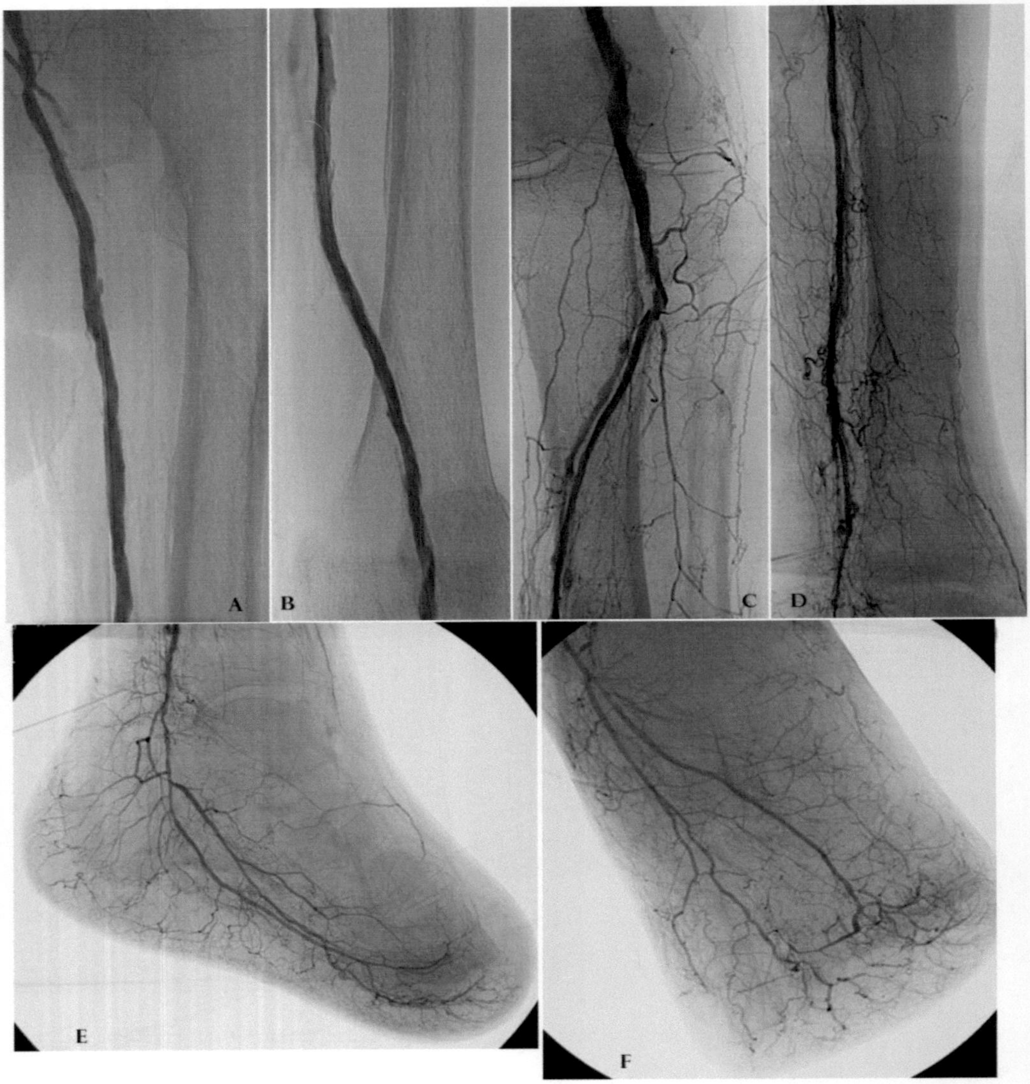

Fig. 9. (A-F) After PTA of the SFA and Popliteal arteries, the angiographic study show patency of the femoro-popliteal tract, patency of the tibio-peroneal trunk and posterior tibial artery with excellent flow for the plantar arteries and for the apical lesion on the foot. Clinical follow up. TcPO2 increased to 33 mmHg with wound healing.

6. Materials

During the last years the development of the BTK techniques and the increasing rate of BTK interventionists have led a continuous expansion of the dedicated materials.

Actually, there are a huge different type of dedicated guide-wire, from 0.014"-in and 0,018"-in to the 0,035"-in or CTO guide-wire, from different manufacturers, all usefully and necessary in the interventional suite.

In the same context, a lot of dedicated catheter balloons are actually available, from long balloons such as 22 cm or longer, to short and coronary-like such as 2 cm; and from 1.25 mm in diameter to 3 mm.
The selection of the guide-wire and the catheter balloons should be done on the personal preferences and experience, but the availability of different materials, from different manufacturer would be useful and necessary to perform very challenging cases.

7. New frontiers and devices

Current results of minimally invasive endovascular techniques, with 2-years patency rate between 40 and 60%, low primary patency and increased repeat intervention rates, has oriented toward new alternative techniques.

7.1 Atherectomy

Percutaneous angioplasty of below-the-knee arteries is an accepted therapy for patients with critical limb ischemia (Buckenham TM, et al. 1993; Hanna GP, et al. 1997; Saab MH, et al. 1992; Soder HK, et al. 2000).
However, below-the-knee interventions are limited by a considerable number of re-stenosis, especially in lesions with heavy calcified plaque. Directional atherectomy may be an alternative option to improve the procedural success and reduce the re-stenosis rate and the re-intervention rate (McKinseyJF, et al. 2008; Zeller T, et al. 2004, 2007).
In our opinion this debulking device is indicated especially in cases of re-stenosis, but also is an excellent option to treat bifurcations and could be used to treat in-stent re-stenosis, despite this indication (in-stent treatment) is contraindicated by the manufacturer.
Atherectomy should be prefer to traditional PTA in the popliteal artery, because of excellent technical results, avoiding dissection and stenting (Fig. 10).
New dedicated BTK devices, with range from 2 to 4 mm in diameter, very small caliber design and excellent push-ability allow the recanalization of long occlusion, involving tibial vessels and/or foot arteries.
The atherectomy cutter catheter usually need a 6F sheath and is designed to track over a 0.014"-in guide-wire. Is recommended to use atherectomy crossing the lesion intraluminally, because of the potential risk of perforation during subintimal debulking. Cases of stenosis can be treated with primary atherectomy whereas occlusions should be pre-dilated with an undersized catheter balloon, to be sure that the guide-wire crosses the occlusion intraluminally and to guaranty the progression of the cutter catheter through the occlusion.
Rotational atherectomy is also a useful technical strategy for calcified vessels. The limits of this technique is the push-ability of the device, that usually require long sheath deployment into the tibial vessel.
After atherectomy, usually, is not necessary perform catheter balloon dilatation, because the atherectomy results are satisfactory when the debulking procedure is performed correctly, cutting in the four faces of the artery wall.
This technique present low rate of complications and could be the option to avoid stent deployment with significant advantage in cases of re-stenosis, allowing the endovascular re-intervention.
Promising acute and long-term clinical results, with a high rate of limb salvage and high rate of primary and secondary patency (McKinsey, et al. 2008), makes this technical strategy an excellent option for endovascular treatment in the below-the-knee district.

7.2 DEB's

The other possible solution to fight re-stenosis in the BTK district could be Drug eluting balloons. This new technology, Paclitaxel-coated balloons should be a potential role in the peripheral district (Manzi M, et al. 2010; Sharma S, et al. 2010; Waksman P, et al. 2009) to avoid re-stenosis due to the antiproliferative effect. The use of DEB is not technically complex and there are, actually, a wide range of different devices. Despite the encouraging data on coronary arteries where drug eluting devices have shown promising antirestenotic effects in experimental and clinical trials, a clinical results in BTK district, early experimental and clinical data are promising but a randomized controlled trials, comparing DEB and traditional angioplasty or DEB and atherectomy must be produced.

The limits of DEB's, in our experience, is the use of this device in a subintimal recanalization. DEB's are preferred to be used in intraluminal recanalization, due to the risk of pseudo-aneurism formation during subintimal recanalization.

7.3 Cryoplasty

The rational to use this technology is based in the presumed more uniform and less traumatic immediate performance of cryoplasty, in synergy with the induction of the apoptotic effect , that would result in less neo-intimal hyperplasia and, as consequence, better immediate and long-term angiographic and clinical results (Sipiliopoulos S, et al. 2010).

The data about 12-months follow-up from the BTK Chill trial (Das TS, et al. 2009), which evaluated cryoplasty in the infra-popliteal district of CLI patients, reported high rates of acute technical success and major amputation-free interval (97.3% and 78.5%, respectively) followed by a low percentage of repeated procedure due to clinically deterioration (21% at 12 months).

We simply report the data published in the actual literature, because we do not have experience with this technical strategy, but the technical and clinical result are encouraging. It seem to avoids stent deployment, with the mentioned benefits in the BTK district. However, more experience are expected and could be useful more data about bigger cohort of patients.

7.4 Laser

The excimer laser technology is based on a cold-tipped laser that delivers intense bursts of energy in the ultraviolet range (308 nm) carried out in ultra-short pulse duration (0.05 nm per pulse vs 0.3-2.0 mm per pulse in the hot-tip laser). The energy delivered elicits photochemical, photothermal and photomechanical actions, which break molecular bonds, and produce vapor bubbles that generate kinetic energy (Serino F, et al. 2010).

This technology has been studied in below-the-knee lesions, with improved results over standard PTA alone and exhibited excellent limb salvage rate (Bosier M, et al 2005; Laird JR, et al.2006). The use of the excimer laser represents a great opportunity to pursue a true endoluminal recanalization with potential long-term efficacy and decreased need for stenting. The LACI and LACI Belgium study have both proven that laser-assisted angioplasty is a low risk, successful treatment strategy in CLI patients. Primary patency rate range from 83% at 6-months to 97.6% at 12-months and the limb salvage rate range from 92.5% at 6-months to 94% at 12-months. However, the reported rate of stent deployment in the mentioned study was in a range from 21% to 52.9%, and this seem to be a contradiction between the opportunity to pursue the reduction of stent deployment that is at the bases of the use of this device and the real data reported about stent placement.

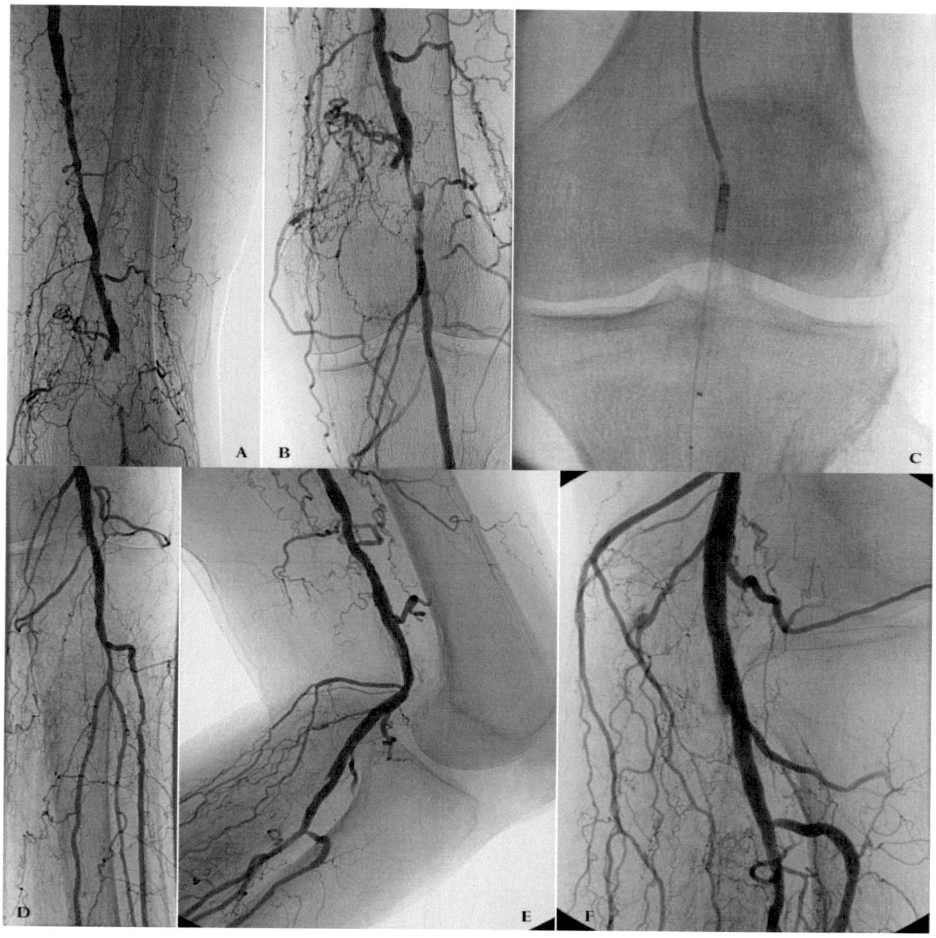

Fig. 10. Case 4. Diabetic patient with claudication intermittens (50 m). (A-B) Diagnostic angiography shows occlusion in the popliteal artery. (C) shows directional atherectomy of the occluded tract. (D-F) angiographic result shows excellent recanalization of the popliteal artery, without dissection, avoiding stenting and patency in flexion position.

8. Stent deployment

Finally, we want to express our opinion about stent deployment in the BTK district. In literature is reported the use of stent for various indications such as dissections, calcified re-stenosis, recoiling and thrombus formation (Tepe G, et al. 2007), with good clinical results. We are in accord with the concept that stent use translates in acute high technical success and good short-term patency rate, but the re-stenosis rate related to neo-intimal hyperplasia is very high and the presence of stent appear as a foreign body in the true or in a subintimal lumen, that makes re-intervention more complex or, sometimes, impossible. Our stent deployment rate in the BTK district in the last year, was less than 3% and it was related to very flow limiting dissection, especially in the bifurcations, thrombus formation with unsuccessful attempts to perform thrombus-aspiration and in 1 case the stent deployment was related to artery perforation with acute bleeding.

The fear that early thrombosis and late luminal loss due to intimal hyperplasia formation potentially leads to insufficient long-term patency rates can explain the reluctance on implanting stents in small diameter below-the-knee (BTK) arteries. Drug-eluting stent (DES) technology was developed to prevent early thrombosis and late luminal loss to potentially improve long-term patency rates (Bosier M, et al. 2011).

Currently, the first level 1 evidence from prospective, randomized, controlled DESTINY and ACHILLES studies indicate that the implantation of DES in short lesion in the infrapopliteal arteries leads to favorable outcomes with high primary patency rates and a published paper (Rosales OR, et al. 2008.) conclude that DES is a safe and effective long-term option for CLI due to severe infrapopliteal arterial disease. Long-term vascular patency led to a high rate of limb preservation and low amputation rate.

May be in the future, a resorbable dedicated stent conceived for the BTK district will change the indications for stent deployment in tibial arteries.

9. Conclusions

Endovascular treatment of critical limb ischemia in diabetics with crural and pedal disease can be an exceedingly challenging and complex problem. Technical success rate and clinical outcomes, with a high rate of limb salvage and amputation-free survival are encouraging, support the endovascular revascularization as the first treatment option and demonstrate that is a reasonable and effective approach. The rapid pace of development of various endovascular devices and techniques often allow the interventionalist to treat increasingly complex and diffuse patterns of disease.

Is essential for endovascular specialist, in order to reach these technical and clinical success, a thorough knowledge of the wide range of endovascular techniques and options.

Usually only one technical strategy is not enough to treat crural and foot arteries and a combination of the previously described techniques improve the results of the procedures and allow to achieve excellent clinical outcomes.

10. References

Adam DJ, Beard JD, Cleveland T, Bell J, Bradbury AW, Forbes JF, et al. (2005). Bypass versus angioplasty in severe ischaemia of the leg (BASIL): multicentre, randomised controlled trial. Lancet. 3;366(9501):1925-34.

Alexandrescu V, Hubermont G, Philips Y, Guillaumie B, Ngongang Ch, Coessens V, et al. (2009). Combined primary subintimal and endoluminal angioplasty for ischaemic inferior-limb ulcers in diabetic patients: 5-year practice in a multidisciplinary 'diabetic-foot' service. Eur J Vasc Endovasc Surg. 37(4):448-56.

Athyros VG, Mikhailidis DP, Papageorgiou AA, Didangelos TP, Ganotakis ES, Symeonidis AN, et al. (2004). METS-GREECE Collaborative Group. Prevalence of atherosclerotic vascular disease among subject with the metabolic syndrome with or without diabetes mellitus: the METS-GREECE Multicentre study. Curr Med Res Opin. 20:1691-701.

Attinger, C. E., Cooper, P. & Blume, P. (1997). Vascular anatomy of the foot and ankle. *Oper. Tech. Plast. Reconstr. Surg.* 4: 183.

Attinger, C. E., Cooper, P., Blume, P. & Bulan, E. (2001). The safest surgical incision and amputations applying the angiosomes principle and using the Doppler to assess the arterialarterial connections of the foot and ankle. *Foot Ankle Clin. North Am.* 6: 745.

Balmer H, Mahler F, Do DD, Triller J & Baumgartner I. (2002). Balloon angioplasty in chronic critical limb ischemia: factors affecting clinical and angiographic outcome. J Endovasc Ther. 9(4):403-10.

Bargellini I, Petruzzi P, Scatena A, Cioni R, Cicorelli A, Vignali C, et al. (2008). Primary infrainguinal subintimal angioplasty in diabetic patients. Cardiovasc Intervent radiol. 31:713-22.

Beckman JA, Creager MA & Libby P. (2002). Diabetes and atherosclerosis. Epidemiology, pathophysiology and management. JAMA 287:2570-81.

Boiser M, Deloose K, Callaert J, Keirse K, Verbist J & Peeters P. (2011). Drug-eluting stents below the knee. J Cardiovasc Surg (Torino) 52(2):231-4.

Boiser M, Peeters P, Elst FV, Vermassen F, Maleux G, Fourneau I, et al. (2005). Excimer laser assisted angioplasty for critical limb ischemia: results of the LACI Belgium study. Eur J Vasc Endovasc Surg 29:613-9.

Bolia A, Miles KA, Brennan J & Bell PR. (1990). Percutaneous transluminal angioplasty of occlusions of the femoral and popliteal arteries by subintimal dissection. Cardiovasc Intervent Radiol. 13(6):357-63.

Bolia A, Sayers RD, Thompson MM & Bell PR. (1994). Subintimal and intraluminal recanalisation of occluded crural arteries by percutaneous balloon angioplasty. Eur J Vasc Surg. 8(2):214-9.

Bolia A. (1998). Percutaneous intentional extraluminal (subintimal) recanalization of crural vessels in lower limb ischemia: long-term results. J Endovasc Ther 9:411-16.

Bolia A. (2005). Subintimal angioplasty in lower limb ischaemia. J Cardiovasc Surg (Torino) 46:385–394.

Bown MJ, Bolia A & Sutton AJ. (2009). Subintimal angioplasty: meta-analytical evidence of clinical utility. Eur J Vasc Endovasc Surg. 38(3):323-37.

Buckenham TM, Loh A, Dormandy JA & Taylor RS. (1993). Infrapopliteal angioplasty for limb salvage. Eur J Vasc Surg 7:21-5.

Calligari, P.R., Taylor, G. I., Caddy, C. M. & Minabe, T. (1992). An anatomic review of the delay phenomenon: I. Experimental studies. *Plast. Reconstr. Surg.* 89: 397.

Chun JY, Markose G & Bolia A. (2010). Developments in subintimal angioplasty in the infrainguinal segment. J Cardiovasc Surg (Torino) 51(2):213-21.

Criqui MH, Fronek A, Barrett-Connor E, Klauber MR, Gabriel S & Goodman D. (1985). The prevalence of peripheral arterial disease in a defined population. Circulation 71(3):510-551.

Criqui MH, Vargas V, Denenberg JO, Ho E, Allison M, Langer RD, et al. (2005). Ethnicity and peripheral arterial disease: the San Diego Population Study. Circulation 112(17):2703-2707.

Das TS, McNamara T, Gray B, Sedillo GJ, Turley BR, Kollmeyer K, et al. (2009). Primary cryoplasty therapy provides durable support for limb salvage in critical limb ischemia patients with infrapopliteal lesions: 12-months follow-up results from chill trial. J Endovasc Ther 16(suppl 2):I119-I130.

Dorros G, Jaff MR, Dorros AM, Mathiak LM & He T. (2001). Tibioperoneal (outflow lesion) angioplasty can be used as primary treatment in 235 patients with critical limb ischemia: five-year follow-up. Circulation 23;104(17):2057-62.

Faglia E, Dalla Paola L, Clerici G, Clerissi J, Graziani L, Fusaro M. et al. (2005). Peripheral angioplasty as the first-choice revascularization procedure in diabetic patients with critical limb ischemia: prospective study of 993 consecutive patients hospitalized and followed between 1999 and 2003. Eur J Vasc Endovasc Surg. 29(6):620-7.

Faglia E, Clerici G, Clerissi J, Gabrielli L, Losa S, Mantero M, et al. (2006). Early and five-year amputation and survival rate of diabetic patients with critical limb ischemia: data of a cohort study of 564 patients. Eur J Vasc Endovasc Surg. 32(5):484-90.

Ferraresi R, Centola M, Ferlini M, Da Ros R, Caravaggi C, Assaloni R, et al. (2009). Long-term outcomes after angioplasty of isolated, below-the-knee arteries in diabetic patients with critical limb ischaemia. Eur J Vasc Endovasc Surg. 37(3):336-42.

Fowkes FG, Housley E, Cawood EH, Macintyre CC, Ruckley CV & Prescott RJ. (1991). Edinburgh Artery Study: prevalence of asymptomatic and symptomatic peripheral arterial disease in the general population. Int J Epidemiol 20(2):384-392

Fusaro M, Agostoni P & Biondi-Zoccai G. (2008). "Trans-Collateral" Angioplasty for a Challenging Chronic Total Occlusion of the Tibial Vessels: A Novel Approach to Percutaneous Revascularization in Critical Lower Limb Ischemia. Catheterization and Cardiovascular Interventions 71:268-72

Fusaro M, Dalla Paola L & Biondi-Zoccai G. (2007). Pedal-Plantar LOOP Technique for a challenging below-the-knee chronic total occlusion: a novel approach to percutaneous revascularization in critical lower limb ischemia. J Invasive Cardiol 19:E34-7.

Fusaro M, Dalla Paola L & Biondi-Zoccai G. (2006). Retrograde posterior tibial artery access for below-the-knee percutaneos revascularization by means of sheathless approach and double wire technique. Minerva Cardioangiol. 54:773-7.

Fusaro M, Dalla Paola L, Brigato C, Marangotto M, Nicolini S, Rripay R, et al. (2007). Plantar to dorsalis pedis artery subintimal angioplasty in a patient with critical foot ischemia: a novel technique in the armamentarium of the peripheral interventionist. J Cardiovasc Med (Hagerstown) 8(11):977-80.

Fusaro M, Tashani A, Mollicheli N, Medda M, Inglese L & Biondi-Zoccai G. (2007). Retrograde pedal artery access for below-the-knee percutaneous revascularisation. J Cardiovasc Med (Hagerstown) 8:216-8.

Gandini R, Pipitone V, Stefanini M, Maresca L, Spinelli A, Colangelo V, et al. (2007). The "Safari" Technique to Perform Difficult Subintimal Infragenicular Vessels. Cardiovasc Intervent Radiol 30:469-73.

Graziani L, Silvestro A, Monge L, Boffano GM, Kokaly F, Casadidio I, et al. (2008). Transluminal angioplasty of peroneal artery branches in diabetics: initial technical experience. Cardiovasc Interv Radiol 31:49–55

Graziani L & Morelli LG. (2011). Combined Retrograde–Antegrade Arterial Recanalization Through Collateral Vessels: Redefinition of the Technique for Below-the-Knee Arteries. Cardiovasc Intervent Radiol 34:S78–S82

Hanna GP, Fujise K, Kjellgren O, GP, Feld S, Fife C, Schroth G, et al. (1997). Infrapopliteal transcatheter interventions for limb salvage in diabetic patients: importance of aggressive interventional approach and role of transcutaneous oximetry. J Am Coll Cardiol 30:664-9.

Häuser H, Bohndorf K, Wack C, Tietze W, Wölfle KD & Loeprecht H. Percutaneous transluminal angioplasty (PTA) of isolated crural arterial stenoses in critical arterial occlusive disease. Rofo. 164(3):238-43.

Hiatt WR, Hoag S & Hamman RF. (1995). Effect of diagnostic criteria on the prevalence of peripheral arterial disease. The San Luis Valley Diabetes Study. Circulation 91(5):1472-1479.

Ingle H, Nasim A, Bolia A, Fishwick G, Naylor R, Bell PR, et al. (2002). Subintimal angioplasty of isolated infragenicular vessels in lower limb ischemia: long-term results. J Endovasc Ther. 9(4):411-6. Erratum in: J Endovasc Ther 9(5):A-6.

Kullo IJ, Bailey KR, Kardia SL, Mosley TH, Jr., Boerwinkle E &Turner ST. (2003). Ethnic differences in peripheral arterial disease in the NHLBI Genetic Epidemiology Network of Arteriopathy (GENOA) study. Vasc Med 8(4):237-242.

Laird JR, Zeller T, Gray BH, Scheinert D, Vranic M, Reiser C, et al. (2006). LACI investigators. Limb salvage following laser-assisted angioplasty for critical limb ischemia: results of the LACI multicenter trial. J Endovasc Ther. 13:1-11.

Manzi M, Cester G & Palena LM. (2010). Paclitaxel-coated balloon angioplasty for lower extremity revascularization: a new way to fight in-stent restenosis. J Cardiovasc Surg 51:567-71.

Manzi M, Fusaro M, Ceccacci T, Erente G, Dalla Paola L & Brocco E. (2009). Clinical results of below-the-knee intervention using pedal-plantar loop technique for the revascularization of foot arteries. J Cardiovasc Surg 50:331-7.

McKinsey JF, Goldstein L, Khan HU, Graham A, Rezeyat C, Morrissey NJ, et al. (2008). Novel Treatment of Patients With Lower Extremity Ischemia: Use of Percutaneous Atherectomy in 579 Lesions. Ann Surg 248:519-28.

Met R, Van Lienden KP, Koelemay MJ, Bipat S, Legemate DA & Reekers JA. (2008). Subintimal angioplasty for peripheral arterial occlusive disease: a systematic review. Cardiovasc Intervent Radiol. 31(4):687-97

Norgren L, Hiatt WR, Dormandy JA, Nehler MR, Harris KA, Fowkes FG, TASC II Working Group et al. (2007). Inter-society consensus for the management of peripheral arterial disease (TASC II). J Vasc Surg 45(Suppl.S):S5-S67.

O'Hare AM, Vittinghoff E, Hsia J & Shlipak MG. (2004). Renal insufficiency and the risk of lower extremity peripheral arterial disease: results from the Heart and Estrogen/Progestin Replacement Study (HERS). J Am Soc Nephrol 15(4):1046- 1051.

Palena LM, Cester G & Manzi M. (2011). Revascularisacion endovascular del pie y de las arterias tibiales a traves de caminos alternativos, utilizando la arcada profunda del pie. Presented at IX SITE- Symposio Internacional sobre Terapeuticas Endovasculares. Barcelona 4-7 May 2011. Published at Tecnicas Endovasculares. 14(1): 3739.

Patel PJ, Hieb RA & Bhat AP. (2010). Percutaneous revascularization of chronic total occlusions. Tech Vasc Interv Radiol. 13(1):23-36.

Reekers JA, Kromhout JG & Jacobs MJ. (1994). Percutaneous intentional extraluminal recanalisation of the femoropopliteal artery. Eur J Vasc Surg. 8(6):723-8.

Romiti M, Albers M, Brochado-Neto FC, Durazzo AE, Pereira CA & De Luccia N. (2008). Meta-analysis of infrapopliteal angioplasty for chronic critical limb ischemia. J Vasc Surg. 47(5):975-81.

Rosales OR, Mathewkutty S & Gnaim C. (2008). Drug eluting stents for below the knee lesions in patients with critical limb ischemia : long-term follow-up. Catheter Cardiovasc Interv. 72(1):112-5.

Saab MH, Smith DC, Aka PK, Browlee RW & Killeen JD. (1992). Percutaneous transluminal angioplasty of tibial arteries for limb salvage. Cardiovasc Intervent Radiol. 15:211–6.

Sarrafian, S. K. (1993). Anatomy of the Foot and Ankle. Philadelphia: Lippincott.. Pp. 294–355.

Selvin E & Erlinger TP. (2004). Prevalence of and risk factors for peripheral arterial disease in the United States: results from the National Health and Nutrition Examination Survey, 1999-2000. Circulation 110(6):738-743.

Selvin E, Marinopoulos S, Berkenblit G, Rami T, Brancati FL, Powe NR, et al. (2004). Meta-analysis: glycosylated hemoglobin and cardiovascular disease in diabetes mellitus. Ann Intern Med. 141(6):421-431.

Senti M, Nogues X, Pedro-Botet J, Rubies-Prat J & Vidal-Barraquer F. (1992). Lipoprotein profile in men with peripheral vascular disease. Role of intermediate density lipoproteins and apoprotein E phenotypes. Circulation. 85(1):30-36.

Serino F, Cao Y, Renzi C, Mascellari L, Toscanella F, Raskovic D, et al. (2010). Excimer laser ablation in the treatment of total chronic obstructions in critical limb ischaemia in diabetic patients. Sustained efficacy of plaque recanalisation in mid-term results. Eur J Vasc Endovasc Surg. 39:234-8.

Sharma S, Kukreja N, Christopoulos C & Gorog DA. (2010). Drug-eluting balloon: new tool in the box. Expert Rev Med Devices. 7:381-8.

Söder HK, Manninen HI, Jaakkola P, Matsi PJ, Räsänen HT, Kaukanen E, et al. (2000). Prospective trial of infrapopliteal artery balloon angioplasty for critical limb ischemia: angiographic and clinical results. J Vasc Interv Radiol. 11(8):1021-31.

Spiliopoulos S, Katsanos K, Karanabatidis D, Diamantopoulos A, Kagadis G, Christeas N, et al. (2010). Cryoplasty versus conventional balloon angioplasty of the femoropopliteal artery in diabetic patients: long-term results from a prospective randomized single-center controlled trial. Cardiovasc Intervent Radiol. 33:929-38.

Spinosa DJ, Leung DA, Hathun NL, Cage DL, Angle JF, Hagspiel KD, et al. (2003). Simultaneous Antegrade and Retrograde access for subintimal recanalization of peripheral arterial occlusion. J Vasc Interv Radiol. 14:1449-54.

Spinosa DJ, Leung DA, Matsumoto AH, Bissonette EA, Cage D, Harthun NL, et al. (2004). Percutaneous intentional extraluminal recanalization in patients with chronic critical limb ischemia. Radiology. 232(2):499-507.

Spinosa DJ, Hathun NL, Bissonette EA, Cage DL, Leung DA, Angle JF, Hagspiel KD, et al.(2005). Subinitmal Arterial flossing with Antegtrade-Retrograde Intervention (SAFARI) for Subinitmal Recanalization to Treat Chronic Critical Limb Ischemia. J Vasc Interv Radiol. 16:37-44.

Taylor, G. I. & Minabe, T. (1992). The angiosomes of the mammals and other vertebrates. *Plast. Reconstr. Surg.* 89: 181.

Taylor, G. I., Corlett, R. J., Caddy, C. M & Zelt, R. G. (1992). An anatomic review of the delay phenomenon: II. Clinical applications. Plast. Reconstr. Surg. 89: 408.

Taylor, G. I. & Pan, W. R. (1998). Angiosomes of the leg: Anatomic study and clinical implications. Plast. Reconstr. Surg. 102: 599.

Tepe G, Zeller T, Heller S, Wiskirchen J, Fischmann A, Coerper S, et al. (2007). Self-expanding nitinol stents for treatment of infragenicular arteries following unsuccessful balloon angioplasty. Eur Radiol. 17:2088-95.

Wack C, Wölfle KD, Loeprecht H, Tietze W & Bohndorf K.(1994). Percutaneous balloon dilatation of isolated lesions of the calf arteries in critical ischemia of the leg. Vasa. 23(1):30-4.

Waksman R & Pakala R. (2009). Drug-eluting balloon: the comeback kid?. Circulation: Cardiovascular Intervention 2:352-8.

Walsh DB, Gilberstone JJ, Zwolajk RM, Besso S, Edelman GC, Schneider JR, et al. (1991). The natural history of superficial femoral artery stenosis. J Vasc Surg. 14:299:304.

Zeller T, Rastan A, Schwarzwälder U, Frank U, Bürgelin K, Amantea P, et al. (2004). Midterm Results after Atherectomy-assisted Angioplasty of Below-Knee Arteries with Use of the Silverhawk Device. J Vasc Interv Radiol. 15:1391-7.

Zeller T, Sixt S, Schwarzwaler U, Schwarz T, Frank U, Burgelin K, et al. (2007). Two-Year Results After Directional Atherectomy of Infrapopliteal Arteries With the SilverHawk Device. J Endovasc Ther. 14:232-40.